Population-Based Nursing

Ann L. Cupp Curley, PhD, RN, is the nurse research specialist at Capital Health in Trenton, New Jersey. In this capacity, she promotes and guides the development of clinical research and facilitates evidence-based practice. She has an extensive background in nursing education at the undergraduate, graduate, and doctoral levels. Her clinical background includes more than 10 years working in community health nursing. Dr. Curley has delivered many papers and presentations on research and evidence-based practice. Her publications include *Urban Health Informatics* and *A Nurse's Perspective on Cuba*. She has served as the principal investigator for several studies, including "The Lived Experience of Nurses Who Move to a New Hospital" and "Ergonomics and the Aging Nursing Workforce." She received her BSN at Boston College, an MSN in community health/CNS track from the University of Pennsylvania, and a PhD in Urban Planning and Policy Development at Rutgers, The State University of New Jersey. She has received many honors, including the Nurse.com, *Nursing Spectrum,* Nursing Excellence Award for Education and Mentorship in 2012 for the Philadelphia and tri-state area.

Patty A. Vitale, MD, MPH, FAAP, is an attending physician in pediatric emergency medicine at Cooper University Hospital in Camden, New Jersey. She holds multiple appointments, including assistant professor of pediatrics and emergency medicine at Cooper Medical School of Rowan University and adjunct assistant professor of epidemiology at Rutgers University School of Public Health. Dr. Vitale teaches and writes medical student curricula in the areas of epidemiology and biostatistics for medical students at Cooper Medical School of Rowan University. For over 8 years, she has taught the course Principles of Epidemiology to graduate and doctoral students in public health, nursing, and biomedical sciences at Rutgers University, formerly the University of Medicine and Dentistry of New Jersey. Dr. Vitale did her residency and postdoctoral training in pediatrics and community pediatrics at the University of California, San Diego. During her fellowship, she obtained her master's in public health from San Diego State University. She is certified by the American Board of Pediatrics and has served on national and statewide committees for the American Academy of Pediatrics in the areas of epidemiology, government affairs, and young physicians. She also sits on the editorial board for *AAP-Grand Rounds,* a publication of the American Academy of Pediatrics. She volunteered as team physician for the U.S. National Gymnastics Team (2003–2008). She is a Junior Olympic National Elite and NCAA women's gymnastics judge and former gymnastics coach and was inducted into the California Interscholastic Hall of Fame for Sports Officials in San Diego, California (2009). Her national and local lectures and publications have focused on family violence, youth violence prevention, pediatric and adolescent health, and homelessness. She has received many honors, including the 2004 AMA Foundation Leadership Award, the 2002 Fellows Award for Excellence in Promoting Children's Health (Academic Pediatric Association), and the 2002 Pediatric Leaders of the 21st Century (American Academy of Pediatrics), among others.

Population-Based Nursing

Concepts and Competencies
for Advanced Practice

Second Edition

Ann L. Cupp Curley, PhD, RN

and

Patty A. Vitale, MD, MPH, FAAP

Editors

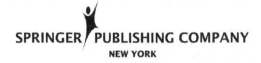

SPRINGER **PUBLISHING COMPANY**
NEW YORK

Springer Publishing Company, LLC
11 West 42nd Street
New York, NY 10036
www.springerpub.com

Acquisitions Editor: Margaret Zuccarini
Production Editor: Kris Parrish
Composition: S4Carlisle Publishing Services

ISBN: 978-0-8261-9613-2
e-book ISBN: 978-0-8261-3049-5
Instructor's Manual ISBN: 978-0-8261-1889-9

Instructor's materials are available to qualified adopters by contacting textbook@springerpub.com.

17 18 19 / 5 4

The author and the publisher of this work have made every effort to use sources believed to be reliable to provide information that is accurate and compatible with the standards generally accepted at the time of publication. The author and publisher shall not be liable for any special, consequential, or exemplary damages resulting, in whole or in part, from the readers' use of, or reliance on, the information contained in this book. The publisher has no responsibility for the persistence or accuracy of URLs for external or third-party Internet websites referred to in this publication and does not guarantee that any content on such websites is, or will remain, accurate or appropriate.

Library of Congress Cataloging-in-Publication Data

Population-based nursing : concepts and competencies for advanced practice / Ann L. Cupp Curley, Patty A. Vitale, editors. — Second edition.
  p. ; cm.
 Preceded by: Population-based nursing / Ann L. Cupp Curley and Patty A. Vitale. c2012.
 Includes bibliographical references and index.
 ISBN 978-0-8261-9613-2—ISBN 978-0-8261-3049-5 (e-book)
 I. Curley, Ann L. Cupp, editor, contributor. II. Vitale, Patty A., editor. III. Curley, Ann L. Cupp. Population-based nursing. Preceded by (work):
 [DNLM: 1. Public Health Nursing. 2. Community Health Nursing. 3. Evidence-Based Nursing. WY 108]
 RT97
 610.73'4—dc23

                                                                                    2015021221

Printed in the United States of America by Bradford & Bigelow.

Contents

Contents

Contributors   ix
Foreword   Nancy J. Rothman, MSN, EdD, RN
   xi
Acknowledgments   xv

Contributors

Barbara A. Benjamin, EdD, RN, Appraiser, American Nurses Credentialing Center, Silver Springs, Maryland

Irina McKeehan Campbell, PhD, MPH, Professor, Department of Community Health, School of Health and Human Services, National University, La Jolla, California

Margaret M. Conrad, DNP, RN, University Correctional Health Care, Rutgers, The State University of New Jersey, Piscataway, New Jersey

Ann L. Cupp Curley, PhD, RN, Nurse Research Specialist, Capital Health, Trenton, New Jersey

Janna L. Dieckmann, PhD, RN, Clinical Associate Professor, School of Nursing, University of North Carolina at Chapel Hill, Chapel Hill, North Carolina

Gloria J. McNeal, PhD, MSN, RN, ACNS-BC, FAAN, Dean, School of Health and Human Services, National University, La Jolla, California

Frances Munet-Vilaró, PhD, RN, Associate Professor, School of Nursing, Division of Nursing Science, Rutgers, The State University of New Jersey, Newark, New Jersey

Barbara A. Niedz, PhD, RN, CPHQ, National Vice President of Quality Improvement, Magellan Health; Contributing Faculty, Walden University School of Nursing, DNP Program, Columbia, Maryland

Sonda M. Oppewal, PhD, RN, APHN-BC, Clinical Associate Professor, School of Nursing, University of North Carolina at Chapel Hill, Chapel Hill, North Carolina

David W. Unkle, MSN, APN, FCCM, Doctoral Student, School of Nursing, The Catholic University of America, Washington, DC; Nurse Practitioner, Mercer Allergy & Pulmonary Associates, LLC, The Center for Allergic & Occupational Contact Dermatitis, Trenton, New Jersey

Patty A. Vitale, MD, MPH, FAAP, Assistant Professor of Pediatrics and Emergency Medicine, Cooper Medical School of Rowan University; Adjunct Assistant Professor of Epidemiology, School of Public Health, Rutgers, The State University of New Jersey, Stratford, New Jersey

Foreword

Population-Based Nursing: Concepts and Competencies for Advanced Practice Second Edition, describes the significance of the role that nurses have played and must continue to play in population health. It addresses the core competencies for population-based nursing, as proposed by the American Association of Colleges of Nursing (AACN) for curricula in doctor of nursing practice (DNP) programs. These competencies, and thus this book, are equally important to nurses in any advanced practice role. The newly added chapter on the global implications of population-based nursing adds an entirely new and interesting dimension to the book.

Evidence-based nursing models for delivering population-based care are essential to achieving the mission of delivering accessible, affordable, high-quality care. Pay for performance based on quality versus quantity is becoming the standard. Quality is being measured by population-based patient outcomes. Patient engagement—through shared decision making, self-management goals, and supported transitions in care—is being recognized as an essential element in evidence-based models of care. All of these important elements are addressed in this text.

Beginning with the recognition of how many famous nurses ensured their place in history by providing population-based care, this book addresses the essential components for designing evidence-based population care: identifying outcomes, epidemiology, evidence at the population level, information systems to improve population outcomes, program design and development, evaluating practice at the population level, engaging communities, and challenges and implications for global health.

Population-Based Nursing: Concepts and Competencies for Advanced Practice Second Edition, challenges advanced practice nurses to design and provide evidence-based care to populations across healthcare settings locally, nationally, and globally. This newly revised text describes what nurses need to know to meet the challenges of providing population-based care in our constantly evolving world.

Nancy L. Rothman, MSN, EdD, RN
Independence Foundation Professor of Urban Community Nursing
Department of Nursing
College of Public Health
Temple University
Philadelphia, Pennsylvania

Preface

The original inspiration for this book grew out of our experience while co-teaching an epidemiology course for students enrolled in a doctorate in nursing practice (DNP) program. We found it difficult to find a textbook that addressed the course objectives and was relevant to nursing practice. We decided a population-based nursing textbook, targeted for use as a primary course textbook in a DNP program or as a supplement to other course materials in a graduate community health nursing program, would be of great benefit and value to students enrolled in these programs. This book is the result of that vision. The chapters address the essential areas of content for a DNP program as recommended by the American Association of Colleges of Nursing (AACN), with a focus on the AACN core competencies for population-based nursing. The primary audience for this text are nursing students enrolled in either a DNP program or a graduate community health nursing program. Each chapter includes discussion questions to help nursing students use and apply their newly acquired skills from each chapter.

In this book, the second edition, our goals were to not only update the content of the existing chapters, but to add a chapter on global health in population-based nursing. We were fortunate that two nurses with extensive experience in global health (Dr. Irina McKeehan Campbell and Dr. Gloria J. McNeal) agreed to write a chapter for us in this emerging field.

Several changes covering a wide range of issues in the healthcare field have occurred over the past few years. These include the implementation of parts of the Affordable Care Act (including the IRS requirement for 501(c)(3) hospitals to conduct community assessments). Pay for performance has been implemented by the Centers for Medicare & Medicaid Services (CMS). The overconsumption of salt in the American diet and increasing usage of electronic cigarettes and hookahs have gained widespread attention. The term *toxic stress* has been coined to describe how exposure to prolonged and severe stressors, such as abuse, neglect, or being a witness or victim of violence, can lead to changes in the brain and to short-term and even long-term poor health outcomes. There is also increasing interest in the use of social media to address population health. This edition addresses these as well as other current issues in population-based nursing.

As in the first edition, this textbook includes successful strategies that nurses have used to improve population outcomes and reinforces high-level application of activities that require the synthesis and integration of information learned. The goal is to provide readers with information that will help them to identify healthcare needs at the population level and improve population outcomes. In particular, Chapter 1 introduces the concept of population-based nursing and discusses examples of successful approaches and interventions to improve population health. In this edition we will use the title "advanced practice registered nurse" (APRN) instead of advanced practice nurse (APN). APRN is the title used in *The Consensus Model for APRN Regulation, Licensure, Accreditation, Certification and Education* (APRN Consensus Workgroup & National Council of State Boards of Nursing APRN Advisory Committee, 2008). This document is the product of the APRN Consensus Work Group and the National Council of State Boards of Nursing (NCSBN). It has been endorsed by more than 30 nursing specialty organizations. The use of this term, and the reason for the change, are addressed in the first chapter.

In order to design, implement, and evaluate interventions that improve the health of populations and aggregates, APRNs need to be able to identify and target outcome measures. Chapter 2 explains how to define, categorize, and identify population outcomes using specific examples from practice settings. The identification of outcomes or key health indicators is an essential first step in planning effective interventions and is a requirement for evaluation. The chapter includes a discussion of nurse-sensitive indicators, Healthy People 2020, national health objectives, and health disparities. Emphasis is on the identification of healthcare disparities and approaches that can be used to eliminate or mitigate them. APRNs can advocate needed change at local, regional, state, or national levels by identifying areas for improvement in practice, by comparing evidence needed for effective practice, and by better understanding health disparities. APRNs have an important collaborative role with professionals from other disciplines and community members to work toward eliminating health disparities.

Epidemiology is the basic science of prevention (Gordis, 2014). Evidence-based practice, as it relates to population-based nursing, combines clinical practice and public health through the use of population health sciences in clinical practice (Heller & Page, 2002). Programs or interventions that are designed by APRNs should be evaluated and assessed for their effectiveness and ability to change or improve outcomes. This is true at an individual or population level. Data from these programs should be collected systematically and in such a manner that can be replicated in future programs. Data collection must be organized and analyzed using clearly defined outcomes developed early in the planning process. Best practice requires that data are not just collected; data must also be analyzed, interpreted correctly, and, if significant, put into practice. Understanding how to interpret and report data accurately is critical as it sets up the foundation for evidence-based practice. With that said, it is important to understand the basics of how to measure disease or outcomes, how to present these measures, and to know what types of measures are needed to analyze a project or intervention.

Chapter 3 describes the natural history of disease and concepts that are integral to the prevention and recognition (e.g., screening) of disease. Basic concepts that are necessary to understand how to measure disease, and design studies that are used in population-based research, are discussed. Disease measures, such as incidence, prevalence, and mortality rates, are covered, and their relevance to practice is discussed. This chapter also includes information on primary, secondary, and tertiary prevention, and the concept of causality is introduced. An additional section on survival and prognosis has been added. This additional material broadens the knowledge of readers with information necessary for advanced practice and interpretation of survival data. The basics of data analysis, including the calculation of relative risk, attributable risk, and odds ratio, are presented with examples of how to use these measures. Study design selection is an important part of the planning process for implementing a program. A portion of Chapter 3 is dedicated to introducing the most common study designs, because correct design selection is an essential part of sound methodology, successful program implementation, and overall success.

In order for APRNs to lead the field of evidence-based practice, it is critical that they possess skills in analytic methods to identify population trends and evaluate outcomes and systems of care (American Association of Colleges of Nursing [AACN], 2006). They need to carry out studies with strong methodology and be cognizant of factors that can affect study results. Identification and early recognition of factors that can affect the results or outcomes of a study, such as systematic errors (e.g., bias), should be acknowledged because they cannot always be prevented. In Chapter 4, the APRN is introduced to the elements of bias with a comprehensive discussion of the complexities of data collection and the fundamentals of developing a database. More in-depth discussion of study designs is covered, as well as a comprehensive review of ways to report on randomized and nonrandomized studies. Critical components of data analysis are discussed, including causality, confounding, and interaction.

In order to provide care at an advanced level, nurses must incorporate the concepts and competencies of advanced practice into their daily practice. This requires that APRNs acquire the knowledge, tools, and resources to know when and how to integrate them into practice. In Chapter 5, the APRN learns how to integrate and synthesize information in order to design interventions that are based on evidence to improve population outcomes. Nurses require several skills to become practitioners of evidence-based care. In this chapter, they learn how to identify clinical problems, recognize patient safety issues, compose clinical questions that provide a clear direction for study, conduct a search of the literature, appraise and synthesize the available evidence, and successfully integrate new knowledge into practice.

Information technologies are transforming the way that information is learned and shared. Online communities provide a place for people to support each other and share information. Online databases contain knowledge that can be assessed for information on populations and aggregates, and many websites provide up-to-date information on health and healthcare. Chapter 6 describes how technology can be used to enhance population-based nursing. It identifies websites that are available and how to evaluate them for quality. It also describes potential ways that technology can be used to improve population outcomes and how to incorporate technology into the development of new and creative interventions. APRNs use data to make decisions that lead to program development, implementation, and evaluation. In Chapter 7, the APRN learns how to design new programs using organizational theory. Nursing care delivery models that address organizational structure, process, and outcomes are described.

Oversight responsibilities for clinical outcomes at the population level are a critical part of advanced practice nursing. The purpose of Chapter 8 is to identify ways and means to evaluate population outcomes and systems changes, as well as to address issues of effectiveness and efficiency and trends in care delivery across the continuum. Strategies to monitor healthcare quality are addressed, as are factors that lead to success. These concepts are explored within the role and competencies of the APRN.

In order for APRNs to make decisions at the community level, APRNs who work in the community need to be part of the higher level of care management and policy decision making, in partnership with the community-based consortium of healthcare policy makers. Chapter 9 describes the tools for successful community collaboration and project development. Emphasis is placed on identifying community needs and assessment of their resources. Specific examples are given to guide APRNs in developing their own community projects.

Chapter 10 identifies barriers to change within communities and the importance of developing and sustaining community partnerships. Specific strategies for program implementation are discussed, as well as the methods to empower the community to advocate for themselves. Specific examples are given in order to guide APRNs in executing a project that has community acceptance and sustainability.

Finally, Chapter 11 explores the implications of global health for the APRN. Theories of global health, population health, and public/community health are differentiated and compared, to further the understanding of how environmental conditions (e.g., poverty, housing, access to care) affect the health status of individuals and groups. Recent patterns in international interdisciplinary collaborations are reviewed, including the global health competencies developed by the Association of Schools of Public Health (ASPH) and the AACN.

Qualified instructors may obtain access to an instructor's manual for this title by contacting *textbook@springerpub.com*.

Ann L. Cupp Curley
Patty A. Vitale

REFERENCES

American Association of Colleges of Nursing. (2006). *The essentials of doctoral education for advanced practice nursing.* Retrieved from http://www.aacn.nche.edu/DNP/pdf/Essentials.pdf

APRN Consensus Workgroup & National Council of State Boards of Nursing APRN Advisory Committee. (2008). *The consensus model for APRN regulation, licensure, accreditation, certification and education.* Retrieved from http://www.aacn.nche.edu/education-resources/APRNReport.pdf

Gordis, L. (2014). *Epidemiology* (5th ed.). Canada: Elsevier Saunders.

Heller, R., & Page, J. (2002). A population perspective to evidence based medicine: "Evidence for population health." *Journal of Epidemiology & Community Health, 56*(1), 45–47.

Acknowledgments

We express our grateful thanks to those professional colleagues who provided direction, guidance, and assistance in writing this book. We also thank our family and friends for their support throughout this process. Thank you to our publisher, Margaret Zuccarini, for her invaluable advice, assistance, and infinite patience, and to Jacob Seifert, assistant editor at Springer, for his assistance and expertise throughout the revision of this book. Thank you also to Kris Parrish, production editor at Springer, for her prompt responses to our questions and requests. And finally, we could not have completed the text without the help of the library staff of the Health Services Library of Capital Health, especially Erica Moncrief, MS, director of library services, and Jennifer Kral, MLS, Capital Health librarian.

Introduction to Population-Based Nursing

Ann L. Cupp Curley

Some of the most significant women in the history of nursing made their reputations by providing population-based care. Their influence on nursing has been such that their names live on and their achievements continue to be recognized because of their important contributions to nursing and to healthcare. A brief look at the stories of some of these women helps to provide a background for understanding population health.

Although she started her career as a teacher, Clarissa (Clara) Barton won her greatest acclaim as a nurse. Horrified by the suffering of wounded soldiers in the American Civil War (many of them former neighbors and students) and struck by the lack of supplies needed to care for them, she worked to obtain various supplies and put herself at great risk by nursing soldiers on the front lines of several major battles. Her experience would eventually lead to her becoming the founder and first president of the American Red Cross (Evans, 2003).

During the Crimean War, Florence Nightingale used statistical analysis to plot the incidence of preventable deaths among British soldiers. She used a diagram to dramatize the unnecessary deaths of soldiers caused by unsanitary conditions and lobbied political and military leaders in London for the need to reform. She worked to promote the idea that social phenomena could be objectively measured and subjected to mathematical analysis. Along with William Farr, she was one of the earliest healthcare practitioners to collect and analyze data in order to persuade people of the need for change in healthcare practices (Dossey, 2000; Lipsey, 2006).

Mary Breckinridge started the Frontier Nursing Service (FNS) in Kentucky in 1925 and remained its director until her death in 1965. Educated as a nurse and midwife, she devoted her life to improving health in rural areas, especially among women and children. She believed in working with the communities that were served by the FNS, and formed and worked with committees composed of community members to help plan and provide care.

Similar to Florence Nightingale, she believed in the use of statistics to measure outcomes. From its onset, the FNS was so successful that there was an immediate drop in infant and maternal deaths in the communities served by the FNS (January, 2009; Frontier Nursing Service, 2014).

These three nurses all worked to improve the health of at-risk populations. They met with political leaders to advocate changes in polices to benefit those populations, and both Nightingale and Breckinridge used statistical analysis to both support the need for change and to evaluate their interventions. Breckinridge was an early advocate of engaging communities to help address community health issues. They were all pioneers of nursing and, although perhaps not in name, certainly in fact, among the first nurses working in advanced practice.

For decades, community health nurses have recognized the importance and the impact of population-based care, but large segments of nursing practice have focused primarily on caring for individual patients. Nursing remains, and should remain, a practice-based and caring profession, but nursing practice is changing. There is a growing awareness of the need to provide evidence-based care and to design interventions that have a broad impact on the populations that nursing serves, no matter the setting. Population health obligates healthcare professionals to implement standard interventions, based on the best research evidence, to improve the health of targeted groups of people. It also obligates nurses to discover new and effective strategies for providing care and promoting health. Although clinical decision making related to individual patients is important, it has little impact on overall health outcomes for populations. Interventions at the population level have the potential to improve overall health across communities.

This book addresses the essential areas of content for a doctorate in nursing practice (DNP) as recommended by the American Association of Colleges of Nursing (AACN), with a focus on the AACN core competencies for population-based nursing. The goal is to provide readers with information that will help them to identify healthcare needs at the population level and to improve population outcomes. Although the focus is on the essential components of a DNP program, the intent is to broadly address practice issues that should be the concern of any nurse in an advanced practice role.

This chapter introduces the reader to the concept of population-based nursing. The reader learns how to identify population parameters, the potential impact of a population-based approach to care, and the importance of designing nursing interventions at the population level in advanced nursing practice.

BACKGROUND

> *For all the scare tactics out there, what's truly scary—truly risky—is the prospect of doing nothing.*
> —President Barack Obama, *The New York Times*, August 16, 2009

The first two decades of the 21st century have been witness to a growing and contentious debate on healthcare reforms. President Barack Obama's stated goals in pushing for reforming health insurance were to extend healthcare coverage to the millions who lacked health insurance, stop the insurance industry's practice of denying coverage on the basis of preexisting conditions, and cut overall healthcare costs.

There is ample evidence of a need for healthcare reform in the United States. The gross domestic product (GDP) is the total market value of the output of labor and property located in the United States. It reflects the contribution of the healthcare sector relative to all other production in the United. In 1960, the health sector's proportion of the GDP was 5% (i.e., $5 of every $100 spent in the United States went to pay for healthcare services). By 1990, this figure had grown to 12% and by 1996, 14%. A report issued by the Committee on the Budget of the U.S. Senate in 2008 warned that unless changes were made in how the United States provides care to its citizens, the GDP for the healthcare sector would grow to 25% by 2025 and 49% by 2089 (Orszag, 2008). In 2014, the Centers for Medicare & Medicaid Services (CMS) published its forecast of healthcare costs for 2013 to 2023. Its estimates are similar to those previously published by the Senate. The CMS has projected that healthcare spending will increase an average of 5.7% each year from 2013 to 2023, about 1.1% faster than the GDP. If accurate, healthcare spending would account for 19.3% of the GDP by 2023. According to the CMS, the state of the economy in the United States, the expansion of the Affordable Care Act (ACA), and the aging of the U.S. population are the three major factors driving healthcare costs at this time (CMS, 2014). The Organization for Economic Cooperation and Development (OECD) provides a global picture of healthcare spending. It reports that U.S. expenditures for healthcare as reflected by GDP are nearly double those of the average for OECD countries. One interesting fact that can be gleaned from that report is that the OECD attributes that the difference in costs (U.S. costs as compared to other countries) is due to private health sector prices, primarily pharmaceuticals (OECD, 2013).

The rising cost of healthcare is reflected in the insurance industry. According to the Henry J. Kaiser Family Foundation (2014a), the average annual premium for employer-sponsored family health coverage in 2014 is $16,834 and the average annual contribution from employees is $4,823. They also report that the average deductible is $1,217. Since 2009, the average deductible has risen 47%.

Unfortunately, although the United States ranks first in spending on healthcare among industrialized nations, it ranks lower than most industrialized countries in important health indicators. Two commonly used indicators for measuring a country's health are infant mortality and life expectancy at birth. Worldwide, the United States is ranked 42nd for life expectancy at birth (life expectancy at birth in the United States is 79.56 years) and 55th for infant mortality (infant mortality rate in the United States is 6.17/1,000 live births; Central Intelligence Agency [CIA], 2014). A report issued by the Institute of Medicine (IOM, 2010a) argues that the system used in the United States for gathering and analyzing health measures is part of the problem. A second problem is the inadequate system used in the United States for gathering, analyzing, and communicating information on the underlying factors that lead to chronic health conditions and other risk factors that contribute to poor health. Readers can refer to Chapter 11 for a more detailed description of how the United States ranks among other countries in relation to health indicators.

Health insurance is an important factor in any discussion about healthcare. The United States is the only industrialized country in the world without universal care. In 2013, 30% of people in the United States who were uninsured went without needed medical care. People who are uninsured are less likely than those who are insured to receive preventive care (Henry J. Kaiser Family Foundation, 2014b). The Commonwealth Fund, a private foundation whose stated mission is to promote a high-performing healthcare system, commissioned a survey of U.S. adults that was conducted by Princeton Survey Research Associates (Collins, Doty, Robertson, & Garber, 2010). The survey looked at the effect of health insurance coverage on healthcare-seeking behaviors. They found that among uninsured women aged 50 to 64, 48% say they did not see a doctor when they were sick, did not fill a prescription, or skipped a test, treatment, or follow-up visit because they could not afford it. The survey results also showed that only 67% of uninsured adult respondents had their blood pressure checked within the past year compared to 91% of insured adults. Additionally, only 31% of uninsured women aged 50 to 64 reported having a mammogram in the past 2 years, compared to 79% of women with health insurance.

Driven by a need for change in how healthcare is paid for, the ACA was signed into law by President Obama in 2010. It went into effect over the span of 4 years beginning in 2011. The public option in the ACA proposed that an insurance plan be offered by the federal government for purchase by consumers and small businesses. This option was eliminated from the reconciled legislation. Currently, there are three different "markets" for insurance through the ACA. The federal marketplace is run solely by the federal government. The state marketplace is run solely by the state, and in partnership marketplaces, states run many of the important functions and make key decisions but the marketplace is operated by the federal government. The ACA includes an option whereby states can expand Medicaid eligibility.

Although it is too early to determine whether the legislation has had an effect on health indicators, there is evidence that the ACA is impacting insurance rates. The Centers for Disease Control and Prevention (CDC) released a report based on the 2014 *National Health Interview Survey* in late 2014 (Cohen & Martinez, 2014). According to this report, 41 million people in the United States were without health insurance in the first 3 months of 2014. This number represents 13.1% of the U.S. population. The lowest uninsured rate (6.6%) is for children 17 years of age and younger as most states have state/federal-funded programs to cover children. (The State Children's Health Insurance Program [SCHIP] was enacted in 1997 as a Medicaid expansion program to insure children whose families made too much to qualify for Medicaid but whose incomes did not permit private insurance coverage.) The report notes that adults younger than 65 were three times more likely to be uninsured (18.4%) than children, a disparity that many hope the ACA will diminish. Almost 10% of the total U.S. population was uninsured for more than a year. Although uninsured rates remain high, the report did find that the number of uninsured adults decreased from 20.4% in 2013 to 18.4% during the first quarter of 2014. A survey conducted by the Gallup Poll in the first quarter of 2014 found that the uninsured rate among adults in the United States for the fourth quarter of 2014 averaged 12.9%, a significant drop from the uninsured rate of 17.1% for the same period 1 year before (Levy, 2014). As noted earlier, it will take time to see whether insured rates for all ages will approach 100%, but the more important goal will be to see whether overall health improves. Of equal importance is to determine whether the ACA improves access to healthcare along with improved insurance rates.

Differences in insurance rates are being observed based on the choices made by states as they relate to the ACA. In the first 3 months of 2014, uninsured rates decreased in states that opted for Medicaid expansion, but not in those states that did not opt for the expansion. In those states that expanded Medicaid, the insurance rate in people younger than 64 dropped from 18.4% to 15.7% in the first quarter of 2014. It did not change in states that did not expand eligibility. During the same time period, there were no decreases in uninsured rates for either state or federal marketplaces, but there was a decrease in the uninsured rate in people aged 64 and younger in partnership marketplaces (Cohen & Martinez, 2014).

There is also evidence that the ACA has impacted the insurance rate of Latinos in the United States. Historically, Latinos have had the highest uninsured rates of any racial or ethnic group in the United States. Less than 1 year after the ACA was implemented, the overall Latino uninsured rate dropped from 36% to 23%, according to the *Commonwealth Fund Affordable Care Act Tracking Survey*, conducted in 2014 (Rasmussen, Collins, Doty, & Beutel, 2014). Notably, the uninsured rate among Latinos in states that did not expand their Medicaid program at the time of the survey remained unchanged. These states are home to about 20 million Latinos, the majority of whom live in Texas and Florida (Doty, Blumenthal, & Collins, 2014).

It is unclear if or how healthcare will be affected in the long term by the ACA, because the law is constantly being challenged by several groups and it is too soon to determine whether it will have an impact on any health indicators. As this book goes to print, Republicans, who have tried repeatedly to strike down the legislation, have taken control of the Senate as well as the House. The Supreme Court's June 2015 decision in *King v. Burwell* preserves federal healthcare subsidies under the ACA for Americans who reside in states that have opted not to create their own health insurance exchanges. In so doing, it removes an immediate uncertainty for those who would have been left without coverage if the federal exchanges had been declared unconstitutional (*King v. Burwell*, June 25, 2015). The ACA currently specifies the maximum amounts people will have to pay in cost sharing based on their incomes, and federal subsidies make up the rest.

Our healthcare system is complex, and there is no simple solution to lowering costs and improving access. The goal of this textbook is not to provide an overarching solution to the issues of cost, but to propose that nurses can contribute to improving the cost-effectiveness and efficiency of care through the provision of evidence-based treatment guidelines to identified populations with shared needs, and by advocating for policies that address the underlying factors that impact health and healthcare. To do this, we must change the way that we deliver healthcare and become politically active. In an ideal world, healthcare policies are created based on valid and reliable evidence and population need and demand. The ideal premise is that there is equitable distribution of healthcare services and that the appropriate care is given to the right people at the right time and at a reasonable cost. For 20 years, the American Nurses Association (ANA) has been advocating for healthcare reforms that would guarantee access to high-quality healthcare for all. The ANA supports the ACA and was an advocate for the public option (ANA, 2014). It is a function of individual choice to either support or not support healthcare reforms. The actions of professional organizations are driven by membership. Regardless of your political alliance, involvement in professional organizations as well as in local, state, and national political activities (even if only minimally as a registered and active voter) is part of the professional responsibility of advanced practice registered nurses (APRNs).

DEFINING POPULATIONS

The AACN definition of advanced practice nursing includes recognizing the importance of identifying and managing health outcomes at the population level (AACN, 2004). In 2006, the AACN specified that graduates of DNP programs have competency in meeting "the needs of a panel of patients, a target population, a set of populations, or a broad community" (AACN, 2006, p. 10). A core component of DNP education is clinical prevention (health promotion and disease prevention at individual and family levels) and population health (focus of care at aggregate and community levels and examination of environmental, occupational, cultural, and socioeconomic dimensions of health) (AACN, 2006; Allan et al., 2004). Regardless of whether DNP graduates practice with a focus on clinical prevention or population health, the ability to define, identify, and analyze outcomes is imperative for improving the health status of individuals and populations (AACN, 2006).

The goal of population-based nursing is to provide evidence-based care to targeted groups of people with similar needs in order to improve outcomes. Population-based nursing uses a defined population or aggregate as the organizing unit for care. *The American Heritage Dictionary of the English Language* ("Population," 2002, p. 1366) defines a population as "all of the people inhabiting a specified area." A second definition is given as "the total number of inhabitants constituting a particular race, class, or group in a specified area" (p. 1366). Subpopulations may be referred to as *aggregates*. Many different parameters can be used to identify or categorize subpopulations or aggregates. They may be defined by ethnicity (e.g., African American or Hispanic), religion (e.g., Roman Catholic or Buddhist), or geographic location (e.g., Boston or San Diego). Aggregates can also be defined by age or occupation. People with a shared diagnosis (e.g., diabetes) or a shared risk factor (e.g., smoking) comprise other identifiable aggregates. Sometimes people may choose to describe themselves as members of a particular group (e.g., Democrat or Socialist). One person may belong to more than one such group (e.g., White, younger than 18 years, current smoker, etc.).

A community is composed of multiple aggregates. The most common aggregate used in population-based nursing is the high-risk aggregate. A high-risk aggregate is a subgroup or subpopulation of a community that shares a high-risk factor among its members, such as a high-risk health condition (e.g., congestive heart failure) or a shared high-risk factor (e.g., smoking and sedentary behavior). The aggregate concept can be used to target interventions to specific aggregates or subpopulations within a community (Porche, 2004). The implementation of standard or proven (evidence-based) strategies to prevent illness and/or improve the health of targeted groups of people can have the effect of ameliorating health problems at the population and/or aggregate level. Making change at the population level may impact the health of a community not only in the present but for generations to come. As we learn how to approach and target populations using evidence, we improve our chance of long-term success and can strive to make lifelong changes in the health of a group of people.

USING DATA TO TARGET POPULATIONS AND AGGREGATES AT RISK

The collection and analysis of data provide healthcare professionals and policy makers with a starting point for identifying, selecting, and implementing interventions that target specific populations and aggregates. Many of the leading causes of death in the United States are preventable. One in three American adults has cardiovascular disease, and it is the leading cause of death among both men and women in the country, killing an average of one American every 37 seconds (American Heart Association [AHA], n.d.). On the basis of data from 2010, the CDC has identified, in descending order, the 10 leading causes of death in the United States They are heart disease, cancer, chronic lower respiratory tract diseases, accidents, stroke, Alzheimer's disease, diabetes, influenza and pneumonia, renal diseases, and intentional self-harm (e.g., suicide) (CDC, 2014a). Several factors, such as the physical environment, healthcare systems, personal behaviors, and the social environment, can have a deleterious impact on individual and community health. The negative consequences of these factors are researched and well documented.

Smoking

Life expectancy for smokers is at least 10 years shorter than for nonsmokers. It is a leading cause of preventable morbidity and mortality, causing nearly one of every five deaths annually in the United States. This figure includes heart attack deaths and lung cancer deaths among nonsmokers who are exposed to secondhand smoke. It is estimated that smoking contributes $96 billion to healthcare costs in the United States (CDC, 2014b).

The CDC used the *2012–2013 National Adult Tobacco Survey* (NATS) to estimate adult smoking prevalence rates in the United States. The findings indicate that 21.3% of U.S. adults use a tobacco product every day or some days. Smoking rates are higher among men, younger adults, non-Hispanic adults, those living in the Midwest and South, those with less education and income, and LGBT (lesbian, gay, bisexual, and transgender) adults (Agaku et al., 2014). Although higher rates are seen in younger adults, a reduction in smoking by school-age children should result in reductions in tobacco-related deaths in the future, and there is good news related to smoking rates among this group. Cigarette smoking rates for high school students have dropped to the lowest levels since the National Youth Risk Behavior Survey (YRBS) began in 1991. The U.S. teen smoking rate of 15.7% has met the national Healthy People 2020 objective of reducing adolescent cigarette usage to 16% or less (CDC, 2014c).

Coupled with this good news related to teen smoking is a new and troubling factor that has emerged, and that is the use of e-cigarettes. Technology has contributed to many positive advances in healthcare. E-cigarettes are not one of them. E-cigarettes are metal tubes that heat liquid into an inhalable vapor that contains nicotine. A study that focused on middle and high school students found that during 2011 to 2013, the number of youth who had never smoked a cigarette but had used e-cigarettes at least once increased by 300%, from 79,000 in 2011 to more than 263,000 in 2013. It is legal for children to purchase e-cigarettes in 10 states, including the District of Columbia. The U.S. Food and Drug Administration (FDA) proposed rules in 2014 that would ban the sale of e-cigarettes to anyone under the age of 18 (Beasley, 2014). APRNs need to keep abreast of new behaviors that can impact health. Being informed about risky behaviors is of primary importance for APRNs to be effective in planning and delivering evidence-based care and in lobbying for changes to protect the public's health.

Another very popular trend is the use of hookahs. Hookahs are water pipes used to smoke specially flavored tobaccos. More and more youth are drawn toward this social trend in which groups of people share a hookah usually in a café setting (American Lung Association, 2007, n.d.). Although hookahs have been around for hundreds of years, they are not a safe alternative to smoking. A Monitoring the Future survey found that as many as 17% of high school seniors have tried hookahs. The numbers are even higher for college-age students (U.S. Department of Health and Human Services, 2012). The tobacco and smoke from hookahs have toxic properties and have been linked to various cancers, including lung and oral cancers. Many of the same effects of cigarette smoking are found with smoking hookahs, and very little is being done to educate youth on the health effects of hookahs (Cobb, Ward, Maziak, Shihadeh, & Eissenberg, 2010). As with any potential threat to health, education of our youth and adult populations regarding the deleterious effects of hookahs is paramount to reducing the potential morbidity and mortality of long-term exposure to these flavored tobaccos. More recently, newer electronic forms of hookahs have been introduced, and little research has been conducted to determine the long-term health effects of these products. Regardless, the use of hookahs is another growing epidemic of health behaviors that an APRN can attempt to modify by evidence-based prevention education. For more on the effects of hookahs, refer to the CDC's site (http://www.cdc .gov/tobacco/data_statistics/fact_sheets/tobacco_industry/hookahs/index .htm#overview).

There is huge potential for cost savings by preventing smoking-related illnesses, and one cannot overlook the effects of secondhand smoking on the health of family members and coworkers. It is well known that secondhand smoke has long-lasting effects on the unborn fetus, infant, and child. These effects can manifest as low birth weight in newborns (Ventura, Hamilton, Mathews, & Chandra, 2003), increased respiratory infections and higher risk of asthma exacerbations (U.S. Environmental Protection Agency [EPA], 2014), sudden infant death (Anderson & Cook, 1997), and a lower intelligence quotient (Yolton, Dietrich, Auinger, Lanphear, & Hornung, 2005). Thus, it is important to recognize not only the direct effects of smoking on health but also the indirect effects on the fetus, infants, children, and family members. The effects of secondhand smoke are not specific to smoking cigarettes. Exposure to hookah smoke is also associated with very similar effects on the fetus, infants, and family members. Education of pregnant mothers is just as important as with other family members as they may not realize the negative effects of secondhand exposure to hookah or cigarette smoke.

As with other smoking-related diseases, the cessation of smoking early on can reverse or ameliorate the potential long-term harmful effects of secondhand smoke exposure. These data provide a starting point for targeting specific high-risk groups for intervention based on parameters such as age, education, income, and geographical location. Another pertinent fact is that many insurance companies are now charging higher premiums for smokers than for nonsmokers. This has led to increasing interest in cessation programs, but whether this will have a long-term impact on smoking rates is unknown. Smoking cessation and smoking prevention programs are not the only areas that offer opportunities for improving the health of people in the United States and for saving money. Other health problems, such as obesity, are also significant public health concerns.

Obesity

In 2009, researchers published their analysis of the cost of obesity in the United States, taking into account separate categories for inpatient, outpatient, and prescription drug spending. They estimated that the medical costs of obesity may have been as high as $147 billion/year by 2008 (including $7 billion in Medicare prescription drug costs). According to their findings, the annual medical costs for people who are obese were $1,429 higher than those for normal-weight people (Finkelstein, Trogdon, Cohen, & Dietz, 2009).

Ogden, Carroll, Kit, and Flegal (2014) studied the prevalence of obesity in children and adults in the United States. They also looked at trends between 2003 and 2012 and found no significant changes in obesity rates for youths or adults between 2003 and 2012. They did find that there was a significant decrease in obesity among children aged 2 to 5 (from 13.9/1,000 to 8.4/1,000). This good news was somewhat tempered by the fact that the rate increased for children aged 2 to 19 (from 16.9/1,000 to 19.34/1,000). They also reported that older non-Hispanic Blacks have the highest age-adjusted rates of obesity (47.8%), followed by Hispanics (42.5%), non-Hispanic Whites (32.6%), and non-Hispanic Asians (10.8%). Among age groups, obesity is higher among middle-age adults (39.5% for people aged 40–59), than among younger adults (30.3% for people aged 20–39), and highest among older adults (35.4% for 60 years or older).

As part of Healthy People 2020, the United States set an objective to decrease the proportion of obese adult Americans (20 years of age or older) to 30.5%. Healthy People 2020 uses the baseline of 33.9%, which was the percentage of persons aged 20 years and older who were obese in 2005 to 2008. The target objective for children (aged 2 to 19 years) is 14.5%. The baseline data for this objective is 16.1%, which was the percentage of children who were considered obese in 2005 to 2008 (HealthyPeople.gov, 2014).

Obesity is associated with increased morbidity and mortality rates. For example, Borrell and Samuel (2014) found that obese adults, when compared with normal-weight adults, had 20% higher all-cause and cardiovascular disease mortality rates, even when controlling for demographic and behavioral characteristics. Although people are familiar with the association between heart disease and obesity, many are just learning about the relationship between obesity and cancer. Obesity is associated with an increased risk for many cancers, including esophageal, pancreatic, colon and rectal, breast (after menopause), endometrial, kidney, thyroid, and gallbladder. It has been estimated that the percentage of cases attributed to obesity (although it varies) may be as high as 40% for some cancers, particularly endometrial and esophageal cancers (National Cancer Institute, 2014).

Jacobs et al. (2010) published a study that helps to illustrate the complexity of understanding risk factors and their relationship to the development of poor health. They studied the association between waist circumference and mortality among 48,500 men and 56,343 women 50 years or older. They determined that waist circumference as a measure of abdominal obesity is associated with higher mortality independent of body mass index (BMI). They note that waist circumference is associated with higher circulating levels of inflammatory markers, insulin resistance, type 2 diabetes, dyslipidemia, and coronary heart disease. In recent years, the constellation of these factors has been described as the *metabolic syndrome*. Metabolic syndrome is a complex syndrome that encompasses many conditions and risk factors, particularly abdominal obesity, high blood pressure, abnormal cholesterol and triglyceride levels, and insulin resistance, and is known to be associated with an increased risk of stroke, heart disease, and type 2 diabetes (Grundy et al., 2005). The increasing prevalence of metabolic syndrome is becoming a tremendous public health concern, and more evidence is appearing in the literature to better define the treatment as well as preventive measures needed to reduce the incidence. Although it is ill defined in children and adolescents, it is clear that early interventions to reduce obesity and sedentary behavior and to improve nutrition can have long-term effects and can improve overall life expectancy. The metabolic syndrome, similar to many conditions, demonstrates the complexity of interactions that occurs in disease development and that no one factor in and of itself can be targeted alone. Our understanding of obesity is also becoming more complex, as new studies have identified independent associations between sitting time/sedentary behaviors and increasing all-cause and cardiovascular disease mortality risk. This phenomenon highlights the importance of avoiding prolonged, uninterrupted periods of sitting time (Dunstan, Thorp, & Healy, 2011). The APRN needs to take into consideration the many facets of health and disease, genetics and environment, including human attitudes, attributes, and behavior when determining how to implement a population-based intervention.

Diabetes Mellitus

One cannot talk about the epidemic of obesity and not mention its concomitant relationship to diabetes mellitus (DM). The number of American adults treated for DM more than doubled between 1996 and 2007 (from about 9 to 19 million). This includes an increase from 1.2 to 2.4 million among people aged 18 to 44 years. During this time period, the treatment costs for DM climbed from $18.5 to $40.8 billion (Soni, 2010). In June 2014, the American Diabetes Association released the results of the *National Diabetes Statistics* report (CDC, 2014d). The report highlights the importance of tracking morbidity rates and the need to be aware of trends in order to target groups for interventions. The percentage of Americans with DM aged 65 and older is estimated to be as high as 25.9% (accounting for over 11 million seniors), which includes those who are undiagnosed. The incidence rate of diabetes in 2012 was 1.7 million new diagnoses per year.

The rise in both incidence and prevalence rates for DM is closely tied to rising obesity levels, which is a preventable risk factor. This upward trend in the incidence rate for DM provides a clear direction for targeting prevention measures toward younger populations. There is, in fact, a huge potential for improving the health of populations by targeting children using primary prevention measures that go well beyond reducing diabetes rates. Implications for early interventions beginning in pregnancy and continuing through infancy and early childhood are clear. Evidence is increasing that early feeding patterns (e.g., breast-feeding versus formula feeding) as well as parental obesity and parental eating patterns are linked to the increased likelihood of developing obesity in children, which puts them at an increased risk for type 2 DM (Owen, Martin, Whincup, Smith, & Cook, 2005). There are many opportunities for APRNs to apply evidence-based, primary prevention interventions to improve the long-term outcomes of children at the beginning of pregnancy and at birth and thereafter. This approach may include targeting high-risk aggregates (e.g., parents with obesity and type 2 DM) and then expanding to communities through educational campaigns or changes in health policy.

Health and the Social Environment

Most of the information discussed earlier exemplifies the biological and environmental factors that contribute to poor health in adults. However, it is becoming more apparent that social (e.g., psychological) factors starting as early as conception (e.g., maternal stress) may play a more significant role in adult health than was once thought. Having a comprehensive understanding of the underlying causes of adult diseases (including social, psychological, biological, and environmental) is necessary to successfully approach the problems seen in populations. Without this comprehensive understanding, it may be difficult to successfully implement a primary prevention program (the goal of which is to prevent disease before it occurs).

Stress is a regular part of day-to-day life, and small amounts of stress are normal and necessary for developing coping skills. However, exposure to prolonged and severe stressors, such as abuse, neglect, or being a witness to or victim of violence, can lead to changes that occur in the brain and can lead to short-term and even long-term poor health outcomes. This type of stress is termed *toxic stress*. The effects of toxic stress are being rigorously studied, and in particular, studies looking at adverse childhood events (ACE) were some of the first to show a correlation between toxic stress exposures and high-risk behaviors and poor health outcomes in adults. The ACE study is an ongoing, joint project of the CDC and Kaiser Permanente that looks retrospectively at the relationships among several categories of childhood trauma. Childhood trauma exposures were broken down into three categories: abuse (e.g., physical or sexual), neglect (e.g., emotional or physical), and household dysfunction (e.g., having an incarcerated household member, family member with mental health issue and/or drug and alcohol problems, domestic violence, or parental divorce or separation). An ACE score is calculated based on past exposures to the subparts of each of the aforementioned categories. The higher the ACE score, the stronger the relationship to high-risk behaviors or poor health outcomes (ACE Study, 2011). In one widely cited ACE study (Felitti et al., 1998), people who experienced a score of four or more categories of ACEs, compared with those who had no history of exposure, had a 4- to 12-fold increased risk for alcoholism, drug abuse, depression, and suicide attempts. They also experienced a 2- to 4-fold increase in smoking and self-reported poor health. Subsequent research provides additional evidence to support the link between childhood trauma and adverse events and poor health outcomes. For additional information on the effects of childhood stress, refer to the CDC publication at www.cdc.gov/ncipc/pub-res/pdf/Childhood_Stress.pdf.

Many additional studies have been conducted that demonstrate the destructive effects of exposure to *toxic stress*. Goodwin and Stein (2004) identified an increased risk of diabetes in adults who were neglected as children and an increased risk of cardiac disease in adults who were sexually abused as children. Smyth, Heron, Wonderlich, Crosby, and Thompson (2008) completed a study of students entering college directly from high school to investigate the association between adverse events in childhood and eating disturbances. They found that childhood adverse events predicted eating disturbances in college. Childhood adverse events have also been linked to drug abuse and dependence (Messina et al., 2008) and greater use of healthcare and mental health services (Cannon, Bonomi, Anderson, Rivara, & Thompson, 2010). Building on earlier studies that linked smoking in adulthood with ACEs, Brown et al. (2010) discovered a relationship between a history of ACEs and the risk of dying from lung cancer. Researchers have identified similar outcomes in studies carried out with populations in other countries. A study conducted in Saudi Arabia, where beating and insults are an acceptable parenting style, identified a correlation between beating and insults (once or more per month) and an increased risk for cancer, cardiac disease, and asthma (Hyland, Alkhalaf, & Whalley, 2012). Scott, Smith, and Ellis (2012) completed a study in New Zealand which found that adults who had a history of child protection involvement had increased odds of a diagnosis of asthma.

More and more studies are being conducted to look at the relationship of sustained exposure to toxic stress to a variety of poor health outcomes and high-risk behaviors. These behaviors include such things as cutting, hypervigilance, promiscuity, eating disorders, poor school performance, depression, violence, suicidal ideation/attempts, and justice system involvement. These are just a few of the many behaviors found to be associated with sustained exposure to toxic stress. Studies such as these illustrate the importance of understanding the social determinants of poor health and the potential for doing good and preventing harm to aggregates and populations by targeting exposures to such things as child abuse and neglect for prevention, early recognition, and intervention.

Population Strategies in Acute Care

Targeting evidence-based interventions toward aggregates in the acute care population also has the potential to improve health outcomes broadly. How can we improve the quality of care for our acute care patients by taking a population-based approach? When nurses apply evidence-based interventions to identified aggregates, they can improve outcomes more effectively than when interventions are designed on a case-by-case (individualized) basis. The following examples illustrate this point.

Several organizations, including the Association for Professionals in Infection Control and Epidemiology and the CDC, have proposed a call to action to move toward elimination of healthcare–associated infections. The CDC and Agency for Healthcare Research and Quality (AHRQ) have published evidence-based recommendations for preventing central venous catheter-related bloodstream infections (CR-BSIs). These recommendations include hand hygiene, use of maximal barrier precautions, use of chlorhexidine gluconate for insertion site preparation, and avoidance of catheter changes. Catheters impregnated with antimicrobial agents are recommended when infection rates are high and/or catheters will be in place for a long time. Using these guidelines, hospitals have made good progress in reducing the incidence rate of CR-BSIs. In a report released by the CDC, CR-BSIs fell 46% between 2008 and 2013 (Steenhuysen, 2015).

Another intervention that uses standard, evidence-based protocols to improve long-term outcomes addresses the treatment of stroke in an acute care setting. It was found that stroke patients taken to hospitals that follow specific treatment protocols have a better chance of surviving than patients taken to hospitals without specific stroke treatment protocols. A study evaluated the outcomes of the first 1 million stroke patients treated at hospitals enrolled in the Get With the Guidelines stroke program that was started by the AHA in 2003. The American Stroke Association guidelines require that hospitals follow seven specific evidence-based steps for treating stroke patients. Between 2003 and 2009, hospitals that followed these protocols lowered the risk of death by 10% for patients with ischemic stroke (Fonarow et al., 2011).

Surveillance of poor health outcomes in acute care facilities is one way in which APRNs can identify causative factors and design interventions to reduce costs and improve care. For example, recognizing the causative factors that lead to increased rehospitalization rates and superutilization of emergency departments could be the first step in designing an intervention. Approximately 25% of all U.S. hospital patients are readmitted within 1 year for the same conditions that led to their original hospitalization. The AHRQ analyzed data from 2006 to 2007 on 15 million patients in 12 states. They found that among Medicare patients, 42% were readmitted to hospitals and 30% had multiple emergency department visits. Among Medicaid patients, 23% had multiple hospital admissions and 50% had multiple emergency department visits. According to the AHRQ, better outpatient care could prevent unnecessary repeat hospital admissions (AHRQ, 2010). Identifying and targeting populations with specific diagnoses for which there are high readmission rates offers great return on investment. Readmissions are costly in dollars to both consumers and hospitals and negatively impact the quality of life for patients.

Chronic Conditions

Noncommunicable diseases (NCDs) are the main cause of illness and disability in the United States and are responsible for the greater part of healthcare costs according to the CDC. About half (50.9%) of U.S. adults have at least one chronic condition, and 26% have two or more chronic conditions. Most chronic conditions result from preventable risk factors such as smoking, poor diet, sedentary behavior, excessive alcohol consumption, high blood pressure, and high cholesterol (Bauer, Briss, Goodman, & Bowman, 2014). In 2000, the U.S. Department of Health and Human Services (HHS) released a report outlining a strategic framework that includes goals to foster healthcare and public health system changes to improve the health of those with multiple chronic conditions. The intention of the framework is to create change in how chronic illnesses are addressed in the United States from an individual approach to one that uses a population-focused approach. The authors of the report point out that 66% of total healthcare spending is directed toward caring for the approximately 20% of Americans with multiple concurrent chronic conditions (e.g., arthritis, heart disease, and DM). One strategy proposed by the HHS is to define and identify populations and subpopulations with multiple chronic conditions broadly and to explore care models to target subgroups at high risk of poor health outcomes. Another proposed strategy addresses the need to develop systems to promote models to address common risk factors and challenges that are associated with many chronic conditions. The framework also addresses the need to create policies and interventions that identify populations and subpopulations at risk and to identify strategies and interventions that target these populations (U.S. Department of Health and Human Services, 2010).

The problem of chronic diseases is not restricted to the United States. The World Health Organization (WHO) has published a report that documents the global problem of NCDs. NCDs now account for more deaths than infectious diseases even in poor countries. Director-General Dr. Margaret Chan of the WHO is quoted as saying, "[F]or some countries, it is no exaggeration to describe the situation is an impending disaster; a disaster for health, society, most of all for national economies" (WHO, 2011, p. v). Chronic diseases, such as heart disease, stroke, cancer, chronic respiratory diseases, and diabetes, are the leading cause of global mortality, representing 60% of all deaths. Out of the 35 million people who died from chronic disease in 2005, half were under 70 years old (WHO, 2014). Millions of people die each year as a result of modifiable risk factors that underlie the major NCDs. The writers of a report by the WHO contend that 8% of premature heart disease, stroke, and diabetes can be prevented. Ten action points, including banning smoking in public places, enforcing tobacco advertising bans, restricting access to alcohol, and reducing salt in food, are listed. All of these actions require a population approach to be effective (WHO, 2011).

A survey conducted by the AHA lends an interesting perspective to this argument. They surveyed 1,000 people in the United States. The AHA found that 76% of the respondents agreed that wine can be good for the heart but only 30% knew the AHA's recommended limits for daily wine consumption. Drinking too much alcohol of any kind can increase blood pressure and lead to heart failure. The survey results also found that most respondents do not know the source of sodium content in their diets and are confused by low-sodium food choices. A majority of the respondents (61%) believe that sea salt is a low-sodium alternative to table salt when in fact it is chemically the same. This survey reinforces the idea that people require more understanding of nutrition and the relationship between nutrition and health. It also reinforces the argument that interventions to improve health must be addressed at the community or population level (AHA, 2011).

Interventions that are evidence based and population appropriate can reduce the underlying causes of chronic disease. This approach has the potential to lower the mean level of risk factors and shift outcomes in a favorable direction. An example that is receiving a lot of recent attention is sodium intake. Excess sodium in the diet can put people at risk for stroke and heart disease. The CDC has reported that 9 of 10 Americans consume more salt than is recommended. Only 5.5% of adults follow the recommendation to limit sodium intake to 1,500 mg a day. Most sodium does not come from salt added to foods at the table but from processed foods. These foods include grain-based frozen meals, soup, and processed meat. In this report, the IOM concludes that reducing sodium content in food requires new government standards for the acceptable level of sodium. Manufacturers and restaurants need to meet these standards so that all sources in the food supply are involved (CDC, 2010; IOM, 2010b). A study published in the *Annals of Internal Medicine* (Smith-Spangler, Juusola, Enns, Owens, & Garber, 2010) estimates that reducing dietary salt 0.3 g/day could greatly reduce the yearly number of U.S. cases of coronary heart disease, stroke, and heart attacks, with a savings of up to $24 billion in healthcare costs each year. Although the IOM has published a report that it finds no evidence that a drastic reduction in reduces the risk of heart attacks, stroke, and mortality, the AHA and the CDC both contend that sodium is associated with high blood pressure, and therefore does put people at risk (Mitka, 2013).

This discussion illustrates the need to promulgate laws and develop policies that can effect positive health outcomes. It also illustrates the difficulty involved in planning interventions when evidence is sometimes contradictory, and causation is not only multifactorial but sometimes outside of the control of the people whose health is compromised. Changing individual behavior is difficult and has little impact on population health. Using the power of legislation and regulation to make changes in the environment, such as banning smoking in public places, improving air quality, and reducing the amount of sodium in processed foods, has enormous potential for improving the overall health of populations.

The basic sciences of public health (particularly epidemiology and biostatistics) provide tools for the APRN working with specialized populations to provide evidence for effective and efficient interventions. The care of specialized groups is the core of advanced practice. *Evidence-based practice* is defined as the conscientious integration of best research evidence with clinical expertise and patient values and needs in the delivery of quality, cost-effective healthcare

(Burns & Grove, 2009). Population-based nursing requires APRNs to plan, implement, and evaluate care in the population of interest. The evaluation of outcome measures in populations begins with an identification of the health problems, the needs of defined populations, and the differences among groups. The rates calculated from these numbers can help the APRN to identify risk factors, target populations at risk, and lay the foundation for designing interventions. Prevention is best carried out at the population level, whether at the level of direct care or through the support and promotion of policies. For example, an evidence-based program to prevent hospital readmissions for congestive heart failure can lead to improved health and decreased health-related costs. The promulgation of policies and regulations to support primary prevention measures, such as decreased sodium in prepared foods, could potentially lead to decreased rates of hypertension and heart disease. Interventions that are appropriate at the individual level and applied at the population level can result in a far-reaching effect.

Outcomes measurement refers to collecting and analyzing data using predetermined outcomes indicators for the purposes of making decisions about healthcare (ANA, 2004). Outcomes research in APRN practice is research that focuses on the effectiveness of nursing interventions. Outcomes measurement in population-based care begins with the identification of the population and the problem, followed by the generation of a clinical question related to outcomes. It is a measure of the process of care. An outcomes measure should be clearly quantifiable, be relatively easy to define, and lend itself to standardization.

In outcomes measurement, the APRN is ultimately concerned with whether or not a population benefits from an intervention. The APRN also needs to be concerned with the question of quality, efficacy (Does the intervention work under ideal conditions?), and effectiveness (Does it work under real-life situations?). Other important considerations are efficiency (cost benefit), affordability, accessibility, and acceptability.

SUMMARY

The Robert Wood Johnson Foundation and the IOM have issued a report to respond to the need to transform the nursing profession. The committee developed four key messages:

1. Nurses should practice to the full extent of their education and should achieve higher levels of education training.
2. The education system for nurses should be improved so that it provides seamless academic progression.
3. Nurses should be full partners with physicians and other healthcare professionals.
4. Healthcare in the Unites States should be redesigned for effective workforce planning and policy making. (IOM, 2011)

To improve population health, APRNs need to practice to the full extent of their education, be active in the political arena, and work collaboratively with other healthcare professionals. To promote health, APRNs can use epidemiological methods to identify aggregates at risk, analyze problems of highest priority, design evidence-based interventions, and evaluate the results. An important concept in the field of population health is attention to the multiple determinants of health outcomes and the identification of their distribution throughout the population. These determinants include medical care, public health interventions, characteristics of the social environment (e.g., income, education, employment, social support, culture), physical environment (e.g., clean air, water quality), genetics, and individual behavior. A final note about the use of "APRN" in this book: *The Consensus Model for APRN Regulation: Licensure, Accreditation, Certification & Education* was completed and published in 2008 by the APRN Consensus Work Group and the National Council of State Boards of Nursing APRN Advisory Committee. The title "APRN" is used throughout this book to refer to certified nurse anesthetists, certified nurse midwives, clinical nurse specialists, and certified nurse practitioners. The model was created through a collaborative effort of more than 40 organizations in order to "align the interrelationships among licensure, accreditation, certification, and education to create a more uniform practice across the country" (American Nurses Credentialing Center [ANCC], 2014, 1st bullet point). The goal is for implementation of the model by 2015 (ANCC, 2014; APRN Consensus Work Group, 2008).

EXERCISES AND DISCUSSION QUESTIONS

Exercise 1.1 Using the following table as an example, list the parameters that describe the population(s) to whom you provide care.

Population	Framing Definitions	Parameters
Patients who have been diagnosed with congestive heart failure (CHF) and who live in the community	Adult (18 years of age and older) patients discharged from an urban medical center with a primary diagnosis of CHF	P1 = diagnosis P2 = age P3 = location/service area
Population of New Jersey	All permanent residents of New Jersey	P1 = geographical location P2 = permanent residency

Exercise 1.2 PolitiFact is a website created by the *St. Petersburg Times* (Now the *Tampa Bay Times*) and a winner of the 2009 Pulitzer Prize (www.politifact.com). It was created to help people find the truth in American politics. Reporters and editors from the newspaper check statements by members of Congress, the White House, lobbyists, and interest groups and rate them on a *Truth-O-Meter*. Find a statement that is being circulated about the ACA, and then check the Truth-O-Meter to determine the veracity of the statement.

Exercise 1.3 Identify two or three population-based and health-related interventions at your institution or in your community. Determine whether the approach has been successful in changing outcomes and/or reducing health-related costs. Identify the aggregate population and what parameters were used in this intervention. Identify any changes in policy associated with these interventions.

Exercise 1.4 This chapter includes a brief description of the health effects of hookahs. Design an educational program that addresses the negative health effects of hookahs. First, research the health effects of hookahs and select three to five health effects to address. Identify your target population and design an educational intervention for your target population. What outcomes will you look at to determine whether your intervention works? What approach will you use to engage your target population?

Exercise 1.5 Toxic stress is described and discussed in this chapter. Conduct a search to answer the following questions. What are the three types (categories) of toxic stress? How does toxic stress affect the brain? Review results from the ACE studies and design a population-based prevention program to reduce exposures to toxic stress. Discuss the barriers to designing such a program. Give examples of prevention programs in your state that reduce or prevent toxic stress exposures. How do they work? Are they effective? If they are not effective, explain why you believe they are not working.

REFERENCES

ACE Study. (2011). *The adverse childhood experiences (ACE) study.* Retrieved from http://acestudy.org/index.html

Agaku, I., King, B. A., Husten, C. G., Bunnell, R., Ambrose, B. K., Hu, S. S., . . . Day, H. R. (2014, June 27). Tobacco product use among adults—United States, 2012–2013. *Morbidity and Mortality Weekly Report (MMWR), 63*(25), 542–547. Retrieved from http://www.cdc.gov/mmwr/preview/mmwrhtml/mm6325a3.htm?s_cid=mm6325a3_w

Agency for Healthcare Research and Quality. (2010). 1 in 4 patients undergoes revolving-door hospitalizations [News Release]. *Health.com.* Retrieved from http://news.health.com/2010/06/04/1-in-4-patients-undergoes-revolving-door-hospitalizations/

Allan, J., Barwick, T., Cashman, S., Cawley, J. F., Day, C., Douglass, C. W., . . . Wood, D. (2004). Clinical prevention and population health: Curriculum framework for health professions. *American Journal of Preventive Medicine, 27*(5), 471–476.

American Association of Colleges of Nursing. (2004). *AACN position statement on the practice doctorate in nursing.* Washington, DC: Author.

American Association of Colleges of Nursing. (2006). *The essentials of doctoral education for advanced practice nursing.* Washington, DC: Author. Retrieved from http://www.aacn.nche.edu/DNP/pdf/Essentials.pdf

American Heart Association. (2011). *Most Americans don't understand health effects of wine and sea salt, survey finds.* Dallas, TX: Author. Retrieved from http://newsroom.heart.org/news/1316

American Heart Association. (n.d.). *American Heart Association facts.* Dallas, TX: Author. Retrieved from http://dept.sfcollege.edu/news/daily/pdf/2008/aha_facts.pdf

American Lung Association. (2007). *An emerging deadly trend: Waterpipe tobacco use.* Chicago, IL: Author. Retrieved from http://www.lung.org/stop-smoking/tobacco-control-advocacy/reports-resources/tobacco-policy-trend-reports/2007-tobacco-policy-trend.pdf

American Lung Association. (n.d.). *Hookah smoking: A growing threat to public health.* Chicago, IL: Author. Retrieved from http://www.lung.org/stop-smoking/tobacco-control-advocacy/reports-resources/cessation-economic-benefits/reports/hookah-policy-brief-updated.pdf

American Nurses Association. (2004). *Nursing: Scope and standards of practice.* Washington, DC: Author.

American Nurses Association. (2014). *Healthcare reform.* Silver Spring, MD: Author. Retrieved from http://www.nursingworld.org/MainMenuCategories/Policy-Advocacy/HealthSystemReform

American Nurses Credentialing Center. (2014). *APRN fact sheet.* Retrieved from: http://www.nursecredentialing.org/Certification/APRNCorner/APRN-Factsheet

Anderson, H. R., & Cook, D. G. (1997). Passive smoking and sudden infant death syndrome: Review of the epidemiological evidence. *Thorax, 52,* 1003–1009.

APRN Consensus Work Group & the National Council of State Boards of Nursing APRN Advisory Committee. (2008). *Consensus model for APRN regulation: Licensure, accreditation, certification & education.* Retrieved from http://www.nursecredentialing.org/Certification/APRNCorner.aspx?gclid=CMqL19D8vMMCFXBp7AodchcAvw

Bauer, U., Briss, P. A., Goodman, R. A., & Bowman, B. (2014). Prevention of chronic disease in the 21st century: Elimination of the leading preventable causes of premature death and disability in the USA. *The Lancet, 384*(9937), 45–52. doi:org/10.1016/S0140-6736(14)60648-6

Beasley, D. (2014, September 11). Ten states, District of Columbia allow minors to buy e-cigarettes—CDC. *Reuters U.S. Edition.* Retrieved from http://www.reuters.com/article/2014/12/11/usa-ecigarettes-minors-idUSL1N0TV2RP20141211

Borrell, L. N., & Samuel, L. (2014). Body mass index categories and mortality risk in U.S. adults: The effect of overweight and obesity on advancing death. *American Journal of Public Health, 104*(3), 512–519. doi:10.2105/AJPH.2013.301597

Brown, D., Anda, R., Felitti, V., Edwards, V., Malarcher, A., Croft, J., & Giles, W. (2010). Adverse childhood experiences are associated with the risk of lung cancer: A prospective cohort study. *BMC Public Health, 10,* 20. Retrieved from EBSCOhost.

Burns, N., & Grove, S. (2009). *The practice of nursing research: Appraisal, synthesis, and generation of evidence* (6th ed.). St Louis, MO: Saunders Elsevier.

Cannon, E., Bonomi, A., Anderson, M., Rivara, F., & Thompson, R. (2010). Adult health and relationship outcomes among women with abuse experiences during childhood. *Violence and Victims, 25*(3), 291–305. Retrieved from EBSCOhost.

Centers for Disease Control and Prevention. (2010). Sodium intake among adults—United States, 2005–2006. *Morbidity and Mortality Weekly Report (MMWR) 59,*(24). Retrieved from http://www.cdc.gov/mmwr/preview/mmwrhtml/mm5924a4.htm?s_cid=mm5924a4_w

Centers for Disease Control and Prevention. (2014a). *FastStats.* Retrieved from http://www.cdc.gov/nchs/fastats/deaths.htm

Centers for Disease Control and Prevention. (2014b).*Tobacco control saves lives and money.* Retrieved from http://www.cdc.gov/Features/TobaccoControlData/

Centers for Disease Control and Prevention. (2014c). *Cigarette smoking among U.S. high school students at lowest level in 22 years* [Press Release]. Retrieved from http://www.cdc.gov/media/releases/2014/p0612-YRBS.html?s_cid=ostltsdyk_cs_506

Centers for Disease Control and Prevention. (2014d). *National diabetes statistics report: Estimates of diabetes and its burden in the United States, 2014.* Atlanta, GA: U.S. Department of Health and Human Services. Retrieved from http://www.cdc.gov/diabetes/pubs/statsreport14/national-diabetes-report-web.pdf

Centers for Medicare & Medicaid Services. (2014). *National health expenditure projections 2013–2023.* Retrieved from http://www.cms.gov/Research-Statistics-Data-and-Systems/Statistics-Trends-and-Reports/NationalHealthExpendData/Downloads/Proj2013.pdf

Central Intelligence Agency. (2014). *The world factbook.* Retrieved from https://www.cia.gov/library/publications/the-world-factbook/rankorder/2091rank.html

Cobb, C. O., Ward, K. D., Maziak, W., Shihadeh, A. L., & Eissenberg, T. (2010). Waterpipe tobacco smoking: An emerging health crisis in the United States. *American Journal of Health Behavior, 34*(3), 275–85.

Cohen, R. A., & Martinez, M. E. (2014). *Health insurance coverage: Early release of estimates from the National Health Interview Survey, January–March 2014* (National Health Interview Survey: Early Release Program). Retrieved from http://www.cdc.gov/nchs/data/nhis/earlyrelease/insur201409.pdf

Collins, S., Doty, M., Robertson, R., & Garber, T. (2010). *How the recession has left millions of workers without health insurance, and how health reform will bring relief: Findings from the Commonwealth Fund Biennial Health Insurance Survey of 2010.* Retrieved from http://www.commonwealthfund.org/~/media/Files/Publications/Fund%20Report/2011/Mar/1486_Collins_help_on_the_horizon_2010_biennial_survey_report_FINAL_v2.pdf

Dossey, B. (2000). *Florence Nightingale: Mystic, visionary, healer.* Springhouse, PA: Springhouse Corporation.

Doty, M., Blumenthal, D., & Collins, S.R. (2014). The Affordable Care Act and health insurance for Latinos. *JAMA, 312*(17), 1735–1736.

Dunstan, D. W., Thorp, A. A., & Healy, G. N. (2011). Prolonged sitting: Is it a distinct coronary heart disease risk factor? *Current Opinion in Cardiology, 26*(5), 412–419. doi:10.1097/HCO.0b013e3283496605

Evans, G. D. (2003). Clara Barton: Teacher, nurse, Civil War heroine, founder of the American Red Cross. *International History of Nursing Journal, 7*(3), 75–82.

Felitti, V., Anda, R., Nordenberg, D., Williamson, D., Spitz, A., Edwards, V., . . . Marks, J. (1998). Relationship of childhood abuse and household dysfunction to many of the leading causes of death in adults: The adverse childhood experiences (ACE) study. *American Journal of Preventative Medicine, 14*, 245–258.

Finkelstein, E., Trogdon, J., Cohen, J., & Dietz, W. (2009). Annual medical spending attributable to obesity: Payer-and service-specific estimates. *Health Affairs, 28*(5). Retrieved from http://content.healthaffairs.org/content/28/5/w822.full.pdf

Fonarow, G., Smith, E., Saver, J., Reeves, M., Bhatt, D., Grau-Sepulveda, M., . . . Schwamm, L. (2011). Timeliness of tissue-type plasminogen activator therapy in acute ischemic stroke: Patient characteristics, hospital factors, and outcomes associated with door-to-needle times within 60 minutes. *Circulation, 123*(7), 750–758. Retrieved from EBSCO*host.*

Frontier Nursing Service. (2014). *Mrs. Mary Breckinridge.* Retrieved from https://www.frontiernursing.org/History/MaryBreckinridge.shtm

Goodwin, R., & Stein, M. (2004). Association between childhood trauma and physical disorders among adults in the United States. *Psychological Medicine, 34*(3), 509–520.

Grundy, S. M., Cleeman, J., Daniels, S. R., Donato, K. A., Eckel, R. H., Franklin, B. A., . . . Costa, F. (2005). Diagnosis and management of the metabolic syndrome: An American Heart Association/National Heart, Lung, and Blood Institute scientific statement. *Circulation, 112*, 2735.

HealthyPeople.gov. (2014). *Nutrition and weight status (Healthy People 2020).* Retrieved from https://www.healthypeople.gov/2020/topics-objectives/topic/nutrition-and-weight-status/objectives

The Henry J. Kaiser Family Foundation. (2014a). *2014 employer health benefits survey.* Retrieved from http://kff.org/health-costs/report/2014-employer-health-benefits-survey/

The Henry J. Kaiser Family Foundation. (2014b). *Employer-sponsored family health premiums rise 3 percent in 2014* [Press Release]. *Retrieved from* http://kff.org/private-insurance/press-release/employer-sponsored-family-health-premiums-rise-3-percent-in-2014/

Hyland, M. E., Alkhalaf, A. M., & Whalley, B. (2012). Beating and insulting children as a risk for adult cancer, cardiac disease and asthma. *Journal of Behavioral Medicine, 36*(6), 632–640. doi:10.1007/s10865-012-9457-6

Institute of Medicine. (2010a). *For the public's health: The role of measurement in action and accountability.* Retrieved from http://iom.edu/~/media/Files/Report%20Files/2010/For-the-Publics-Health-The-Role-of-Measurement-in-Action-and-Accountability/For%20the%20Publics%20Health%202010%20Report%20Brief.pdf

Institute of Medicine. (2010b). *Strategies to reduce sodium intake in the United States.* Retrieved from http://www.iom.edu/Reports/2010/Strategies-to-Reduce-Sodium-Intake-in-the-United-States/Report-Brief-Strategies-to-Reduce-Sodium-Intake-in-the-United-States.aspx

Institute of Medicine. (2011). *Initiative on the future of nursing.* Retrieved from http://www.thefutureofnursing.org/recommendations

Jacobs, E., Newton, C., Wang, Y., Patel, A., McCullough, M., Campbell, P., . . . Gapster, S. (2010). Waist circumference and all-cause mortality in a large U.S. cohort. *Archives of Internal Medicine, 170*(15), 1293–1301.

January, A. M. (2009). Friday at Frontier Nursing Service. *Public Health Nursing, 26*(2), 202–203. doi:10.1111/j.1525-1446.2009.00771.x King v Burwell, No. 14-114, (Supreme Court of the United States. June 25,1015).

Levy, J. (2014). *In U.S., uninsured rate holds at 13.4%*. Retrieved from http://www.gallup.com/poll/178100/uninsured-rate-holds.aspx

Lipsey, S. (2006). *Mathematical education in the life of Florence Nightingale*. Retrieved from http://www.agnesscott.edu/lriddle/women/night_educ.htm

Messina, N., Marinelli-Casey, P., Hillhouse, M., Rawson, R., Hunter, J., & Ang, A. (2008). Childhood adverse events and methamphetamine use among men and women. *Journal of Psychoactive Drugs* (Nov. Suppl. 5), 399–409. Retrieved from EBSCO*host*.

Mitka, M. (2013). IOM report: Evidence fails to support guidelines for dietary salt reduction. *JAMA, 309*(24), 2535.

National Cancer Institute. (2014). *Obesity and cancer risk*. Retrieved from http://www.cancer.gov/cancertopics/factsheet/Risk/obesity

Obama, B. (2009, August 16). Why we need healthcare reform. *The New York Times*, WK9.

OECD Health Systems. (2013). Health at a glance 2013: OECD indicators. Retrieved from http://www.oecd.org/els/health-systems/Health-at-a-Glance-2013.pdf

Ogden, C. L., Carroll, M. D., Kit, B. K., & Flegal, K. M. (2014). Prevalence of childhood and adult obesity in the United States. *JAMA, 311*(8), 806–814.

Orszag, P. R. (2008). *Growth in healthcare costs. Statement before the Committee on the Budget United States Senate*. Retrieved from http://www.cbo.gov/ftpdocs/89xx/doc8948/01-31-HealthTestimony.pdf

Owen, C. G., Martin, R. M., Whincup, P. H., Smith, G. D., & Cook, D. G. (2005). Effect of infant feeding on the risk of obesity across the life course: A quantitative review of published evidence. *Pediatrics, 115*(5), 1367–1377.

Population. (2002). In *The American heritage dictionary of the English language* (4th ed., p. 1366). Boston, MA: Houghton Mifflin.

Porche, D. J. (2004). *Public and community health nursing practice*. Thousand Oaks, CA: SAGE.

Rasmussen, P., Collins, S., Doty, M., & Beutel, S. (2014). *Are Americans finding affordable coverage in the health insurance marketplace? Results from the Commonwealth Fund Affordable Care Act Tracking Survey*. Retrieved from http://www.commonwealthfund.org/publications/issue-briefs/2014/sep/affordable-coverage-marketplace.

Scott, K., Smith, D., & Ellis, P. (2012). A population study of childhood maltreatment and asthma diagnosis: Differential associations between child protection database versus retrospective self-reported data. *Psychosomatic Medicine, 74*(8), 817–823. doi:10.1097/PSY.0b013e3182648de4

Smith-Spangler, C., Juusola, J., Enns, E., Owens, D., & Garber, A. (2010). Population strategies to decrease sodium intake and the burden of cardiovascular disease: A cost-effectiveness analysis. *Annals of Internal Medicine, 152*(8), 481. Retrieved from EBSCO*host*.

Smyth, J., Heron, K., Wonderlich, S., Crosby, R., & Thompson, K. (2008). The influence of reported trauma and adverse events on eating disturbance in young adults. *International Journal of Eating Disorders, 41*(3), 195–202. Retrieved from EBSCO*host*.

Soni, A. (2010, December). *Trends in use and expenditures for diabetes among adults 18 and older, U.S. civilian noninstitutionalized population, 1996 and 2007*. Agency for Healthcare Research and Policy. Retrieved from http://www.meps.ahrq.gov/mepsweb/data_files/publications/st304/stat304.pdf

Steenhuysen, J. (2015, January 14). U.S. hospitals make strides in cutting key infections: CDC report. *Reuters U.S. edition*. Retrieved from http://www.reuters.com/article/2015/01/14/us-usa-hospitals-infections-idUSKBN0KN22O20150114

U.S. Department of Health and Human Services. (2010). *Multiple chronic conditions—A strategic framework: Optimum health and quality of life for individuals with multiple chronic conditions*. Washington, DC: Author.

U.S. Department of Health and Human Services. (2012). *Preventing tobacco use among youth and young adults: A report of the Surgeon General*. Retrieved from http://www.surgeongeneral.gov/library/reports/preventing-youth-tobacco-use/index.html

U.S. Environmental Protection Agency. (2014). *Fact sheet: National survey on environmental management of asthma and children's exposure to environmental tobacco smoke*. Retrieved from http://www.epa.gov/smokefre/pdfs/survey_fact_sheet.pdf

Ventura, S. J., Hamilton, B. E., Mathews, T. J., & Chandra, A. (2003). Trends and variations in smoking during pregnancy and low birth weight: Evidence from the birth certificate, 1990–2000. *Pediatrics, 111*, 1176–1180. Retrieved from http://pediatrics.aappublications.org/content/111/Supplement_1/1176.full.pdf+html

World Health Organization. (2011). *Global status report on NCDs*. Retrieved from http://www.who.int/nmh/publications/ncd_report2010/en/

World Health Organization. (2014). *Chronic diseases and health promotion*. Retrieved from http://www.who.int/chp/en/

Yolton, K., Dietrich, K., Auinger, P., Lanphear, B. P., & Hornung, R. (2005). Exposure to environmental tobacco smoke and cognitive abilities among U.S. children and adolescents. *Environmental Health Perspectives, 113*(1), 98–103.

T · W · O

Identifying Outcomes

Frances Munet-Vilaró and Sonda M. Oppewal

Nurses have a long and rich history of wanting to do the most good for the most people. Today, it is imperative that advanced practice registered nurses (APRNs) continue that tradition by delivering care that improves the health of populations. By assessing community, aggregate, family, and individual factors and conditions that have a strong influence on health, APRNs are better equipped to deliver effective and evidence-based care. Identifying population-level healthcare needs and healthcare disparities can help to improve equality in health outcomes at all levels.

The American Association of Colleges of Nursing's (AACN) definition of advanced practice nursing includes the importance of identifying and managing health outcomes at the population level (AACN, 2004). In 2006, the AACN specified that graduates of doctorate in nursing practice (DNP) programs have competency in meeting "the needs of a panel of patients, a target population, a set of populations, or a broad community" (p. 10). A core component of DNP education is clinical prevention (health promotion and disease prevention at individual and family levels) and population health (focus of care at aggregate and community levels and examination of environmental, occupational, cultural, and socioeconomic dimensions of health) (AACN, 2006; Allan et al., 2004). Regardless of whether DNP graduates practice with a focus on clinical prevention or population health, the ability to define, identify, and analyze outcomes is imperative for improving the health status of individuals and populations (AACN, 2006; Department of Health and Human Services [HHS], 2014).

The purpose of this chapter is to explore how APRNs can identify determinants of health and define population outcomes. Specific examples from various settings, such as acute care, subacute care, long-term care, and the community, are given, as well as outcomes related to health disparities and national health objectives. The identification of factors that lead to certain outcomes or key health indicators is an essential first step in planning effective interventions and is used later in the evaluation process. By comparing outcomes, APRNs can advocate needed resources and changes in policies at local, regional, state, and/or national levels by identifying areas for improvement in practice, by comparing evidence needed for effective practice, and by better understanding health disparities. Health disparities are not fair or socially just. They are preventable. They reflect an uneven distribution of social determinants and environmental, economic, and political factors. Health disparities can be defined as the differences identified in incidence or prevalence of illness, health outcomes, mortality, injury, or violence, or differences in opportunities to reach optimal health equity due to disadvantages based on ethnicity, socioeconomic status, gender, sexual orientation, geographic location, or other reasons (Meyer, Yoon, & Kaufmann, 2013). APRNs play an important collaborative role with professionals from other disciplines and community members to work toward eliminating health disparities.

IDENTIFYING AND DEFINING POPULATION OUTCOMES

Background

One of the earliest records of observed outcomes by nurses dates back to 1854 during the Crimean War at the Scutari Hospital in Turkey when Florence Nightingale, credited as the founder of modern nursing, documented a decrease in mortality among the British soldiers after providing more nutritious food, cleaning up the environment, and improving the sewage system (Fee & Garofalo, 2010). Despite the leadership and pioneering work that Nightingale provided in outcomes documentation, the nursing literature revealed variation in the documentation of nursing outcomes (Hill, 1999; Lang & Marek, 1991; van Maanen, 1979). Griffiths (1995) observed that the literature from the mid-1960s to the mid-1990s was not very progressive in documenting nursing outcomes but showed promise of improving. Health reform efforts to improve quality and access and reduce costs spurred more work to examine outcomes while examining their relationship to indicators of structure and process. Although earlier work in nursing outcomes focused on costs, it was clear that a more comprehensive model that reflected other types of outcomes was needed to advance healthcare and reflect the various outcomes that resulted from nursing interventions (Nelson, Mohr, Batalden, & Plume, 1996). More recently, nursing interventions are based on evidence using models of practice that include standards and synchronization with other systems to deliver quality of care, patient safety, and optimal population health outcomes (Institute of Medicine [IOM], 2013; Kurtzman & Corrigan, 2007; Patrician et al., 2013).

Defining, Categorizing, and Identifying Outcomes

Health outcomes are usually defined as an end result that follows some kind of healthcare provision, treatment, or intervention and may describe a patient's condition or health status (Kleinpell, 2007; Kleinpell & Gawlinski, 2005; Oermann & Floyd, 2002). Using a population perspective, a health outcome can be measured using public health metrics, such as mortality and life expectancies, that are used to demonstrate the contribution of certain diseases to population mortality. New trends also emphasize the inclusion of qualitative metrics that are based on subjective data, such as self-perceived health status, psychological state, or ability to function, that can illustrate collective social well-being (Boothe, Sinha, Bohm, & Yoon, 2013; Parrish, 2010). Evaluating population-based outcomes and their impact on population health involves looking at what to assess and how to assess it. Establishing the impact takes time and requires using an evaluation that is able to link interventions to long-term outcomes such as reducing disease morbidity and mortality at the population level. APRNs can best determine the effectiveness of an intervention and long-term impact by focusing on an accurate assessment and interpretation of data that are generated or collected using individual, population, and community health indicators (Anderson & McFarlane, 2010). Classifying and categorizing outcomes can be done in several ways. For example, outcomes may be classified into categories by describing "who" is measured, such as individuals, aggregates, communities, populations, or organizations; by identifying the "what" or the type of outcome, such as care, patient, or performance-related outcomes (Kleinpell, 2001, 2003; Kleinpell & Gawlinski, 2005); and by determining the "when" or the time it takes to achieve an outcome, such as short-term, intermediate, or long-term outcomes (Rich, 2009). Table 2.1 provides examples of various outcomes using these different classification systems. Each outcome type is listed by beneficiary and has a related example of the type of measurement, the potential outcome, and the potential impact of that outcome. Many of them also include a time frame for the outcome.

TABLE 2.1 • Examples of Outcomes, Measures, and Impact by Beneficiary, Type, and Time Frame

Beneficiary (Who?)	Measure	Potential Outcome	Impact
Individual outcomes	Blood pressure (BP) measurement	Decreased BP	The degree to which perceived health status is improved by BP management
Aggregate outcomes	Weekly weights of participants in an exercise class	Reduced mean weight for exercise class members each week	Sustained weight maintenance using body mass index (BMI) parameters
Community outcomes	A town's seat belt usage per 100 drivers ≥ 18 years of age computed yearly	Increased yearly rate of a town's seat belt usage per 100 drivers ≥18 years of age	Decrease in the town's percentage of automobile accident injuries/fatalities in drivers ≥18 years of age
Population outcomes	Reported number of infant deaths within 1 year of birth per 1000 infants	Decreased infant mortality rate compared to previous year	Five-year decrease in infant mortality rate

(continued)

TABLE 2.1 • Examples of Outcomes, Measures, and Impact by Beneficiary, Type, and Time Frame (*continued*)

Type (What?)	Measure	Potential Outcome	Impact
Care-related outcomes	Annual rate of hospital-acquired infections determined from hospital infectious disease reports	Decreased hospital-acquired infections rate from previous year	Decreased length of stay and decreased mortality in patients with hospital-acquired infections
Patient-related outcomes	Observation of insulin injection administration technique	Correct demonstration by patient of safe insulin administration technique	Decreased hospital admissions for uncontrolled diabetes
Performance-related outcomes	Chart review for completed checklist of asthma best practices protocol	Nursing staff adherence to asthma best practices protocol	Decreased hospital readmissions due to asthma

Time Frame (When?)	Measure	Potential Outcome	Impact
Short-term outcomes	Self-report of nipple discomfort among first-time breast-feeding mothers in a postpartum unit	Absence of nipple discomfort among first-time breast-feeding mothers 1 week after hospital discharge from a postpartum unit	Improved breast-feeding rates among women discharged from a postpartum unit
Intermediate outcomes	Self-report of tobacco usage by first-time outpatient clinic users during the calendar year	An increase in smoking-cessation rates among outpatient clinic users during the calendar year	Decrease in smoking-related illnesses among outpatient clinic users during the calendar year
Long-term outcomes	Incidence rate of HIV in an urban African American population	Annual reduction of incidence rate of HIV in an urban African American population	Annual reduction of morbidity and mortality related to HIV in an urban African American population

One of the early frameworks that nurses used to categorize outcomes and that is still used today is based on four dimensions that correspond to points on a compass. Known as the *Clinical Value Compass*, the four dimensions or categories are *clinical* (e.g., disease-specific outcomes), *functional* (e.g., ability to participate in activities of daily living, overall well-being), *cost* (e.g., number of encounters, length of stay, finances, and resources), and *satisfaction* (e.g., patient and family satisfaction) (Nelson, Batalden, Plume, & Mohr, 1996; Nelson et al., 1996; Oermann & Floyd, 2002).

Another framework used frequently in nursing and healthcare to evaluate quality of care relies on the examination of three components: *structure, process,* and *outcome. Structure* refers to healthcare resources, such as the number and type of health and social service agencies, and can also include utilization indicators. *Process* describes how the healthcare is delivered, and *outcome* refers to the change in health status related to the intervention provided (Donabedian, 1980). This framework is particularly useful in describing the health of a community. It is based on the concept of community as client and focuses on the health of the collective or population instead of the individual (Shuster, 2014). Using this framework, a community's health can be described in terms of its structure by the number and type of health and social agencies present, its healthcare workforce, health services utilization indicators, and the community's educational and socioeconomic levels in relation to demographic measures of ethnicity, gender, and age. A community's health process can measure healthcare delivery methods and how well community members work together to build capacity and solve their problems, which reflects the ability to share power and resources, and to respond to needs and changes (Chaskin, Brown, Venkatesh, & Vidal, 2001; Minkler & Wallerstein, 2007). Community health outcomes can include measures associated with vital statistics (e.g., births, deaths, marriages, divorces, fetal deaths, and induced termination of pregnancies); morbidity or illness data and trends; social determinants of health such as housing, unemployment, and poverty rates; health risk profiles of aggregates by specific areas, neighborhood safety, access to fresh fruits and vegetables, as well as physical activity venues such as parks, playgrounds, and neighborhood sports fields (Anderson & McFarlane, 2010). Other indicators of a community's health status may include the number of premature deaths, quality of life, disabilities, risk factors, and injuries. Community health outcomes models are used to assess the interaction between the physical and the social environments (the built environment) and its impact on health at the individual, population, and community levels (DeGuzman & Kulbok, 2012). Guided by these models of practice and research, APRNs can work in partnership with community members to identify what community members see as relevant and important, build social capital, use outcome data to advocate for changes in policy, and then continue to work in partnership to identify strategies to intervene, monitor, and improve those outcomes (Bigbee & Issel, 2012; Hunter, Neiger, & West, 2011; Loyo et al., 2012; Mahadevan & McGinnis, 2013).

Vital statistics provide important outcome measures that APRNs can monitor and compare over time and analyze by demographic variables to detect such things as health disparities. In the United States, the National Center for Health Statistics (NCHS) collects the official records of births, deaths, marriages, divorces, fetal deaths, and induced terminations of pregnancies from state and local health departments (Aschengrau & Seage, 2013). Personnel from local health departments review the data from death certificates, including demographic data, looking at the immediate cause of death and any contributing factors of death, and recording multiple causes of death. Local data are sent to a state office for collation and then sent to the NCHS, which provides this information to the public on its website (http://www.cdc.gov/nchs) and in an annual publication, *Vital Statistics of the United States* (Friis & Sellers, 2009). APRNs can access national and global health statistics from multiple agency sources, including government agencies, to identify health trends and patterns (Partners, 2014). However, due to the lack of agencies and/or resources in certain populations or regions, health information might not be available or might be limited in scope.

In the early 1980s, personal health behaviors became a key source of information that paved the way to understanding risk behavior and its impact on morbidity and mortality. The Behavioral Risk Factor Surveillance System (BRFSS; http://www.cdc.gov/brfss/), a system established to collect state-level data, also allows states to estimate prevalence for regions that can be compared across states (CDC, 2013). The data generated by this surveillance system have been pivotal in assessing and addressing emerging health issues and other urgent health concerns. Examples of emergent health issues include man-made and natural disasters, vaccine shortages (e.g., influenza, MMR [measles, mumps, and rubella]), and increasing incidence of preventable diseases such as influenza, measles, and so on. The use of cell phone technology has expanded BRFSS's accessibility to populations that were not accessible by prior data-collection methods and has increased representation and generated higher quality information.

Social determinants of health and inequalities data are areas that APRNs can also use to inform and guide their practice to develop socioculturally appropriate interventions. Social determinants that lead to health inequalities are recognized situations related to where people are born, grow up, work, live, and the systems of care available to them to deal with illness and disease (HHS, 2014; World Health Organization [WHO], 2008). To expand our understanding of the association between social determinants and health outcomes, theoretical models are being tested to examine the interaction between the social environment (physical, chemical, biological, behavioral, and/or life events) and genetics and its application to population health (Reiss, Leve, & Neiderhiser, 2013). For example, in some immigrant populations, factors such as fear of deportation (immigration stress), limited financial resources, perceived racism, and limited social capital and political power can have a negative impact on their health (Agency for Healthcare Research and Quality [AHRQ], 2013). These social conditions may limit a person's ability to be employed, access healthcare services, and receive timely quality care. This is globally evident with ethnic populations of immigrants that have an expired visa, or an unauthorized or undocumented status (United Nations, 2008). A problem encountered repeatedly by healthcare practitioners is the lack of available census data and statistics about key issues in the health and healthcare of people with unauthorized status. APRNs may be able to access health information needed by working together with other sectors outside of health, such as housing, labor, education, and community-based or faith-based organizations that offer services to immigrant communities. This involves the collection, documentation, and use of data that can be used to monitor health inequalities in exposures, opportunities, and outcomes. Examples of social determinants that are related to health inequalities include poverty, educational level, racism, income, and poor housing. These inequalities can lead to poor quality of life, poor self-rated health, multiple morbidities, limited access to resources, premature death, and unnecessary risks and vulnerabilities.

APRNs are often responsible for reviewing morbidity and mortality trends and can use this information to advocate improved health policy and additional resources, or to develop innovative interventions. For example, if an APRN notices an increase over the past year of closed head injuries in teenagers because of motor vehicle crashes (MVCs), she or he can design a plan of care that targets risk factors associated with teenage driving and MVCs. The APRN may review emergency department (ED) records of teenage drivers in car accidents to assess factors such as seat belt usage, distracted driving behaviors, blood alcohol levels, drug screening, prior ED visits for accidents, and age at the time of the incident. The APRN may also approach high schools in order to collaborate with school nurses for the purpose of developing peer training programs. High school students could be trained as peer teachers to encourage classmates to wear seat belts, avoid entering a car with an impaired driver, say no to drug and alcohol usage, and eliminate use of electronic devices, such as cellular phones, while driving. Nurse educators could encourage teachers to integrate the importance of wearing seat belts in their classes by discussing the potential for traumatic brain injury in MVCs, especially in unrestrained drivers. Review of the biomechanics of accidents in a physics or science class might provide teens with knowledge that is both beneficial and relatable and may reinforce the dangers of unrestrained driving. Additionally, the use of web-based simulation education regarding the use of cellular phones and its similarities to driving under the influence could also be integrated into this type of curriculum (Buckley, Chapman, & Sheehan, 2014). Finally, school nurses could lead spot surveillance of seat belt usage as teenagers enter and exit school parking lots. After developing and implementing appropriate interventions, the APRN should reassess (e.g., in 6 months, 1 year) seat belt usage and repeat ED visits for motor vehicle accidents, and revaluate whether there have been any positive drug screens or elevated blood alcohol concentrations in relation to MVCs. Reevaluation of these data can help to identify those interventions that work. It may also lead to changes in school policy and/or curriculum to modify behavior, thereby reducing MVCs among teens. Statewide policy changes that the APRN can advocate include legislation whereby any detectable blood alcohol concentration is illegal, more stringent and enforced driving fines for unrestrained passengers and drivers, and graduated driving license laws that increase driving supervision time and/or call for limits with driving past 9 p.m. until the driver is of a certain age (Mirman et al., 2014). Although this is just one example of how surveillance by an APRN could lead to the development of interventions to improve outcomes in a population, one can see the potential value of community collaboration and the use of such outcomes to identify a need for change and to evaluate the impact of interventions.

Morbidity data are less standardized in general than mortality data because state legislatures and local agencies decide what illnesses must be reported to the Centers for Disease Control and Prevention (CDC). Reporting of cases of infectious diseases and related conditions is an important step in controlling and preventing the spread of communicable disease. The list of reportable or notifiable diseases can change as some diseases may become eradicated and other, new diseases and conditions are discovered or felt to be preventable and/or treatable. The accuracy of morbidity data is diminished if healthcare providers fail to report a disease or illness for fear of invading the individual's privacy or because they may not be aware of reporting requirements or because the healthcare provider misdiagnosed the illness (Macha & McDonough, 2012). It is imperative that APRNs educate themselves on the reporting requirements in their state. Certain diseases with easy and/or rapid transmission are more likely to harm a population's health. Infectious or communicable diseases, such as certain sexually transmitted infections (STIs) or other diseases such as rabies, rubella, plague, measles, tetanus, and food-borne illnesses, can lead to more significant morbidity and mortality if not reported promptly (Friis & Sellers, 2009). Provisional weekly updates of reportable diseases can be accessed electronically through the *Morbidity and Mortality Weekly Report (MMWR)*, published by the CDC.

Another way to evaluate population morbidity other than relying on the list of reportable diseases is derived from population surveys that are conducted to determine the frequency of acute and chronic illnesses and disability as well as other population characteristics. The U.S. National Health Survey (NHS) is an example of a morbidity survey that was first authorized by Congress in 1956 for the purpose of informing the U.S. population about various health measures and indicators. In 1960, the NHS and the National Office of Vital Statistics merged to form the NCHS, which has been part of the CDC since 1987. The NCHS works with public and private partners to collect data that provide reliable and valid evidence on a population's health status, influences on health, and health outcomes (CDC, 2014a). APRNs can review these data to identify health disparities among subgroups based on ethnicity and/ or socioeconomic status, monitor trends with health status and with healthcare delivery systems, support research endeavors, identify health problems, evaluate health policies, and access important information that can be used to improve policies and health services.

The NCHS collects data in four main ways, each method yielding information that is readily available on the Internet for use by healthcare providers, researchers, and educators. First, the *National Vital Statistics System* provides information about state and local vital statistics, including teen birth rates, prenatal care, birth weights, risk factors related to poor pregnancy outcomes, infant mortality rates, life expectancy, and leading causes of death (www.cdc .gov/nchs/nvss.htm). Second, the *National Health Interview Survey* (NHIS) provides health information from household interviews conducted by Census Bureau personnel. Data on health status, access to care, use of health services, immunization rates, risk factors and health-related behaviors, and health insurance coverage can be gleaned from the NHISs (www.cdc.gov/nchs/nhis .htm). The *National Health and Nutrition Examination Survey* (NHANES) is the third major survey source conducted through mobile examination centers held at randomly selected sites throughout the United States. Data are obtained from interviews (e.g., environmental exposures, risk factors), and additional data are collected from physical examinations, diagnostic procedures, laboratory tests, and indicators of growth and development, including weight, diet, and nutrition (www.cdc.gov/nchs/nhanes.htm). The fourth major method of data collection from the NCHS is the *National Healthcare Surveys* (www.cdc .gov/nchs/dhcs.htm). Information is obtained using a collection of surveys targeted toward various healthcare providers and healthcare settings. A variety of data are collected, including information regarding patient safety and safety indicators, clinical management of specific health conditions, disparities in healthcare utilization and health quality, and information about the use of healthcare innovations. All these survey data are collated and made available for policy makers, practitioners, and researchers. Each of the four key methods conducted by the NCHS provides useful outcome information. Additional surveys can be found on the CDC's website (www.cdc.gov/nchs), but the aforementioned surveys are most useful for analyzing outcomes data.

How do APRNs decide what outcomes to study? There are a variety of outcomes that exist in relation to cost, clinical and functional data, social conditions, and community and environmental indicators. Often, outcomes will reflect the desired or anticipated effects of the intervention that are related to the problem or population of interest. Another way to select outcomes is by reviewing available epidemiological and social epidemiological data for outcomes that may be of interest or relevance to an APRN's intervention or study (Krieger, 2001; Macha & McDonough, 2012; Minkler & Wallerstein, 2007). Using the earlier example of designing an intervention to reduce teenage MVCs, an APRN could seek out epidemiological data from the *National Annenberg Risk Survey of Youth* conducted by researchers at the University of Pennsylvania. This survey includes teen attitudinal risk factors and protective factors, and identifies several factors that could potentially be identified as outcomes of interest for an APRN working on reducing teen MVCs (www.annenbergpublicpolicycenter.org/teen-drivers-need-better-training-to-counter-inexperience-and-inattention). In addition, an Internet application known as the Community Health Status Indicators (CHSI) uses the Geographic Information Systems (GIS) Analyst, a user-friendly web-based data source, to map geographical areas, which allow the visualization, exploration, and understanding of the indicators (wwwn.cdc.gov/CommunityHealth/homepage.aspx?j=1). Indicators can be mapped and compared visually with those in other areas, counties, and neighboring counties (Heitgerd et al., 2008).

There is no shortage of usable resources for identifying outcomes. *The Guide to Community Preventive Services* is a helpful resource (available at www.thecommunityguide.org). It provides evidence-based recommendations about public health interventions, analyses from systematic reviews to determine program and policy effectiveness, information on whether an intervention might work in one's community, and information about the intervention's costs and benefits. APRNs can review topics or areas of focus and strategies that work for various outcomes. For example, systematic reviews are available on adolescent health. By spending a few minutes exploring the website, one can find numerous outcomes such as number of self-reported risk behaviors, including engagement in any sexual activity, frequency of sexual activity, number of partners, frequency of unprotected sexual activity, use of protection to prevent STIs, use of protection to prevent pregnancy, and self-reported or clinically documented STIs. Other community-guide topics are listed in Table 2.2 with example outcomes adapted from the website.

Outcome monitoring has become increasingly important over the years and, in many cases, is a necessity to justify program implementation or program funding. For example, outcome monitoring is used to assess quality of healthcare by examining the association between the level of improved health

TABLE 2.2 • Community Guide Topics and Outcome Examples

Topics	Outcome Examples
Adolescent health	Alcohol, tobacco, and drug usage; injury, violence, and suicide rates; body mass index (BMI), physical activity, and educational attainment
Alcohol	Daily alcohol intake (ounces per day), type of alcohol intake (beer, wine, etc.), binge drinking, underage drinking, attendance at community-based rehabilitation programs
Asthma	Symptom-free days, quality-of-life scores, school absenteeism, environmental mold remediation, medication usage, hospital admissions
Birth defects	Folic acid daily intake, daily alcohol consumption, medications, vaccinations
Cancer	Cigarette smoking, physical activity, nutrition, screening test results
Diabetes	Hemoglobin A1c, incidence of skin infections, obesity, peripheral neuropathy, renal insufficiency
Health communication and social marketing	Use of reliable digital and mobile technology for health information (HI) or appointment reminders; health literacy level; communication by provider of understandable HI; difficulty using HI
HIV/AIDS, STIs, and pregnancy	Abstinence, condom use, incidence of STIs or pregnancy
Mental health	Depression scale scores, hospital admissions, attendance at school or work, suicidal ideation or attempts
Motor vehicle	Use of child safety seats, use of seat belts, blood alcohol concentration, use of phone while driving, moving violations
Nutrition	Daily intake of fruits and vegetables, BMI, soda intake, fat intake, fiber intake
Obesity	Daily physical activity, sedentary time in front of the TV, computer or electronic screen, weight loss, BMI
Oral health	Dental caries; incidence of oral or throat cancer; use of helmets, face masks, and mouth guards in contact sports; reduced or discontinued use of chewing tobacco
Physical activity	Muscle strength and endurance activities, moderate- or vigorous-intensity aerobic physical activity
Social environment	Surroundings such as neighborhoods or workplace, involvement in church, politics, or social networks
Tobacco	Out-of-pocket costs for cessation therapies, creation of smoke-free policies, retail tobacco sales to youth

(*continued*)

TABLE 2.2 • Community Guide Topics and Outcome Examples (*continued*)

Topics	Outcome Examples
Vaccines	Number of infectious cases, hospitalizations, deaths from vaccine-preventable disease, immunization rates, immunization failures
Violence	Number of violence-related hospitalizations and deaths, participation in therapeutic foster care, school-based violence prevention programs, reduction of nonaccidental trauma in infants and toddlers
Worksite health promotion	Stair usage by employees, gym membership by employees, use of weight management counseling by employees

Adapted from U.S. Department of Health and Human Services, Community Preventative Services Task Force. (2015a).

services and the desired health outcomes of individuals and populations (IOM, 2013). This is best done by having a quality-improvement plan that systematically and consistently implements improvement strategies to address areas that are deficient and not meeting benchmarks. Electronic health records help to simplify the recording and monitoring of outcomes over time, between patient groups and populations. Outcomes are an expected part of what APRNs must collect when their focus is on populations. When combined with an evidence-based practice approach, outcomes can help provide standards or parameters for developing innovative interventions, instituting approaches more likely to impact the problem, and/or developing new practice guidelines or protocols (Robert Wood Johnson Foundation, 2009). For example, an APRN working in a community-based clinic with a lesbian, gay, bisexual, and transgender (LGBT) population may gather information about factors that contribute to documented risk behaviors, such as smoking and excessive drinking, in this community. An assessment can be made to determine whether differences in health outcomes exist based on age, perceived differential treatment by healthcare providers due to sexual orientation, access to LGBT support networks, barriers to access services that address the specific health needs of this diverse population, and other variables of interest (Fredriksen-Goldsen, Kim, Barkan, Muraco, & Hoy-Ellis, 2013). Once these outcomes are assessed, action can be taken to address those issues that may be contributing to high-risk behaviors. Interventions can be designed or policy changed to better address those factors, with a reassessment of outcomes after the intervention to see whether there is a reduction in high-risk behaviors.

Outcomes can also be used to measure quality of care in an outpatient setting. APRNs in an outpatient pediatric oncology practice who administer chemotherapy through a central venous catheter may set a goal to reduce catheter-related bloodstream infections by employing a before and after hands-on simulation education program for parents and nurses emphasizing aseptic techniques before, during, and after infusion. The success of the intervention can be measured by comparing outcomes such as number of positive cultures and prolonged hospitalizations, and rates of bloodstream infection before and after implementation of the educational intervention.

Nurse-Sensitive Quality Indicators

As documented evidence of patient safety concerns grew in the United States and at a time when healthcare costs were increasing and healthcare quality was being questioned, various nursing organizations started to focus on establishing a coordinated system for evaluating patient safety. In 1994, the American Nurses Association (ANA) developed Nursing's Safety and Quality Initiative, which initiated studies of patient safety with the goal of advocating healthy change. It was clear that nurse managers and administrators needed sound data for comparing their hospital units with similar units across the nation as a means of improving quality by developing and refining quality-improvement initiatives and monitoring progress. The indicators needed to be specific or sensitive to nursing care rather than ones that reflected medical care or institutional care. The indicators would have to be highly correlated with nursing quality and be measurable with a high degree of reliability and validity, and must not pose undue hardships on personnel tasked with collecting the data. Donabedian's (1982) framework of focusing on structure, process, and patient-centered outcomes was used for identifying and honing the indicators. By 2003, there was a set of 10 indicators that could be placed in Donabedian's framework (AHRQ, 2005). *Structure* indicators included staff mix and nursing care hours per patient day; *process* indicators included maintenance of skin integrity and nurse satisfaction; and patient-focused *outcomes* included nosocomial infections, patient fall rates, patient satisfaction with pain management, patient education, nursing care, and overall care (Dunton, 2008; Gallagher & Rowell, 2003; Montalvo, 2007).

The National Database of Nursing Quality Indicators® (NDNQI®) was created in 1998 by the ANA as part of the initiative to make changes to improve safety and quality of care, to help educate nurses about measurement, and to invest in research studies that examined safe and high-quality patient care. The NDNQI helped standardize information that was submitted by hospital units throughout the United States on indicators related to nursing structure (staffing level, educational level), process measures, and outcome measures. Hospitals use these results to compare their performance with those of other hospitals with similar demographic makeup and patient population. The database is invaluable for preparing for accreditation or certification by The Joint Commission or the American Nurses Credentialing Center because nurse executives can compare staffing patterns and methods of care delivery with clinical outcomes (Quigley, 2003). Originally housed and managed by the University of Kansas Medical Center (KUMC) School of Nursing through a contractual agreement with the American Nurses Credentialing Center (ANCC), NDNQI was purchased by Press Ganey in June 2014. Technical assistance and continuing education are provided by liaisons to ensure that reliable and valid data-collection methods are used by hospital personnel. This database provides a wealth of information on a quarterly and annual basis of more than 1,200 facilities in the United States. This allows for the comparison and evaluation of nursing care at the unit level of structure, process, and outcomes with other institutions that share similar characteristics (Dunton, 2008; Montalvo, 2007).

The ANA broadened the identification of nurse-sensitive indicators from acute care hospital settings to community-based, nonacute care settings such as long-term care facilities, schools, and home healthcare settings. This work began in 1998, and by 2000, 10 indicators were identified: pain management, consistency of communication, staff mix (combination and number of RNs, LPNs, nursing assistants), client satisfaction, prevention of tobacco use, cardiovascular disease prevention, caregiver activity, identification of primary caregiver, activities of daily living (ADL), independent activities of daily living (IADL), and psychosocial interaction (Gallagher & Rowell, 2003; Press Ganey Associates, 2014). The ability to collect and compare data on nurse-sensitive indicators and the ability to develop new indicators over time enhance the NDNQI initiative and provide APRNs with important information to help measure, compare, and improve the health and safety of populations.

Standardized Language in Nursing

The use of standardized language is important in any field to ensure a level of communication that is both consistent and effective in ensuring quality outcomes. Specifically, in nursing and other health professions, standardized language is critical for patient safety and quality of care. By establishing a uniform nursing language in electronic health records, research, and the development of evidence-based practice, APRNs will have a stronger foundation to communicate and improve patient outcomes and standards of care. The North American Nursing Diagnosis Association (NANDA) was developed in the 1970s to classify and standardize nursing diagnoses. Now referred to as NANDA International or NANDA-I, the nursing diagnoses include a name or label, signs and symptoms or defining characteristics, and risk factors associated with the diagnosis. The NANDA definitions and classifications have been recently updated to reflect new trends in nursing healthcare (www.nanda .org). Members of NANDA worked with nursing researchers at the University of Iowa to develop the Nursing Interventions Classification (NIC) and the Nursing Outcomes Classification (NOC). NANDA, NIC, and NOC, now referred to as NNN, collectively reflect a standardized way of communicating with defined terms within and across various national and international settings (Smith & Craft-Rosenberg, 2010). As APRNs contribute to the body of evidence-based practice and collaborate with others to generate more evidence of effective practice, their work may benefit from reviewing and using the NNN language for diagnoses, nursing interventions, and patient outcomes (Kautz & Van Horn, 2008). It is imperative that APRNs use standardized language in their research and in their practice so that outcomes can be compared in similar ways with larger databases for evaluation and research purposes.

NATIONAL HEALTHCARE OBJECTIVES

Healthy People 2020

Healthy People 2020, released by the U.S. Department of Health and Human Services (HHS) in early December 2010, serves as a blueprint or road map for the United States to achieve health promotion and disease prevention objectives that are designed to improve the health of all Americans. The Healthy

People initiative started in 1979 when the surgeon general released a report that focused on promoting health and preventing disease for all Americans. It was followed by Healthy People 2000 in 1989 and, 10 years later, Healthy People 2010. With leadership provided by the HHS, an appointed Advisory Committee and numerous public and private groups, local and state policy makers and officials, and numerous organizations (voluntary, advocacy, faith-based, and for-profit businesses), input is solicited regionally, statewide, and nationally to help craft the vision, mission, and overarching goals. These groups and organizations also develop strategies to improve health and prevent disease with the ultimate goal of helping Americans live longer and healthier lives. The resulting objectives, whether on the county, state, or national level, are intended for use by broad audiences and stakeholders to help motivate, guide, and focus action for a healthier nation.

Compared to previous national health promotion blueprints, the Healthy People 2020 framework emphasizes the importance of a variety of influences on health, such as personal (e.g., genetic, biological, psychological), organizational or institutional (e.g., Head Start or employee health programs), environmental (e.g., social and physical), and policy level (e.g., smoking bans in public places, seat belt laws). It moves beyond an individual-level approach to interventions and guides the creation of policies to promote the social and physical environments that are conducive to health. Another change in the 2020 version is the reorganization of objectives so that they can be retrieved by three broad categories: interventions, determinants, and objectives and information (with a feature for users to be able to retrieve information by local, state, or national level). Some of the 2020 objectives have been retained from Healthy People 2010 because they were not met, some objectives have been modified, and some are entirely new to Healthy People 2020. A major difference with Healthy People 2020 is that it is intended to be web-user-friendly such that users can easily retrieve, search, and interact with the database easily and effectively. Hence, APRNs and other users are able to tailor information available from Healthy People 2020 for their specific use and according to their specific needs in ways that were not available with earlier versions of Healthy People.

Table 2.3 provides a summary of the Healthy People 2020 initiatives with its vision, mission, goals, foundation health measures, and topic areas. Each topic area has a list of objectives with data sources, baseline, and target measures to achieve. The new features of Healthy People 2020 are additional topic-related clinical recommendations, evidence-based interventions, and other resources and links with consumer health information. Information about Healthy People 2020 can be found at www.healthypeople.gov/2020/default.aspx.

The website has useful information that APRNs can use to identify and monitor outcomes. Other tools, referred to as indicators, exist that APRNs can use for determining outcomes or measures of the quality of healthcare. These tools are available from the AHRQ Indicators website at www.quality indicators.ahrq.gov, along with software used to compute the quality-indicator rates, users' guides, reports, and other technical assistance and support.

TABLE 2.3 • Vision, Mission, Goals, Foundation Health Measures, and Topic Areas of Healthy People 2020

Vision	A society in which all people live long, healthy lives.
Mission	Healthy People 2020 strives to: • Identify nationwide health-improvement priorities • Increase public awareness and understanding of the determinants of health, disease, and disability and the opportunities for progress • Provide measurable objectives and goals that can be used at the national, state, and local levels • Engage multiple sectors to take actions to strengthen policies and improve practices that are driven by the best available evidence and knowledge • Identify critical research, evaluation, and data-collection needs
Overarching goals	Attain high-quality, longer lives free of preventable disease, disability, injury, and premature death • Achieve health equity, eliminate disparities, and improve the health of all groups • Create social and physical environments that promote good health for all • Promote quality of life, healthy development, and healthy behaviors across all life stages
Foundation Health Measures	
General health status	• Life expectancy • Healthy life expectancy • Physical and mental unhealthy days • Limitation of activity • Chronic disease prevalence • International comparison (where available)
Disparities and inequity	Disparities/inequity to be assessed by the following: • Race/ethnicity • Gender • Socioeconomic status • Disability status • LGBT status • Geography
Social determinants of health	Determinants can include the following: • Social and economic factors • Natural and built environments • Policies and programs
Health-related quality of life and well-being	Well-being/satisfaction • Physical, mental, and social health-related quality of life • Participation in common activities category

(continued)

TABLE 2.3 • Vision, Mission, Goals, Foundation Health Measures, and Topic Areas of Healthy People 2020 (*continued*)

Healthy People 2020 Topic Areas
• Access to health services
• Adolescent health
• Arthritis, osteoporosis, and chronic back conditions
• Blood disorders and blood safety
• Cancer
• Chronic kidney diseases
• Dementias, including Alzheimer's disease
• Diabetes
• Disability and health
• Early and middle childhood
• Educational and community-based programs
• Environmental health
• Family planning
• Food safety
• Genomics
• Global health
• Healthcare-associated infections
• Health communication and health information technology
• Health-related quality of life and well-being
• Hearing and other sensory or communication disorders
• Heart disease and stroke
• HIV
• Immunization and infectious diseases
• Injury and violence prevention
• LGBT health
• Maternal, infant, and child health
• Medical product safety
• Mental health and mental disorders
• Nutrition and weight status
• Occupational safety and health
• Older adults
• Oral health
• Physical activity
• Preparedness
• Public health infrastructure
• Respiratory diseases
• Sexually transmitted diseases
• Sleep health
• Social determinants of health
• Substance abuse
• Tobacco use
• Vision

LGBT, lesbian, gay, bisexual, and transgender
Adapted from: U.S. Department of Health and Human Services (2015b).

The inpatient quality indicators were designed to help hospitals identify possible issues and problems in need of quality improvement by using hospital administrative data to analyze morbidity and mortality rates for specific conditions and procedures, hospital- and area-level procedure utilization rates, and number of procedures (for select procedures). In addition to the inpatient quality indicators, other sets of quality indicators are available, including preventative quality indicators, patient safety indicators, and pediatric quality indicators.

AHRQ's National Healthcare Quality Report

Since 2003, the AHRQ has partnered with members of the HHS to report on healthcare quality improvement by publishing the *National Healthcare Quality Report (NHQR)*. The intent of this report is to respond to the status of healthcare quality in the United States, identify where improvement is most needed, and describe how the quality of healthcare that is given to Americans changes over time. This report includes more than 200 health measures placed in four categories that reflect quality measures: effectiveness, patient safety, timeliness, and patient centeredness (AHRQ, 2013). Findings from the 2013 report revealed that healthcare for Americans is improving in some areas and worsening in others. Populations with disabilities, including children, were added to the list of populations with priority in this report. Some areas of care that improved included colon cancer screening and treatment, adolescents receiving booster vaccinations for the prevention of certain diseases, and patients with heart failure being discharged with treatment-management instructions. Examples of areas where the quality of care is worsening include annual inspection of feet to check for sores in diabetic patients over 40 years of age, maternal deaths per 100,000 live births, and people with asthma using daily preventive medication. A key finding was that some populations had improved access to care, but there was no improvement in access to private health insurance coverage. Additional access to healthcare and quality of healthcare received did not improve for ethnic minority populations, poor people, or people with disabilities. A second key finding was in the differences in quality-of-care outcomes based on geography, with West South Central and East South Central states performing poorly in delivering quality care compared to New England and West North Central states. A third key finding was that the pace of improving quality was slow for ambulatory care but was improving more quickly in hospital settings, nursing homes, and hospice care. Hospital care has been improving since the Centers for Medicare & Medicaid Services (CMS) started reporting on quality measures, which can be found on the Hospital Quality Compare website (www.hospitalcompare.hhs.gov). A fourth key finding was in the area of quality measures that have been retired or removed or have the most rapid pace of change. Quality measures that were removed included hospital patients with heart attacks or heart failure who received immediate appropriate treatment and were discharged home with a management and counseling plan, patients who received hemodialysis, diabetic patients who were screened for cholesterol, hospital patients with pneumonia who received antibiotic treatment and management, and surgical patients who received prophylactic antibiotics prior to surgery and monitoring for antibiotic need postsurgery. The report recommends that healthcare providers take time to communicate with patients to facilitate understanding of treatment intervention. In addition, people with the skills, authority, and commitment to change healthcare need to receive information quicker in order to improve access to care, reduce disparities, and accelerate the pace of quality improvement (AHRQ, 2013).

Health Disparities

Healthy People 2010 included two overarching goals: to increase years of healthy living and to eliminate health disparities. These goals have been retained for Healthy People 2020 as evidence continues to mount that the United States has issues related to equity of healthcare access, quality of care, and health status. The midcourse review of Healthy People 2010 as well as many governmental and nongovernmental reports and independent studies document these disparities (AHRQ, 2013; Daniel, 2010; IOM, 2013; Koci, 2010; Mac-Mullen, Tymkow, & Shen, 2006; Schaffer, Goodhue, Stennes, & Lanigan, 2012; Sentell, Zhang, Davis, Baker, & Braun, 2014; Stoodley & Wung, 2014).

Healthy People 2010 differs from Healthy People 2000 in that it included a feature for monitoring objectives and subobjectives in relation to ethnicity, income, education, and/or gender. Healthy People 2020 builds on these efforts and will continue to monitor inequities and health disparities in the United States. By monitoring potential differences among groups, health professionals will have the tools to recognize why and where population disparities are occurring. This in turn will (one hopes) lead to creative strategies to reduce health disparities and improve equity in health and the delivery of healthcare.

There are numerous dimensions of disparities or differences related to health that can adversely affect groups of people because of specific characteristics or obstacles. It is widely recognized now that the social determinants of health, such as housing, education, access to public transportation, access to safe water, access to fresh food, and the built environment, are all related to a population's health. In addition to ethnicity, other characteristics also contribute to the presence of disparities or the achievement of good health such as gender, sexual orientation, geographic location, working environment, cognitive, sensory, or physical disability, and socioeconomic status. The outcomes identified in the objectives of Healthy People 2020 are intended to improve the health of all groups of people and bridge those gaps. Healthy People 2020 will assess health disparities in U.S. populations in future years by tracking morbidity and mortality outcomes in relation to factors found to be associated with disparities.

APRNs have numerous resources they can access to improve quality and timely access to quality healthcare, and decrease health disparities. The National Partnership for Action (NPA) to End Health Disparities (minorityhealth.hhs.gov/npa) was started by the Office of Minority Health to mobilize individuals and groups to work to improve quality and eliminate health disparities. The National Priorities Partnership (www.qualityforum .org/Setting_Priorities/NPP/National_Priorities_Partnership.aspx) includes key private and public stakeholders who have agreed to work on major health priorities of patients and families, palliative and end-of-life care, care coordination, patient safety, and population health. The Quality Alliance Steering Committee (www.healthqualityalliance.org) is another partnership of healthcare leaders who work to improve healthcare quality and costs. Various strategies to bridge the gaps in healthcare quality are available at the national level and may be applied or considered at the state, regional, or local level in collaboration with stakeholders as a means of decreasing health disparities. Another excellent resource can be found on the site of the Association of American Medical Colleges (AAMC). It has compiled the report *The State of Health Equity Research: Closing Knowledge Gaps to Address Inequities* (available at www.aamc .org/initiatives/research/healthequity/402654/closingknowledgegaps.html). The AAMC and AcademyHealth worked together to review all U.S. health disparities–focused health services research funded during the 5-year period between 2007 and 2011. Their purpose was to determine where such research is taking place and who is funding it, identify gaps in populations and health outcomes, and assess trends in the funding of solution-focused health equity research (AACM, 2014).

Established in 1988, the Office of Minority Health and Health Disparities (OMHD) is housed within the CDC. Resources available from this office may be used by APRNs to obtain data that demonstrate how minority populations compare with the U.S. population as a whole. Such disparities are complicated to analyze and explain as they go beyond differences in genetics, biological characteristics, and health behaviors (microlevel properties). Racist and discriminatory behaviors and policies, cultural barriers, lack of access to care, and interaction with the environment (macrolevel properties) play a major role in creating the problem (see Chapter 11).

Another resource available to APRNs can be found at Quick Health Data Online (www.healthstatus2020.com/index.html). This site has several valuable components, including the Quick Health Data Online system, the Health Disparities Profile, and the Women's Health and Mortality Chartbook. The Quick Health Data Online system provides information on state- and county-level data from all 50 states, the District of Columbia, and U.S. territories. The data can be analyzed by stratifying them into various categories, including demographic characteristics, disease type, and insurance status. This resource is invaluable for identifying a state's health disparities. The Health Disparities Profile examines key health indicators by state level and by race and ethnicity (www.healthstatus2020.com/disparities/ChartBookData_search.asp). Such information is very important to APRNs who wish to develop or implement interventions to target vulnerable community members and those who are most at risk of having poor health outcomes.

The National Institutes of Health (NIH) awards grants to Centers for Population Health and Health Disparities (CPHHD) that are selected to address disparities and inequities associated with cancer and heart disease, the two leading causes of death in U.S. adults. This program involves numerous partnerships, including NIH's National Cancer Institute (NCI), the National Heart, Lung, and Blood Institute (NHLBI), and the Office of Behavioral and Social Sciences Research (OBSSR). Ten centers were awarded funds in May 2010 to promote transdisciplinary research in the areas of cancer and heart disease with a goal to reduce disparities and inequities in the health of underserved populations. These grants will also train researchers to work together across disciplines to advance our understanding of the factors that contribute to health disparities. The website http://cancercontrol.cancer.gov has a variety of resources available, including funding opportunities, reports and health surveys, data sets, tool kits for research projects, and cross-cutting areas such as health disparities, patient-centered communication, and care coordination. There is also a health disparities calculator (HD*Calc). HD*Calc is statistical software that can be downloaded and used to generate and calculate 11 disparity measurements (http://seer.cancer.gov/hdcalc). Additional information about CPHHD, including information about each individual center's goals, can be easily located at the aforementioned website. APRNs can contact the principal investigators or other research staff to obtain information, to explore collaborative endeavors with researchers, to participate with community-based participatory research, to assist with translational research studies, and to share expertise with the aim of decreasing health disparities among vulnerable populations.

Examples of Health Disparities

Even a cursory review of reports and studies available through government agencies and various other organizations as well as peer-reviewed journals reveals many examples of healthcare disparities in the United States. The following are just a few examples.

Despite advances in diabetes prevention and treatment, Native Americans/Alaska Natives have a higher age-adjusted percentage of people with diabetes mellitus (as compared to Whites), followed by non-Hispanic Blacks and Hispanics (CDC, 2014b; Jiang et al., 2013). African Americans have a higher annual incidence of lung cancer (86.8 per 100,000 people) than Whites (73.7 per 100,00 people), with the highest incidence occurring in the South (CDC, 2010). Protective service workers (police, fire fighters) had the lowest awareness, treatment, and control of hypertension when compared with workers in executive and managerial occupations (Davila et al., 2012). Even though the infant mortality rate in the United States has declined in recent years, and even when controlling for socioeconomic factors, African American infants, compared to White infants, are more than twice as likely to die in their first year of life, and the African American fetal mortality rate is more than double that of Whites (Alio et al., 2010; HHS, 2013; MacDorman, Kirmeyer, & Wilson, 2012). Examples of studies that explore gender inequities include a study by an APRN who explored a framework of female marginalization and found that women were more likely to die from cardiovascular disease when compared with men (Koci, 2010). Researchers in the area of health literacy have found disparities based on the literacy level of the client and the ability of the provider to facilitate patient understanding of treatment and management of a disease. Studies on the impact of health literacy on health outcomes have found that there is poor utilization of primary healthcare services, increased use of EDs to access immediate care, and perceived poor health among people with low health literacy (Berkman, Sheridan, Donahue, Halpern, & Crotty, 2011; Schumacher et al., 2013).

Evidence-based nursing interventions can be successful in addressing such disparities. A research team was successful in helping clients manage their diabetes by tailoring a diabetes self-management intervention for older, rural African American women (Leeman et al., 2008). Another research team with Home Care of Rochester (HCR) designed a theory-based outcomes improvement model based on the Sunrise Enabler approach to deliver home nursing care to Hispanic patients (Leininger, 2006). According to the 2010 National Healthcare Disparities Report published by the AHRQ, Hispanics receive a poorer quality of care than non-Hispanic Whites in 23 of the 38 core quality measures (AHRQ, 2011). In addition to paying attention to culturally and linguistically appropriate services (CLAS) and healthcare standards, the team recognized the problem that Hispanics had with accessing healthcare. By creating a model of care based on Leininger's Theory of Culture Care and Universality, team members developed a plan for delivering culturally congruent care. They recruited and oriented Hispanic nurses to provide home care and developed educational information in a way the population appreciated by using a telenovela or soap opera video format. HCR used the Outcome and Assessment Information Set (OASIS) to evaluate the model. They found that the acute hospitalization rate for Hispanic patients dropped almost by half following the intervention when previously it had been twice that of the overall population before the program was implemented, and there were some small gains seen in the Hispanic patients' adherence to medications and a reduction in the usage of emergency services (Woerner, Espinosa, Bourne, O'Toole, & Ingersoll, 2009). Policies are also being written and adopted at all levels of government to address healthcare disparities. For example, a new federal policy to address the literacy gap requires that healthcare delivery systems have a plan in place to address literacy issues at all levels (Koh et al., 2012).

In summary, health disparities are deplorable, and effective strategies to reverse this trend are urgently needed. Although much research has been done to better understand healthcare disparities, researchers suggest that a multidimensional approach is needed; a history of institutionalized racism and individual racism that is embedded in every aspect of life of ethnic minorities must be recognized and properly addressed (Klawetter, 2014). For the purpose of eliminating health disparities, the National Stakeholder Strategy for Achieving Health Equity, a product of the National Partnership for Action, established guidelines for the development and continuous assessment of the impact of policies and programs to improve the health of vulnerable populations and achieve health equity. Healthcare workers need cultural competency training, communication needs to improve between providers and patients, strategies to improve community relations are needed, and adherence to nondiscriminatory health policies is also necessary to bridge the gaps in providing equity and quality care to eliminate health disparities (http://minorityhealth.hhs.gov/npa/files/Plans/NSS/NSSExecSum.pdf).

It is critical that APRNs advocate for the elimination of health disparities, as this work is of vital importance and urgently needed. And from an ethical standpoint, working to eliminate health disparities is the right thing to do. By recognizing health disparities and developing a better understanding of how process and status impact the outcome of interest, APRNs are better prepared to develop effective interventions to eliminate or reduce health disparities. Such strategies may include advocating better health insurance coverage for poor and immigrant populations; ensuring that sufficient services exist in underserved areas; assessing the interaction among social environments, genetics, and population health; encouraging minority participation in research studies with community-based participatory research and specifically with practice-based research networks; using linguistically and culturally appropriate communication and written handouts; promoting and facilitating community partnerships; and implementing strategies to encourage people from minority populations to become healthcare professionals (Daniel, 2010; Geronimus, 2013; Radwin, Cabral, & Woodworth, 2013; Sentell et al., 2014).

APRNs have successfully tested interventions to decrease health disparities, and by careful and thorough review of the current literature and resources available, they have the tools to develop additional effective and culturally sensitive interventions and to identify outcomes in order to achieve better and more equitable health outcomes.

SUMMARY

APRNs have a critical role in improving population health by intervening at every level from the individual to the community. Before an effective intervention can take place, it is imperative that realistic and measureable outcomes are first identified and defined so that they can be measured and analyzed. Outcomes may be classified by the beneficiary of the health intervention and by type such as care, patient, or performance-related, and also by time frame of achievement. Outcomes may also be categorized by clinical or disease-specific outcomes, function, cost-effectiveness, self-perception health status, and satisfaction outcomes. A commonly used framework to classify outcomes is Donabedian's framework of structure, process, and outcomes. This framework has been used for describing a community's health as well as for classifying nurse-sensitive indicators. Outcomes are an important part of the standardized language that nursing leaders and researchers continue to refine and operationalize as a means of improving healthcare and are particularly relevant as electronic health records grow in usage throughout the United States (AHRQ, 2005).

The national healthcare objectives as released in Healthy People 2020 provide a blueprint of health promotion and disease prevention objectives that are designed to improve the health of all people in the United States. Building on the goal of Healthy People 2010, APRNs can use these web-based resources to identify outcomes and compare them with national and state data that can be further analyzed by stratifying for a population's ethnicity, race, income, education, and/or gender. Federal agencies, such as the AHRQ, the CDC Office of Minority Health and Health Disparities, and the NIH Centers for Population Health and Health Disparities, provide ready access to a plethora of information and resources that can be used to identify and define outcomes.

APRNs have a tremendous opportunity to access and use available data to contribute to the current body of knowledge that forms the basis for evidence-based practice. By selecting and using well-defined indicators and comparing those to national norms, APRNs can provide important information on trends or patterns of quality of care. This information has the potential to stimulate the development of creative and innovative programs or interventions to improve health outcomes. Evidence of improved outcomes will help APRNs to justify and advocate for change through policy, practice, and research, with the ultimate goal of providing quality care for all.

EXERCISES AND DISCUSSION QUESTIONS

Exercise 2.1 Poor infant mortality rates for African American babies in the United States are an example of a glaring health disparity.
- Where would you go to find information about this problem?
- How would you obtain information regarding infant mortality rates from your local, state, or regional community?
- What factors must be considered when interpreting epidemiological data on health disparities?
- What interventions have been designed to reduce infant mortality rates, and specifically the infant mortality rates of specific groups with the highest mortality rates?
- How might an APRN participate in local efforts to reduce infant mortality rates?

Exercise 2.2 An APRN is interested in trying to prevent mortality from acute stroke and decides to develop an online continuing education program to teach RNs, APRNs, and physician assistants about stroke protocols, including administration of tissue plasminogen activator (tPA), a thrombolytic therapy.
- What outcomes might the APRN monitor to determine the effectiveness of this program?
- The APRN takes a closer look at identifying subgroups in his or her community with the highest risk of stroke. In what ways can he or she tailor the educational intervention to better reach these groups at the community level? At the state level?

Exercise 2.3 An APRN is volunteering in a homeless shelter and is caring for a young woman who is withdrawn and not making eye contact. The APRN observes bruising on the woman's arms and cheek.
- What information should the APRN assess that can be used to provide the appropriate health intervention(s)?
- The likelihood that youths who are homeless will experience health inequalities depends mainly on what types of determinants?
- What health indicators should the APRN monitor as a measure of health outcomes?

Exercise 2.4 A recent conference you attended included a session on ways that hospitals in the Southeast are using the NDNQI. You do not know very much about nursing indicators but recognize this would be helpful to you in the new role you will have as a nurse manager.
- Where can you obtain information about the NDNQI?
- You later learn that the hospital where you work has just started collecting data on 5 of the NDNQI nursing indicators. You ask to review the data and find that the nursing care hours per patient day on your unit are low in comparison with the national data provided from the database. How can you use this information to improve patient care on your unit?

Exercise 2.5 Diabetes affects a growing number of Americans. You have been invited to join a collaborative of community agencies interested in tackling diabetes from a community perspective.
- What resources will you use to identify different outcomes related to diabetes?
- What outcomes related to diabetes are of most interest to community members?

- How will you compare the outcomes you select to monitor at the local level with state and national outcomes?

Exercise 2.6 APRNs should not only recognize but also make it part of their practice to develop strategies to reduce or eliminate health disparities. Review information from Healthy People 2020 and the CDC Office of Minority Health and Health Disparities websites.
- What health disparities can you find that are relevant to your community?
- How can you better advocate for minority groups who have poorer health outcomes?
- What specific objectives in Healthy People 2020 can help this effort?

Exercise 2.7 You are a psychiatric clinical nurse specialist interested in improving mental health services in your community. You decide to review the Guide to Community Preventive Services to identify a evidence-based intervention that will help older adults who live at home better manage depression.
- What information is in the guide that may be relevant to your practice?
- What other government-sponsored websites may have useful information?
- What types of outcomes would you measure to assess the problem of depression in older adults?

REFERENCES

AHRQ. (2005). *The Donabedian Model of patient safety: Medical teamwork and patient safety: The evidence-based relation.* Retrieved July 15, 2014, from http://www.ahrq.gov/research/findings/final-reports/medteam/figure2.html

AHRQ. (2011). *Disparities in health care quality among racial and ethnic minority groups: Selected findings from the AHRQ 2010 NHQR and NHDR.* Retrieved August 7, 2014, from http://www.ahrq.gov/research/findings/nhqrdr/nhqrdr10/minority.pdf

AHRQ. (2013). *National healthcare quality & disparities reports.* Retrieved July 23, 2014, from http://www.ahrq.gov/research/findings/nhqrdr/index.html

Alio, A. P., Richman, A. R., Clayton, H. B., Jeffers, D. F., Wathington, D. J., & Salihu, H. M. (2010). An ecological approach to understanding black–white disparities in perinatal mortality. *Maternal Child Health Journal, 14,* 557–566. doi:10.1007/s10995-009-0495-9

Allan, J., Agar Barwick, T., Cashman, S., Cawley, J. F., Day, C., Douglass, C. W., Evans, C. H., … Wood, D. (2004). Clinical prevention and population health: Curriculum framework for health professions. *American Journal of Preventive Medicine, 27*(5), 471–476. doi:10.1016/S0749-3797(04)00206-5

American Association of Colleges of Nursing. (2004). *AACN position statement on the practice doctorate in nursing.* Washington, DC: Author.

American Association of Colleges of Nursing. (2006). *The essentials of doctoral education for advanced nursing practice.* Retrieved from http://www.aacn.nche.edu/DNP/pdf/Essentials.pdf

Anderson, E. T., & McFarlane, J. (2010). *Community as partner: Theory and practice in nursing* (6th ed.). New York, NY: Lippincott Williams & Wilkins.

Aschengrau, A., & Seage, G. R. (2013). Sources of public health data. *Essentials of epidemiology in public health* (3rd ed.). Burlington, MA: Jones & Bartlett Learning.

Association of American Medical Colleges. (2014). *The state of health equity research: Closing knowledge gaps to address inequities.* Retrieved from https://www.aamc.org/initiatives/research/healthequity/402654/closingknowledgegaps.html

Berkman, N. D., Sheridan, S. L., Donahue, K. E., Halpern, D. J., & Crotty, K. (2011). Low health literacy and health outcomes: An updated systematic review. *Annual of Internal Medicine, 155*(2), 97–107. doi:10.7326/0003-4819-155-2-201107190-00005

Bigbee, J. L., & Issel, L. M. (2012). Conceptual models for population-focused public health nursing interventions and outcomes: The state of the art. *Public Health Nursing, 29*(4), 370–379. doi: 10.1111/j.1525-1446.2011.01006.x

Boothe, V. L., Sinha, D., Bohm, M., & Yoon, P. W. (2013). Community health assessment for population health improvement; resource of most frequently recommended health outcomes and determinants. CDC Stacks Public Health Publications. Retrieved July 14, 2014, from http://stacks.cdc.gov/view/cdc/20707

Buckley, L., Chapman, R. L., & Sheehan, M. (2014). Young driver distraction: State of the evidence and directions for behavior change programs. *Journal of Adolescent Health, 54*(5 Suppl.), S16–S21. doi:10.1016/j.jadohealth.2013.12.021

Centers for Disease Control. (2010). Racial/ethnic disparities and geographic differences in lung cancer incidence—38 states and the District of Columbia, 1998–2006. *Morbidity and Mortality Weekly Report (MMWR), 59*(44), 1434–1438. Retrieved from http://www.cdc.gov/mmwr/preview/mmwrhtml/mm5944a2.htm?s_cid=mm5944a2_w

Centers for Disease Control. (2013). *Behavioral Risk Factor Surveillance System (BRFSS).* Retrieved July 22, 2014, from http://www.cdc.gov/brfss/about/about_brfss.htm

Centers for Disease Control. (2014a). *National health care surveys.* Retrieved August 3, 2014, from http://www.cdc.gov/nchs/dhcs.htm

Centers for Disease Control. (2014b). *National diabetes statistics report, 2014.* Retrieved August 2014, from http://www.cdc.gov/diabetes/pubs/estimates14.htm#4

Chaskin, R. J., Brown, P., Venkatesh, S., & Vidal, A. (2001). *Building community capacity.* New York, NY: Walter de Gruyter.

Daniel, M. (2010). Strategies for targeting health care disparities among Hispanics. *Family & Community Health, 33*(4), 329–342. doi:10.1097/FCH.0b013e3181f3b292

Davila, E. P., Kuklina, E. V., Valderrama, A. L., Yoon, P. W., Rolle, I., & Nsubuga, P. (2012). Prevalence, management, and control of hypertension among U.S. workers: Does occupation matter? *Journal of Occupational and Environmental Medicine, 54*(9), 1150–1156. doi:10.1097/JOM.0b013e318256f675

DeGuzman, P. B., & Kulbok, P. A. (2012). Changing health outcomes of vulnerable populations through nursing's influence on neighborhood built environment: A framework for nursing research. *Journal of Nursing Scholarship, 44*(4), 341–348. doi:10.1111/j.1547-5069.2012.01470.x

Donabedian, A. (1980). *Explorations in quality assessment and monitoring.* Ann Arbor, MI: Health Administration Press.

Donabedian, A. (1982). *The criteria and standards of quality.* Ann Arbor, MI: Health Administration Press.

Dunton, N. E. (2008). Take a cue from the NDNQI. *Nursing Management, 39*(4), 20–23. doi:10.1097/01.NUMA.0000316054.35317.b

Fee, E., & Garofalo, M. E. (2010). Florence Nightingale and the Crimean war. *American Journal of Public Health, 100*(9), 1591. doi:10.2105/AJPH.2009.188607

Fredriksen-Goldsen, K. I., Kim, H. J., Barkan, S. E., Muraco, A., & Hoy-Ellis, C. P. (2013). Health disparities among lesbian, gay, and bisexual older adults: Results from a population-based study. *American Journal of Public Health, 103*(10), 1802–1809. doi: 10.2105/AJPH.2012.301110

Friis, R. H., & Sellers, T. A. (2009). *Epidemiology for public health practice* (4th ed.). Boston, MA: Jones & Bartlett.

Gallagher, R. M., & Rowell, P. A. (2003). Claiming the future of nursing through nursing-sensitive quality indicators. *Nursing Administration Quarterly, 27*(4), 273–84.

Geronimus, A. T. (2013). Deep integration: Letting the epigenome out of the bottle without losing sight of the structural origins of population health. *American Journal of Public Health, 103*(Suppl. 1), S56–S63. doi:10.2105/AJPH.2013.301380

Griffiths, P. (1995). Progress in measuring nursing outcomes. *Journal of Advanced Nursing, 21*, 1092–1100. doi:10.1046/j.1365-2648.1995.21061092.x

Heitgerd JL, Dent AL, Holt JB, Elmore KA, Melfi K, Stanley JM, & al., e. (2008). Community health status indicators: adding a geospatial component, 5(3). Retrieved from http://www.cdc.gov/pcd/issues/2008/jul/07_0077.htm.

Hill, M. (1999). Outcomes measurement requires nursing to shift to outcome-based practice. *Nursing Administration Quarterly, 24*(1), 1–16.

Hunter, B. D., Neiger, B., & West, J. (2011). The importance of addressing social determinants of health at the local level: The case for social capital. *Health & Social Care in the Community, 19*(5), 522–530. doi:10.1111/j.1365-2524.2011.00999.x

Institute of Medicine. (2013). *Toward quality measures for population health and the leading health indicators.* Washington, DC: National Academies Press.

Jiang, L., Manson, S. M., Beals, J., Henderson, W. G., Huang, H., Acton, K. J., . . . Special Diabetes Program for Indians Diabetes Prevention Demonstration Project. (2013). Translating the Diabetes Prevention Program into American Indian and Alaska Native communities: Results from the Special Diabetes Program for Indians Diabetes Prevention demonstration project. *Diabetes Care, 36*(7), 2027–2034. doi:10.2337/dc12-1250

Kautz, D. D., & Van Horn, E. R. (2008). An exemplar of the use of NNN language in developing evidence-based practice guidelines. *International Journal of Nursing Terminologies and Classifications 19*(1), 14-19. Retrieved from http://findarticles.com/p/articles/mi_qa4065/is_200801/ai_n25138588/?tag=content;col1

Klawetter, S. (2014). Conceptualizing social determinants of maternal and infant health disparities. *Affilia: Journal of Women and Social Work, 29*(2), 131–141.

Kleinpell, R., & Gawlinski, A. (2005). Assessing outcomes in advanced practice nursing practice: The use of quality indicators and evidence-based practice. *AACN Clinical Issues, 16*(1), 43–57. doi:10.1097/00044067-200501000-00006

Kleinpell, R. M. (2001). Measuring outcomes in advanced practice nursing. In R. Kleinpell (Ed.), *Outcome assessment in advanced practice nursing* (pp. 1–50). New York, NY: Springer.

Kleinpell, R. M. (2003). Measuring advanced practice nursing outcome, strategies and resources. *Critical Care Nurse,* (Suppl.), 6–10.

Kleinpell, R. M. (2007). APRNs: Invisible champions? *Nursing Management, 38*(5), 18–22. doi:10.1097/01.LPN.0000269815.74178.de

Koci, A. (2010). Care of women and marginalized populations in the critical care setting. *Critical Care Nursing Quarterly, 33*(3), 244–247. doi: 10.1097/CNQ.0b013e3181e65fb4

Koh, H. K., Berwick, D. M., Clancy, C. M., Baur, C., Brach, C., Harris, L. M., & Zerhusen, E. G. (2012). New Federal Policy Initiatives To Boost Health Literacy Can Help The Nation Move Beyond The Cycle Of Costly 'Crisis Care'. *Health Aff (Millwood).* doi: 10.1377/hlthaff.2011.1169

Krieger, N. (2001). Theories for social epidemiology in the 21st century: An ecosocial perspective. *International Journal of Epidemiology, 30*(4), 668–677. doi:10.1093/Ije/30.4.668

Kurtzman, E. T., & Corrigan, J. M. (2007). Measuring the contribution of nursing to quality, patient safety, and health care outcomes. *Policy Politics & Nursing Practice, 8*(1), 20–36. doi:10.1177/1527154407302115

Lang, N. M., & Marek, K. D. (1991). The policy and politics of patient outcomes. *Journal of Nursing Quality Assurance, 5*(2), 7–12.

Leeman, J., Skelly, A. H., Burns, D., Carlson, J., & Soward, A. (2008). Tailoring a diabetes self-care intervention for use with older, rural African American women. *Diabetes Educator, 34*(2), 310–317. doi:10.1177/0145721708316623

Leininger, M. M. (2006). Culture care diversity and universality theory and evolution of the ethnonursing method. In M. M. Leininger & M. R. McFarland (Eds.), *Cultural care diversity and universality: A worldwide nursing theory* (2nd ed., pp. 1–41). Boston, MA: Jones & Bartlett.

Loyo, H. K., Batcher, C., Wile, K., Huang, P., Orenstein, D., & Milstein, B. (2012). From model to action: Using a system dynamics model of chronic disease risks to align community action. *Health Promotion Practice, 14*(1), 53–61. Retrieved from http://hpp.sagepub.com/content/14/1/53.full.pdf+html

MacDorman, M. F., Kirmeyer, S. E., & Wilson, E. C. (2012). Fetal and perinatal mortality, United States, 2006. *National Vital Statistics Report, 60*(8), 1–22.

Macha, K., & McDonough, P. (Eds.). (2012). *Epidemiology for advanced nursing practice* (1st ed.). Sudbury, MA: Jones & Bartlett.

MacMullen, N. J., Tymkow, C., & Shen, J. J., (2006). Adverse maternal outcomes in women with asthma: Differences by race. *MCN. The American Journal of Maternal/Child Nursing, 31*(4), 263–268. doi:10.1097/00005721-200607000-00012

Mahadevan, R., & McGinnis, T. (2013). Considerations for building partnerships between provider practices and community organizations. In Robert Wood Johnson Foundation (Ed.), *Improving health care quality and equity: Considerations for building partnerships between provider practices and community organizations* (pp. 1–14). Princeton, NJ: Robert Wood Johnson Foundation.

Meyer, P. A., Yoon, P. W., & Kaufmann, R. B. (2013). Introduction: CDC health disparities and inequalities report—United States, 2013. *Morbidity and Mortality Weekly Report Surveillance, 62*(Suppl. 3), 3–5.

Minkler, M., & Wallerstein, N. (2007). Improving health through community organization and community building: A health education perspective. In M. Minkler (Ed.), *Community organizing and community building for health* (2nd ed., pp. 30-52). Piscataway, NJ: Rutgers University Press.

Mirman, J. H., Curry, A. E., Winston, F. K., Wang, W., Elliott, M. R., Schultheis, M. T., . . . Durbin, D. R. (2014). Effect of the teen driving plan on the driving performance of teenagers before licensure: A randomized clinical trial. *JAMA Pediatrics, 168*(8), 764–771. doi:10.1001/jamapediatrics.2014.252

Montalvo, I. (2007). The National Database of Nursing Quality Indicators® (NDNQI®). *Online Journal of Issues in Nursing, 12*(3). Retrieved from EBSCO*host*.

Nelson, E. C., Batalden, P. B., Plume, S. K., Mihevc, N. T., & Swartz, W. G. (1995). Report cards or instrument panels: Who needs what? *The Joint Commission Journal on Quality Improvement, 21*(4), 155–166.

Nelson, E. C., Batalden, P. B., Plume, S. K., & Mohr, J. J. (1996). Improving health care, Part 2: A clinical improvement worksheet and users' manual. *Joint Commission Journal on Quality Improvement, 22*(8), 531–548.

Nelson, E. C., Mohr, J. J., Batalden, P. B., & Plume, S. K. (1996). Improving health care, part 1: The clinical value compass. *Joint Commission Journal for Quality Improvement, 22*(4), 243–258.

Oermann, M., & Floyd, J. A. (2002). Outcomes research: An essential component of the advanced practice nurse role. *Clinical Nurse Specialist, 16*(3), 140–144. doi:10.1097/00002800-200205000-00007

Parrish, R. G. (2010). Measuring population health outcomes. *Preventing Chronic Disease, 7*(4), A71.

Partners, P. H. (2014, July 22). *Health data tools and statistics.* Retrieved from http://phpartners.org/health_stats.html

Patrician, P. A., Dolansky, M. A., Pair, V., Bates, M., Moore, S. M., Splaine, M., & Gilman, S. C. (2013). The Veterans Affairs National Quality Scholars program: A model for interprofessional education in quality and safety. *Journal Nursing Care Quality, 28*(1), 24–32. doi:10.1097/NCQ.0b013e3182678f41

Press Ganey Associates. (2014). National Database of Nursing Quality Indicators® (NDNQI®). Retrieved July 2014, from http://www.nursingquality.org/#intro

Quigley, E. (2003). Contributions of the professional, public, and private sectors in promoting patient safety. *Online Journal of Issues in Nursing, 8*(3), Manuscript 1. Retrieved from www.nursingworld.org/MainMenuCategories/ANAMarketplace/ANAPeriodicals/OJIN/TableofContents/Volume82003/No3Sept2003/ContributionsinPromoting.aspx

Radwin, L. E., Cabral, H. J., & Woodworth, T. S. (2013). Effects of race and language on patient-centered cancer nursing care and patient outcomes. *Journal of Health Care Poor Underserved, 24*(2), 619–632. doi:10.1353/hpu.2013.0058

Reiss, D., Leve, L. D., & Neiderhiser, J. M. (2013). How genes and the social environment moderate each other. *Americal Journal of Public Health, 103*(Suppl. 1), S111–121.

Rich, K. A. (2009). Evaluating outcomes of innovations. In N. A. Schmidt & J. M. Brown (Eds.), *Evidence-based practice: Appraisal and application of research.* Sudbury, MA; Jones & Bartlett.

Schaffer, M. A., Goodhue, A., Stennes, K., & Lanigan, C. (2012). Evaluation of a public health nurse visiting program for pregnant and parenting teens. *Public Health Nursing, 29*(3), 218–231. doi: 10.1111/j.1525-1446.2011.01005.x

Schumacher, J. R., Hall, A. G., Davis, T. C., Arnold, C. L., Bennett, R. D., Wolf, M. S., & Carden, D. L. (2013). Potentially preventable use of emergency services: The role of low health literacy. *Medical Care, 51*(8), 654–658. doi:10.1097/MLR.0b013e3182992c5a

Sentell, T., Zhang, W., Davis, J., Baker, K. K., & Braun, K. L. (2014). The influence of community and individual health literacy on self-reported health status. *Journal of General Internal Medicine, 29*(2), 298–304. doi:10.1007/s11606-013-2638-3

Shuster, G. F. (2014). Community as client: Assessment and analysis. In M. Stanhope & J. Lancaster (Eds.), *Public health nursing: Population-centered health care in the community* (8th ed., pp. 396–419). St. Louis, MO: Mosby.

Smith, K. J., & Craft-Rosenberg, M. (2010). Using NANDA, NIC, and NOC in an undergraduate nursing practicum. *Nurse Educator, 35*(4), 162–166. doi:10.1097/NNE.0b013e3181e33953

Stoodley, L., & Wung, S. F. (2014). Hyperglycemia after cardiac surgery: Improving a quality measure. *AACN Advanced Critical Care, 25*(3), 221–227. doi:10.1097/NCI.0000000000000028

United Nations. (2008). Unequal health outcomes in the United States. (U.N. Committee on the Elimination of Racial Discrimination). Retrieved July 23, 2014, from http://www.prrac.org/pdf/CERDhealthEnvironmentReport.pdf

U.S. Department of Health and Human Services (HHS). (2013). *Child health USA 2013*. Retrieved August, 2014, from http://mchb.hrsa.gov/chusa13/perinatal-health-status-indicators/p/fetal-mortality.html

U.S. Department of Health and Human Services (HHS). (2014). *Healthy People 2020: Social determinants of health.* Retrieved July 25, 2014, from http://www.healthypeople.gov/2020/topicsobjectives2020/overview.aspx?topicid=39

U.S. Department of Health and Human Services (HHS), Community Preventive Services Task Force. (2015a). The community guide. Retrieved from http://www.thecommunityguide.org/index.html

U.S. Department of Health and Human Services (HHS). (2015b). *Healthy People 2020.* Retrieved from http://www.healthypeople.gov/

van Maanen, H. M. T. (1979). Perspectives and problems on quality of nursing care: An overview of contributions from North America and recent developments in Europe. *Journal of Advanced Nursing, 4*(4), 377–389. doi: 10.1111/j.1365-2648.1979.tb00872.x

Woerner, L., Espinosa, J., Bourne, S., O'Toole, M., & Ingersoll, G. L. (2009). Project ¡ÉXITO!: Success through diversity and universality for outcomes improvement among Hispanic home care patients. *Nursing Outlook, 57*, 266–273. doi:10.1016/j.outlook.2009.02.001

World Health Organization. (2008). Closing the gap in a generation: Health equity through action on the social determinants of health. Retrieved rom http://www.who.int/social_determinants/thecommission/finalreport/en/

Epidemiological Methods and Measurements in Population-Based Nursing Practice: Part I

Patty A. Vitale and Ann L. Cupp Curley

Evidence-based practice as it relates to population-based nursing combines clinical practice and public health through the use of population health sciences in clinical practice (Heller & Page, 2002). Epidemiology is the science of public health. It is concerned with the study of the factors determining and influencing the frequency and distribution of disease, injury, and other health-related events and their causes (Gordis, 2014). In addition to epidemiology, an understanding of other scientific disciplines, such as biology and biostatistics, is also important for identifying associations and determining causation when looking at exposures and outcomes as they relate to population health.

Population-based care focuses on populations at risk, analysis of aggregate data, evaluation of demographic factors, and recognition of health disparities. It is concerned with the patterns of delivery of care and outcome measurements at the population or subpopulation level. The purpose of this chapter is to provide readers with an understanding of the natural history of disease and the approaches that are integral for the prevention of disease. We introduce basic concepts that are necessary to understand how to measure disease outcomes and select study designs that are best suited for population-based research. Emphasis is placed on measuring disease occurrence with a fundamental discussion of how to calculate incidence, prevalence, and mortality rates. Successful advanced practice nursing in population health depends on the ability to recognize the difference between the individual and population approaches to the collection and use of data, and the ability to assess needs and evaluate outcomes at the population level. Concepts surrounding survival data are also discussed along with strategies to guide advanced practice registered nurses (APRNs) on how to calculate and interpret survival data.

THE NATURAL HISTORY OF DISEASE

The natural history of disease refers to the progression of a disease from its *preclinical state* (prior to symptoms) to its *clinical state* (from onset of symptoms to cure, control, disability, or death). Disease is not something that occurs suddenly, but rather, it is a multifactorial process that is dynamic and occurs over time. It evolves and changes and is sometimes initiated by events that take place years, even decades, before symptoms first appear. Many diseases have a natural life history that can extend over a very long period of time. The natural history of disease is described in stages. Understanding the different stages allows for a better understanding of the approach to the prevention and control of disease.

Stage of Susceptibility

The stage of susceptibility refers to the time prior to disease development. In the presence of certain risk factors, genetics, or environment, disease may develop and the severity can vary among individuals. Risk factors are those factors that are associated with an increased likelihood of disease developing over time. The idea that individuals could modify "risk factors" tied to heart disease, stroke, and other diseases is one of the key findings of the Framingham Heart Study (National Heart, Lung, and Blood Institute and Boston University, 2010). Started in 1948 and still in operation, this study is one of the most important population studies ever carried out in the United States. Before Framingham, for example, most healthcare providers believed that atherosclerosis was an inevitable part of the aging process. Although not all risk factors are amenable to change (e.g., genetic factors), the identification of risk factors is important and fundamental to disease prevention.

Preclinical Stage of Disease

During the preclinical phase, the disease process has begun but there are no obvious symptoms. Although there is no clear manifestation of disease, because of the interaction of biological factors, changes have started to occur. During this stage, however, the changes are not always detectable. Screening technologies have been developed to detect the presence of some diseases before clinical symptoms appear. The Papanicolaou (Pap) smear is an example of an effective screening method for detecting cancer in a premalignant state to improve mortality related to cervical cancer. The use of the Pap smear as a screening tool facilitates early detection and treatment of premalignant changes of the cervix prior to development of malignancy.

Clinical Stage of Disease

In the clinical stage of disease, sufficient physiologic and/or functional changes occur, leading to the development of recognizable symptoms of disease. It might also be accurately referred to as the treatment stage. For some people, the disease may completely resolve (either spontaneously or with medical intervention), and for some it will lead to disability and/or death. It is for this reason that the clinical stage of disease is sometimes subdivided for better medical management. Staging systems used in malignancies to better define the extent of disease involvement are an example of a system that can help guide the type of treatment modality selected based on stage. In many cases, staging can provide an estimate of prognosis. Another example is the identification of disability as a specific subcategory of the treatment stage. Disability occurs when a clinical disease leaves a person either temporarily or permanently disabled. When people become disabled, the goal of treatment is to mitigate the effects of disease and to help these individuals to function to their optimal abilities. This is very different from the goal for someone who can be treated and restored to the level of functioning that he or she enjoyed prior to the illness.

The Nonclinical Disease Stage

This nonclinical or unapparent disease stage can be broken into four subparts. The first subpart is the *preclinical stage*, which, as mentioned earlier, is the acquisition of disease prior to development of symptoms and is destined to become disease. The second subpart is the *subclinical stage* that occurs when someone has the disease but it is not destined to develop clinically. The third subpart is the *chronic or persistent stage of disease*, which is disease that persists over time. And finally, there is the fourth subpart or *latent stage* in which one has disease with no active multiplication of the biologic agent (Gordis, 2014).

The Iceberg Phenomenon

For most health problems, the number of identified cases is exceeded by the number of unidentified cases. This occurrence, referred to as the "iceberg phenomenon," makes it difficult to assess the true burden of disease. Many diseases do not have obvious symptoms, as stated earlier, and may go unrecognized for many years. Unrecognized diseases, such as diabetes, hypertension, and mental illness, create a significant problem with identifying populations at risk and estimating service needs. Complications also arise when patients are not recognized or treated during an early stage of a disease when interventions are most effective. Additionally, patients who do not have symptoms or do not recognize their symptoms do not seek medical care and, in many cases, even if they do have a diagnosis, will not take their medications as they perceive that they are healthy when they are asymptomatic.

PREVENTION

Understanding the natural history of disease is as important as understanding the causal factors of disease because it provides the APRN with the knowledge that is required to design programs or interventions that target populations at risk. Understanding how disease develops is fundamental to the concept of prevention and provides a framework for disease prevention and control.

The primary goal of prevention is to prevent disease before it occurs. The concept of prevention has evolved to include measures taken to interrupt or slow the progression of disease or to lessen its impact. There are three levels of prevention.

Primary Prevention

Primary prevention refers to the process of altering susceptibility or reducing exposure to susceptible individuals and includes general health promotion and specific measures designed to prevent disease prior to a person getting disease. Interventions designed for primary prevention are carried out during the stage of susceptibility and can include such things as providing immunizations to change a person's susceptibility. Actions taken to prevent tobacco usage are another example of primary prevention. Tobacco use is one of the 12 leading health indicators used by Healthy People 2020 to measure health. Cigarette smoking is the leading cause of preventable morbidity and mortality in the United States (Centers for Disease Control and Prevention [CDC], 2014a), and prevention or cessation of smoking can reduce the development of many smoking-related diseases. Taxes on cigarettes, education programs, and support groups to help people stop smoking and the creation of smoke-free zones are all examples of primary prevention measures. The CDC linked a series of tobacco control efforts by Minnesota to a decrease in adult smoking prevalence rates. From 1999 to 2010, Minnesota implemented a series of antismoking initiatives, including a statewide smoke-free law, cigarette tax increases, media campaigns, and statewide cessation efforts. Adult smoking prevalence decreased from 22.1% in 1999 to 16.1% in 2010 (CDC, 2011). This is an excellent example of a statewide primary prevention effort to reduce smoking prevalence through a variety of initiatives.

Secondary Prevention

The early detection and prompt treatment of a disease at the earliest possible stage are referred to as *secondary prevention*. The goals of secondary prevention are to either identify and cure a disease at a very early stage or slow its progression to prevent complications and limit disability. Secondary prevention measures are carried out during the preclinical or presymptomatic stage of disease. Screening programs are designed to detect specific diseases in their early stages while they are curable and to prevent or reduce morbidity and mortality related to a later diagnosis of disease. Examples of secondary prevention include the Pap smear, mentioned earlier, as well as annual testing of cholesterol levels, mammography, and rapid HIV testing of asymptomatic individuals.

Tertiary Prevention

Tertiary prevention strategies are implemented during the middle or late stages of clinical disease and refer to measures taken to alleviate disability and restore effective functioning. Attempts are made to slow the progression or to cure the disease. In cases in which permanent changes have taken place, interventions are planned and designed to help people lead a productive and satisfying life by maximizing the use of remaining capabilities (rehabilitation). Cardiac rehabilitation programs that provide physical and occupational therapies to postoperative cardiac patients are an example of tertiary prevention.

CAUSATION

The Epidemiological Triangle

The relationship between risk factors and disease is complex. Research studies may describe a relationship between a risk factor and disease, but how do we know this relationship is causal? An understanding of causation is important if APRNs want to effectively impact the health of populations. The *epidemiological triangle* is a model that has historically been used to explain causation. The model consists of three interactive factors: the causative agent (those factors for which presence or absence cause disease—biologic, chemical, physical, nutritional), a susceptible host (such things as age, gender, race, immune status, genetics), and the environment (including such diverse elements as water, food, neighborhood, pollution). A change in the agent, host, and environmental balance can lead to disease (Harkness, 1995). The underlying assumptions of this model are that causative factors can be both intrinsic and extrinsic to the host and that the cause of disease is related to interaction among these three factors. This model initially was developed to explain the transmission of infectious diseases and was particularly useful when the focus of epidemiology was on acute diseases. It is less helpful for understanding and explaining the more complicated processes associated with chronic disease. With the rise of chronic diseases as the primary cause of morbidity and mortality, a model that recognizes multiple causative factors was needed to better understand this complex interaction.

The Web of Causation

The dynamic nature of chronic diseases calls for a more sophisticated model for explaining causation than the epidemiological triangle. Introduction of the *web of causation* concept first appeared in the 1960s when chronic diseases overtook infectious diseases as the leading cause of morbidity and mortality in the United States. The foundation of this concept is that disease develops as the result of many antecedent factors and not as a result of a single, isolated cause. Each factor is itself the result of a complex pattern of events that can be best perceived as interrelated in the complex configuration of a web. The use of a web is helpful for visualizing how difficult it is to untangle the many events that can precede the onset of a chronic illness.

Critics have argued that this model places too much emphasis on epidemiological methods and too little on theories of disease causation. As theories evolved about the relationship between smoking and cancer, the U.S. surgeon general appointed a committee to review the evidence. This committee developed a set of guidelines for judging whether an observed association is causal. These guidelines include temporal relationship, strength of the association, dose–response relationship, replication of the findings, biologic plausibility, consideration of alternate explanation, cessation of exposure, consistency with other knowledge, and specificity of the association (Gordis, 2014). For a more detailed discussion on this model, see Chapter 4.

METHODS OF ANALYSIS

Successful population-based approaches depend on the ability to recognize the difference between the collection and use of data from individuals and populations and the ability to assess needs and evaluate outcomes at the population level. Several of the more recent theories of causation can be helpful in determining whether an exposure is causally related to the development of disease. In particular, calculating the strength of association using statistics is one of several criteria that can be used to determine causality. However, statistics must be used with caution. Health is a multidimensional variable: factors that affect health, and that interact to affect health, are numerous. Many relationships are possible. There are problems inherent in the use of statistics to explain differences among groups. Although statistics can describe disparities, they cannot explain them. It is left to the researchers to explain the differences. In addition to statistics, one must also be aware of the validity and reliability of the data. There are problems associated with the categorizing and gathering of statistics during the research process that can have an effect on how the data should be interpreted. In order to be successful in research, one must do more than just collect data: One must look at the theoretical issues associated with explaining the relationship among the variables. Additionally, even if a relationship is found to be statistically significant, that does not assure that it is clinically significant. Recognizing limitations in research and in practice are the most important steps prior to making conclusions in any setting. Therefore, it is important that APRNs have a commitment to higher standards with an emphasis placed on adherence to careful and thorough procedural and ethical practice.

Methods derived from epidemiology can be useful in identifying the etiology or the cause of a disease. Among the important steps in this process are the identification of risk factors and their impact in a population, determining the extent of a disease and/or adverse events found in a population, and evaluating both existing and new preventive and therapeutic measures and modes of healthcare delivery. Applying strong epidemiologic methods with a sound application and interpretation of statistics are the foundation for evidence-based practice. The integration of evidence can lead to the creation of sound public policy and regulatory decisions.

Descriptive Epidemiology

Rates

Knowledge of how illness and injury are distributed within a population can provide valuable information on disease etiology and can lay the foundation for the introduction of new prevention programs. It is important to know how to measure disease in populations, and rates are a useful method for measuring attributes over time such as disease and injury in any population. Rates can also be used to identify trends and evaluate outcomes and can allow for comparisons within and between groups. The *Morbidity and Mortality Weekly Report* (*MMWR;* located at www.cdc.gov/mmwr) is a publication of the CDC and contains updated information on incidence and prevalence of many diseases and conditions. These rates provide healthcare providers with up-to-date information on the risks and burdens of various diseases and conditions (CDC, 2014b). The information obtained from the *MMWR* can be used to identify trends and provide policy makers with information for designating resources. The following is an example of how such information can be used:

> Hypertension is a major risk factor for heart disease and stroke. Heart disease and stroke occur in approximately 30% of adults aged 18 years and older in the United States. A comparison of rates between 2007 and 2010 revealed that Hispanic Blacks had a higher rate of hypertension (41.3%) than non-Hispanic Whites (28.6%) and Hispanics (27.7%). Adults born in the United States had a higher rate of hypertension (30.6%) than non-U.S.-born adults (25.7%). Adults younger than 65 years with public insurance had a higher rate of hypertension (28.3%) than those with private insurance (20.0%) and those with no insurance (20.4%).

This excerpt is adapted from an issue of *MMWR* published on November 22, 2013 (Gillespie & Hurvitz, 2013). By publishing rates in percentages and comparing those rates among groups, it highlights both the burden of heart disease and stroke and the disparity between different demographic profiles related to hypertension. This information can be useful to both clinicians and policy makers who make decisions about interventions and services.

When calculating rates, the numerator is the number of events that occur during a specified period of time and is divided by the denominator, which is the average population at risk during that specified time period. This number is multiplied by a constant—either 100, 1,000, 10,000, or 100,000—and is expressed as per that number. The purpose of expressing rates as per 100,000, for example, is to have a constant denominator, and it allows investigators to compare rates among groups with different population sizes. Simply put, the rate is calculated as follows:

Rate = Numerator/denominator × Constant multiplier

In order to calculate rates, the APRN must first have a clear and explicit definition of the patient population and of the event. An important consideration when calculating rates is that anyone represented in the denominator must have the potential to enter the group in the numerator, and all persons represented in the numerator must come from the denominator.

Rates can be either crude or specific. Crude rates apply to an entire population without any reference to any characteristics of the individuals within it. For example, to calculate the crude mortality rate, the numerator is the total number of deaths during a specific period of time divided by the denominator, which is the average number of people in the population during that specified period of time (including those who have died). Typically, the population value for a 1-year period is determined using the midyear population.

Specific rates can also be calculated for a population that has been categorized into groups. Suppose that an APRN wants to calculate the number of new mothers who initiate breastfeeding in a specific hospital in 2015. The formula would be:

$$\frac{\text{Total number of breastfeeding infants in community hospital in 2015}}{\text{Total number of live births in the same community hospital in 2015}} \times \text{Constant multiplier}$$

In order to compare rates in two or more groups, the events in the numerator must be defined in the same way, the time intervals must be the same, and the constant multiplier must be the same. Rates can be used to compare two different groups, or one group during two different time periods. Returning to the example about breastfeeding, the breastfeeding rates could be compared in the same hospital, but at two different times, before and after implementation of a planned intervention to increase breastfeeding rates.

Formulas for the rates discussed in this chapter can be found at the end of the chapter (Exhibit 3.1).

Incidence and Prevalence

Incidence rates describe the occurrence of new events in a population over a period of time relative to the size of the population at risk. *Prevalence* rates describe the number of all cases of a specific disease or attribute in a population at a given point in time relative to the size of the population at risk. Incidence provides information about the rate at which new cases occur and is a measure of risk. For example, the formula for the incidence rate for HIV is:

$$\frac{\text{Total number of people who are diagnosed with HIV in a community during 2015}}{\text{Population in that community at midyear of 2015}} \times 1,000 = \text{Rate per 1,000}$$

Incidence rates provide us with a direct measure of how often new cases occur within a particular population and provide some basis on which to assess risk. By comparing incidence rates among population groups that vary in one or more risk factors, the APRN can begin to get some idea of the association between risk factors and disease. If in the earlier example of breastfeeding, the APRN discovers breastfeeding rates are significantly different among different ethnic groups, the characteristics of the groups can be compared and the causes for this disparity can be hypothesized and tested.

Period prevalence measures the number of cases of disease during a specific period of time and is a measure of burden. The formula for the period prevalence rate for HIV in 2015 is:

$$\frac{\text{Total number of people who are HIV positive in a community during 2015}}{\text{Population in that community at midyear of 2015}} \times 1,000 = \text{Rate per 1,000}$$

In the formula given here, all newly diagnosed cases for the year plus existing cases are included. *Point prevalence* is defined as the number of cases of disease at a specific point in time divided by the number of people at risk at that specific point in time multiplied by a constant multiplier. An example of the use of point prevalence would be the information gathered from a survey in which an investigator asks such questions as who has diabetes, hypertension, epilepsy, or any other disease or event at that specific point in time. Prevalence, whether point or period, cannot give us an estimate of the risk of disease; it can only tell us about the burden of disease for a specified period of time. Prevalence is useful when comparing rates between populations but should be interpreted with caution. Diseases that are chronic will have a higher prevalence, because at any given time, those with chronic disease will always have that disease. This can make it challenging to interpret prevalence rates as they don't tell us the risk of developing disease but they can be helpful when trying to determine resource needs for chronic diseases. With diseases that are short in duration, prevalence may not capture the true burden of disease for that population. Additionally, it is important to note that unidentified cases are not captured in either prevalence rates or incidence rates. Rates can only estimate the burden of disease, but they are the best way to draw comparisons using a common denominator.

An example of how prevalence rates are used in the literature is as follows:

> The CDC (2010, 2014c) revealed that in 2013, no state had a prevalence of obesity less than 20% (in 2009, 28 states had a prevalence of obesity less than 20%). Also in 2013, 18 states had a prevalence of obesity between 30% and 35% (in 2009, 9 states had prevalence rates over 30%). Regionally, the South had the highest prevalence of obesity (30.2%), followed by the Midwest (30.1%), the Northeast (26.5%), and the West (24.9%).

Information on the rising prevalence of adult obesity in the United States has led to increased attention to factors that cause obesity (especially in children). This has led to the development of new programs aimed at primary and secondary prevention.

Mortality Rates

Mortality rates, also known as death rates, can be useful when evaluating and comparing populations. As stated earlier, there are many factors that can affect the natural history of disease, and measuring mortality allows investigators to compare death rates among and within populations. The formula for mortality rate is:

$$\frac{\text{Number of deaths in a population during a specified time}}{\text{Average population estimate during the specified time}} \times \text{Constant multiplier}$$

Mortality rates can be specific or broad in definition and can include any qualifiers for time, age, or disease type. It is important to include those specifics in your denominator to ensure the population value used is the best estimate of the population at risk. For example, to look at the number of deaths in 2015 due to breast cancer in women aged 18 to 40, the denominator should *only* include the midyear population of women aged 18 to 40 in 2015. It is also important to include those women who died during that year in the denominator. Again, it is impossible to know exactly how many women in that age group are at risk using a midyear population, but the key is to use similar sources of measurement so that comparisons can be made assuming similar sources are used to estimate the denominator.

Standardization of crude rates is an important consideration when comparing mortality rates among populations. Standardization is used to control for the effects of age and other characteristics in order to make valid comparisons between groups. Age adjustment is an example of rate standardization and perhaps the most important one. No other factor has a larger effect on mortality than age. Consider the problem of comparing two communities with very different age distributions. One community has a much higher mortality rate for colon cancer than the other, leading investigators to consider a possible environmental hazard in that community, when in fact, that community's population is older, which could account for the higher mortality. Direct age adjustment or standardization allows a researcher to eliminate the age disparities between two populations by using a standardized population. This allows the researcher to compare mortality or death rates between groups by eliminating age differences between populations and comparing actual age-adjusted mortality rates to determine whether age truly plays a role in the crude unadjusted mortality rates.

There are two methods of age adjustment: direct, as mentioned earlier, and indirect. The direct method applies observed age-specific mortality or death rates to a standardized population. The indirect method applies the age-specific rates of a standardized population to the age distribution of an observed population and is used to determine whether one population has a greater mortality because of an occupational hazard or risk compared to the general population (to learn how to perform age adjustment, refer to an advanced epidemiology text).

The *case fatality rate* (CFR) is a measure of the severity of disease (such as infectious diseases) and can be helpful when designing programs to reduce the rate or disparity in the population. It should be noted that CFR is not a true rate as it has no explicit time implication but rather is a proportion of persons with disease who died from that disease after diagnosis. It is a measure of the probability of death among diagnosed cases. Its usefulness for chronic diseases is limited because the length of time from diagnosis to death can be long. The CFR is also useful in determining when to use a screening test. Screening tests identify disease early so that an intervention or treatment can be initiated in the hopes of lessening the morbidity or mortality of that disease. Those diseases that are rapidly fatal may not necessarily be beneficial to screen unless the screening will allow for a cure or treatment to change the overall outcome or to prevent unnecessary spread of the disease. Screening is useful in identifying disease in asymptomatic individuals in whom further transmission of disease can be prevented or reduced, such as in HIV. CFRs, therefore, can be helpful for comparisons between study populations and can provide useful information that could help determine whether an intervention or treatment is working. The formula for the *CFR* is as follows:

$$\text{Case fatality rate \%} = \frac{\text{Number of individuals with the specified disease after disease onset or diagnosis}}{\text{Number of cases of that specific disease}} \times 100$$

The CFR is usually expressed as a percentage; so in this case, one would multiply this rate by a constant multiplier of 100 to obtain the percentage of disease that is fatal. It is important in all of these rates to include those who have died from the disease in the denominator. Removing those who have died from the denominator falsely increases the CFR, making the disease appear more fatal or severe (Gordis, 2014).

The *proportionate mortality ratio* is useful for determining the leading causes of death. The formula for proportionate mortality ratio is as follows:

$$\frac{\text{Number of deaths from a specified cause during specified time period}}{\text{Total deaths from all causes during the same specified time period}} \times 100$$

Again, this measure is usually reported as a percentage and reflects the burden of death due to a particular disease. This information is useful for policy makers who make decisions about the allocation of resources. (See Exhibit 3.1 for a list of these formulae.)

Survival and Prognosis

Mortality rates are very helpful when comparing groups and looking at disparities among populations. One cannot discuss mortality without having an understanding of survival and prognosis. Many diseases, particularly cancer, are studied over time, with attention placed on survival. Ideally, survival should be measured from the onset of disease until death, but the true onset of disease is generally unknown. Survival rates are usually calculated at various intervals from diagnosis or initiation of treatment. Prognosis is calculated using collected data to estimate the risk of dying or surviving after diagnosis or treatment begins. As mentioned earlier, case fatality rates give a good estimate of prognosis or severity of disease. However, they are best suited for acute diseases in which death occurs relatively soon after diagnosis. Survival analysis is better suited for chronic diseases or those diseases that take time to progress.

Survival time is generally calculated from the time of diagnosis or from the start of treatment. This can vary from patient to patient as some patients may seek care immediately after symptoms present or may wait months to seek care. Some patients are diagnosed prior to symptom presentation after they screened positive on a screening test. Some may obtain a diagnosis immediately, whereas others may have poor access to care and diagnosis is delayed by weeks to months or even years. Once a diagnosis is made, treatment may or may not occur immediately. Additionally, some patients may die before diagnosis or treatment. Because these individuals are not represented in survival analysis, this can lead to a falsely increased survival time. With that said, one can see how difficult it is to establish a true survival time after diagnosis. However, we can estimate survival if we use a common denominator and consistent criteria for measurement.

Before we discuss how to calculate and interpret survival data, we must touch on two important concepts, *lead time bias* and *overdiagnosis bias*. Lead time bias is a phenomenon whereby a patient is diagnosed earlier by screening and appears to have increased survival due to screening but rather dies at the same time he or she would regardless of screening. In other words, the time from which a patient is diagnosed earlier from screening is the lead time and the bias is the error that occurs as a result of concluding that screening leads to a longer survival after diagnosis. As can be seen in the following timeline, the survival time is longer when screening is implemented, but the ultimate time of death is unchanged. Although this is not true for all screening tests, it is important to recognize the phenomenon of lead time bias as it can affect the conclusions that are made regarding survival, which ultimately can affect a patient's perceived prognosis.

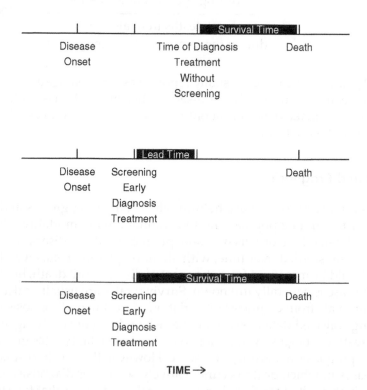

Overdiagnosis bias occurs as a result of making a diagnosis from screening for a disease or cancer that would not have manifested clinically or has a slow progression, such that the person dies from another etiology. This type of bias has the potential to increase undue stress in individuals and can also falsely increase survival times, especially for diseases with slow progression. In both these types of biases, there is no difference in overall mortality in those screened versus those who were not screened. With that said, considerations must also be made for those screening tests in which a false-negative test reassures a patient who may not seek care and ultimately develops cancer and potentially has decreased survival due to delay in diagnosis. All of these biases need to be taken into consideration when interpreting survival data.

Prognosis is calculated using survival rates. There are two methods of conducting survival analysis and estimating prognosis that are discussed. The first is the *actuarial method*, which measures the likelihood of surviving after each year of treatment (or a predetermined interval). This is calculated as follows: the probability of surviving 2 years if one survived 1 year, or the probability of surviving 3 years if one survived 2 years, and so on. Prognosis is most commonly described in the literature as the probability of surviving 1, 2, 3, or more years. Generally, survival is calculated as a probability P1, P2, P3, and so on. The survival after 1 year is designated as P1; if patients survived 1 year after treatment, those who survived to 2 years = P2; if patients survived 2 years after treatment, those who survived to 3 years = P3; and so on. To calculate P1, divide the number of survivors over the number of patients with the disease at the start of the study or treatment. It is important to note that those who are lost to follow-up (also known as withdrawals) or who are no longer studied must be removed from the denominator. When a study ends or is terminated, those patients are no longer followed and must be taken into consideration in your analysis, and this is called *censorship*. For simplicity, the following examples will assume no losses to follow-up, but it is important to recognize that those who are lost to follow-up or those who are censored must be taken into account in your calculations. Of note, in a more advanced epidemiology textbook, you will find that those who are lost to follow-up will be subtracted out of the denominator and multiplied by ½ to account for the chance they were at risk for half the interval. Again for the purposes of this text, we will use a hypothetical example in which no patients are lost to follow-up. By definition, here is how to calculate P1, P2, and so on:

- P1 = (Number alive after 1 year of treatment)/(Number who started treatment)
- P2 = (Number alive after 2 years of treatment)/(Number who survived first year of treatment − Those who dropped out or were lost to follow-up)
- P3 = (Number alive after 3 years of treatment)/(Number who survived second year of treatment − Those who dropped out or were lost to follow-up)

To calculate the probability of surviving 1, 2, 3, or more years, the calculation is as follows:

P1 = probability of surviving 1 year
P1 × P2 = probability of surviving 2 years
P1 × P2 × P3 = probability of surviving 3 years
P1 × P2 × P3 × P4 = probability of surviving 4 years
P1 × P2 × P3 × P4 × P5 = probability of surviving 5 years

Using data from Table 3.1 we can calculate and interpret these probabilities.

TABLE 3.1 • Survival Rates After Treatment (Hypothetical Life Table of 100 Patients With No Patients Lost to Follow-Up)

	Number Survived				
	After 1 Year	At 2 Years	At 3 Years	At 4 Years	At 5 Years
Cohort (N = 100)	88	76	55	47	33

In this example:

P1 = 88/100 = 0.88
P2 = 76/88 = 0.86
P3 = 55/76 = 0.72
P4 = 47/55 = 0.85
P5 = 33/47 = 0.70
Probability of surviving 1 year = 0.88
Probability of surviving 2 years = $0.88 \times 0.86 = 0.76$
Probability of surviving 3 years = $0.88 \times 0.86 \times 0.72 = 0.54$
Probability of surviving 4 years = $0.88 \times 0.86 \times 0.72 \times 0.85 = 0.46$
Probability of surviving 5 years = $0.88 \times 0.86 \times 0.72 \times 0.85 \times 0.70 = 0.32$

It is important to distinguish between the probability of surviving 5 years and the probability of surviving 5 years given that someone survived 4 years. Generally, the longer someone survives after treatment, the more likely that person will make it to the next year. Overall survival after 5 years is always a smaller number as the probability of surviving each year is multiplied against each year (Gordis, 2014).

Note that the actuarial method can be used to look at outcomes other than survival or death as it can estimate probabilities of an outcome or event occurring such as a treatment side effect (e.g., vomiting, headache) or recurrence of disease. Another important consideration is survival over time. When looking at survival rates measured over years, it is important that an APRN take into account the improvements and advances in treatments over time. APRNs should consider comparing survival rates for earlier treatment regimens with those for newer regimens, as this can affect the validity of the overall survival if not taken into consideration. In addition, certain confounders (e.g., age, gender, ethnicity, socioeconomic status) may contribute to differences in survival rates and should be examined when performing a survival analysis (see Chapter 4 for more on confounding). Recognition of these differences is a critical step for the evaluation of potential health disparities and is a perfect opportunity for an APRN to develop strategies to address the underlying issue causing those disparities.

In the literature, survival analysis using the actuarial method is plotted on a curve in which the x-axis represents time and the y-axis represents the number of survivors at each time interval. This is called a *survival curve* and represents the pattern of survival over predetermined time intervals. Using the data from the earlier example, the probabilities are plotted in a standardized survival curve (Figure 3.1).

The second type of survival analysis is the *Kaplan–Meier method*. This method is commonly used in medicine and is well suited for analyses of small

FIGURE 3.1 • **Hypothetical Example of a Survival Curve Using Data From the Earlier Example**

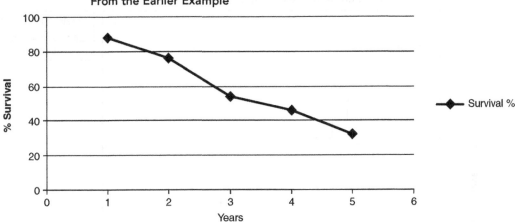

and large populations, as well as comparisons between treatments or interventions. Although beyond the scope of this book, statistical analyses can be performed to compare treatments or interventions using tests of significance (log-rank test) and logistic regression (proportional hazard models [Cox models]). As with any comparison trial, it is important to take into consideration the characteristics of those patients who are lost to follow-up because if they occur more frequently in one treatment group compared to another, this can affect the results. For example, if the majority of patients lost to follow-up are receiving treatment A and most of them can be characterized as impoverished with poor access to care, then this could skew the results of the remaining patients receiving treatment A. Thus, minimizing loss to follow-up or censored patients and/or maintaining similar losses with similar characteristics in each group is paramount to reducing bias and improving the strength of the study conclusions. This reiterates the importance of randomization, which will be discussed more thoroughly in Chapter 4.

Kaplan–Meier curves are used to plot survival, and these plots represent a stepwise pattern of survival in which the increments of time are not standardized (e.g., 1 year, 5 years), but rather each step represents an event (e.g., time to death or an outcome of interest). Kaplan–Meier curves are seen more commonly in the literature and are a better estimate of survival as they also take into consideration patients who are lost to follow-up or are censored. These curves also allow for comparisons between different treatment regimens (Figure 3.2).

Kaplan–Meier curves are different from traditional survival curves, in that they do not slope downward after each event but rather maintain a horizontal line until the next event (e.g., death) occurs, and then a downward vertical line is drawn until the new cumulative survival is reached and the steps are continued until the study is completed. At the time in which no deaths are occurring (also known as the death-free period), the cumulative survival is maintained; however, hatch marks can be seen in these plots, which represent

FIGURE 3.2 • Hypothetical Example of a Kaplan–Meier Curve—Comparison of Treatment A To Treatment B

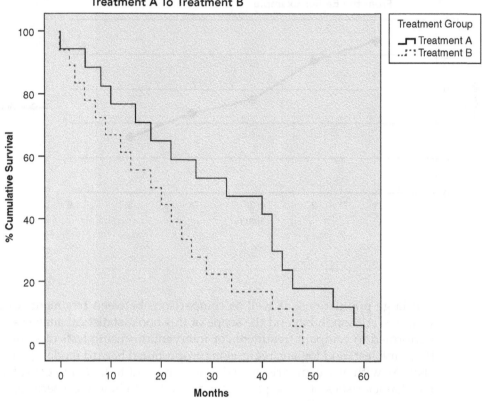

those lost to follow-up or censored during that interval (Jekel, Katz, Elmore, & Wild, 2007).

The importance of having the knowledge and skills to interpret and calculate survival data cannot be underscored. APRNs can use survival data or outcome data in various ways. Most important, the evidence obtained from survival or outcome data can help APRNs to design and justify interventions to improve the quality of life for diseases such as cancer. Comparisons to other groups can be made by addressing outcomes of interest to determine whether certain interventions make a difference in the quality of life and ultimately impact the survival of those involved.

Health Impact Assessment

As mentioned previously, rates can be used to describe the distribution of disease and other health-related states and events, but sometimes the APRN may be more concerned with knowing how data can be used to describe the relevancy of clinical practice. *Health impact assessment* (HIA) is the assessment of the potential health effects, positive or negative, of a particular intervention on a population. HIAs can evaluate population-directed programs or interventions before they are implemented and can provide recommendations on how those programs can potentially affect the health of a population whether positive or negative (see www.cdc.gov/healthyplaces/hia.htm). Certain calculations can be performed to determine the efficacy of a treatment or intervention. The number needed to treat (NNT), the disease impact number (DIN), and the population impact number (PIN) are formulae that are used in HIAs. NNT is the number of patients needed to receive a treatment to prevent one bad outcome, and the lower the NNT, the better for assessing superiority of treatments. However, the NNT takes into account only those patients being treated rather than all those with disease in the population. The DIN, on the other hand, uses the number of those with the disease in question among whom one event will be prevented by the intervention. Similarly, the PIN is the number of those in the whole population among whom one event will be prevented by the intervention (Heller & Dobson, 2000). Another calculation commonly used is the years of potential life lost (YPLL), which measures premature mortality, and the productive years that are lost related to early death (Gordis, 2014). Each of these measurements is helpful in determining the benefits or risks of new interventions or treatments. Specifically, the DIN and the PIN provide a better population-based estimate of treatment or intervention impacts on the population as a whole. (See Exhibit 3.1 for a list of these formulae.)

Fontaine, Redden, Wang, Westfall, and Allison (2003) published a study conducted to estimate the YPLL because of overweight and obesity. They found that the risk for YPLL is greatest for the youngest age groups. They also report, "The maximum YPLL for White men aged 20 to 30 with a severe level of obesity (BMI > 45) is 13 years and is 8 years for White women. For men this would represent a 22% reduction in expected remaining life span" (p. 187). Information on YPLL helps to magnify the importance of primary prevention measures designed to address such diseases as obesity and other risk factors such as smoking.

More extensive information on HIA formulae and standardization can be found in most advanced epidemiology texts. It is important for the APRN who is involved in population-based evaluation to be aware of these concepts.

DESCRIPTIVE STUDIES

Descriptive epidemiology is used to describe the distribution of disease and other health-related states and events in terms of personal characteristics, geographical distribution, and time. There are four types of descriptive studies: case reports, case series, cross-sectional studies, and correlation or ecologic studies. The data used in descriptive studies are often readily available and can be retrieved from such sources as hospital records, census data, or vital statistics records.

Case Reports and Case Series

Case reports are succinct written accounts of generally rare or unusual cases in which the treatment or management of the disease or condition is worth reporting. These are usually published to assist healthcare providers in the management of rare, unresearched, or undocumented cases. A case series is merely a report of a series of patients with similar diseases or conditions that describes their management or treatment in order to identify new strategies that may be helpful to treat patients with similar conditions. They also lead to future studies and can be helpful for APRNs as they can use these cases to build a case for future research of treatments or interventions that have not yet been rigorously studied.

Correlation Studies

Correlation studies are also referred to as ecologic studies and are used to conduct studies of aggregate or population characteristics. In ecologic studies, rates are calculated for characteristics that describe populations and are used to compare frequencies between different groups at the same time or the same group at different times. They are useful for identifying long-term trends, seasonal patterns, and event-related clusters. Because data are collected on populations instead of individuals, an event cannot be linked to an exposure in individuals, and the investigator cannot control for the effect of other variables. These types of studies lead to more rigorous studies that can control for variables of interest and look at individual data to determine whether an association truly exists. Correlational studies can only report that a correlation exists and cannot show an association exists as they compare population or aggregate data. An example of a correlation study would be one that shows a correlation between high fat content and breast cancer. Countries with a high fat content correlate to countries with higher rates of breast cancer. Without knowing individual data, one cannot determine whether women with breast cancer actually also have a high fat consumption (Gordis, 2014).

A study by Tresserras, Canela, Alvarez, Sentis, and Salleras (1992) provides another example of a correlational study. The authors used data from 95 countries to study the relationship between infant mortality and the prevalence of adult illiteracy. The results of these analyses indicate that adult illiteracy correlates positively with infant mortality, such that populations with a higher prevalence of illiteracy have higher infant mortality rates and populations with a lower prevalence of illiteracy have lower infant mortality rates. The authors point out, "In interpreting the results, the possible presence of some biases has to be taken into account" (p. 436). These data show that a correlation exists between the variables, but not necessarily a causal one. There are many possible explanations for the relationship, including (but not exclusively) demographic and economic differences among the countries. Correlation studies must be interpreted with caution, but important information can be obtained from the trends that could identify disparities and lead to further studies and hypothesis testing.

Cross-Sectional Studies

In *cross-sectional* studies, also known as prevalence studies, both exposures and outcomes are collected simultaneously. These studies provide a "snapshot" at one point in time and thus exclude people who have died or who chose not to participate, which can introduce bias. Temporal relationships are difficult to determine in these studies as only prevalence can be determined and the risk of developing disease cannot be estimated. Many cross-sectional studies are surveys that sample a population and its various characteristics. They can be inexpensive and can provide timely descriptive data about a group under study, but again, they do not tell us about causality or the true risk of developing a certain outcome such as disease.

Spoelstra, Given, von Eye, and Given (2010) conducted a cross-sectional study to determine whether individuals with a history of cancer fall at a higher rate than those without cancer. They also examined whether or not the occurrence of falls in the elderly was influenced by individual characteristics. The study population consisted of 7,448 community-dwelling elderly who were 65 years or older living in one state in the Midwestern United States. The analysis of the data revealed that having cancer was not a predictor of falls in this study. Further analysis revealed that predictors of falls in this population included race, sex, activities of daily living, incontinence, depression, and pain. Although cancer was not found to be a predictor of falls, the authors did find a high frequency of falls in that study population. The findings led the authors to conclude that it is important to develop a predictive model for fall risk in the community-dwelling elderly.

This study serves to illustrate both the advantages and disadvantages of cross-sectional studies. The study was carried out at one point in time using an existing data set (the Minimum Data Set). One limitation of the study was that it missed people whose falls were not reported. Another limitation the authors cited was that they could not determine whether a specific cancer diagnosis, stage, or treatment was a risk factor for falls. Finally, they were unable to determine whether or not comorbidities may have placed individuals at a higher risk for falls. The inability to control for or identify the significance of potentially important variables is a disadvantage of using a cross-sectional study design. With that said, a cross-sectional study is a fairly quick method to obtain descriptive data and can be useful in identifying prevalence rates for specified populations.

ANALYTIC EPIDEMIOLOGY

Analytic epidemiology looks at the origins and causal factors of diseases and other health-related events. Analytic designs are often carried out to test hypotheses formulated from a descriptive study. The goal of analytic epidemiology is to identify factors that increase or decrease risk. Risk is the probability that an event will occur. For example, a patient who is obese might ask, "What is the likelihood that I will develop diabetes if I do not lose weight?"

Although descriptive studies allow a basis for comparison and can provide the APRN with data to identify potential risk factors and differences among groups, study designs, such as a prospective cohort, need to be carried out in order to determine whether there is an association between an exposure and a disease and to determine the strength of that association. To do this, the APRN can compare exposed and nonexposed groups and follow them over time to see who develops an outcome (such as a specific disease) and who does not. Comparison is an essential component of population studies. Case-control studies can also allow for comparisons by retrospectively looking back in time to see what exposure or risk factors are associated with being a case or a control. Comparisons can also be made by following a group using treatment A compared to treatment B or treatment A can be compared to no treatment at all. There are multiple study designs, but we will focus only on the most common study designs and discuss the advantages and disadvantages that each one poses in practice.

Cohort Studies

Cohort designs can be either prospective or retrospective. In a prospective cohort design, the investigator begins with a defined population and then follows a group of individuals who were either exposed or nonexposed to a factor of interest and then follows both groups to compare the incidence of an outcome or disease. In a cohort study, one can look at multiple outcomes that develop from an exposure. In a retrospective cohort design, exposure is ascertained from past records and outcome is ascertained at the time the study begins. If an association exists between the exposure and the outcome, then the incidence rate in the exposed group will be greater than the incidence rate in the nonexposed group. The ratio of these is the *relative risk* (RR), which is the incidence rate in the exposed group divided by the incidence rate in the nonexposed group. RR is a measure of the strength of an association between an exposure and an outcome or disease (Table 3.2).

If the RR = 1 (the numerator equals the denominator), then the risk to the two groups is equal. If the RR >1 (the numerator is greater than the denominator), the risk in the exposed group is greater than the risk in the nonexposed group and can be considered a positive association. If the RR <1 (the denominator is greater than the numerator), the risk in the exposed group is less than the risk in the nonexposed group and can be considered protective.

TABLE 3.2 • Calculation of Relative Risk and Attributable Risk in a Cohort Study

	Disease	No Disease	Totals	
Exposure	a	b	a + b	Incidence in the exposed (Inc exp) = a/a + b
No Exposure	c	d	c + d	Incidence in the nonexposed (Inc nonexp) = c/c + d
Relative risk (RR) = Inc exp/Inc nonexp				
Attributable risk (AR) = Inc exp − Inc nonexp				
AR proportion in the exposed population = $\dfrac{\text{Inc exp} - \text{Inc nonexp}}{\text{Inc exp}}$				
AR proportion in the total population = $\dfrac{\text{Incidence in total population} - \text{Inc nonexp}}{\text{Incidence in total population}}$				

An example of a protective association may be the association between exercise and heart disease. Exercise can actually reduce the risk of heart disease and has a RR <1. Thus, it is considered a protective exposure.

Attributable risk (AR), absolute risk, or risk difference is the amount of risk that can be attributed to an exposure. For example, it is well known that smoking can cause lung cancer, but lung cancer can also occur in nonsmokers. The amount of disease that is associated with risks/exposures other than smoking is called the *background risk*. In order to calculate the risk attributable to a particular exposure, subtract the incidence of disease (lung cancer) in the exposed group (smokers) minus the incidence of disease (lung cancer) in the nonexposed group (background risk). This value is considered the AR due to exposure (see Table 3.2). If an APRN wants to know how much risk of disease can be reduced by removing a risk factor, one can calculate the absolute risk reduction (ARR), which is synonymous with the AR. The relative risk reduction (RRR) is calculated the same as the AR proportion. This can be confusing as these terms are interchanged in medicine and epidemiology, but it is important to recognize and understand how these terms are used and interpreted. An example of RRR would be described as: What percentage of motor vehicle deaths could be reduced if we could eliminate texting while driving? This RRR percentage is what is commonly reported in the news and can be very helpful for policy makers and for justification of funding. The AR can also be calculated as a proportion of the total population. For example, to determine the amount of lung cancer attributable to smoking in the total population (AR proportion), one would have to know the incidence in the total population (to review how to calculate the incidence in the total population, please refer to an advanced epidemiology textbook). APRNs should be familiar with how to calculate and interpret RR and AR, as these values are reported commonly in the literature and reports such as the *MMWR*.

Cohort studies are best carried out when the investigator has good evidence that links an exposure to an outcome, when the time interval between exposure and the outcome is short, and when the outcome occurs relatively often. One of the major problems with cohort studies is that they can be time-consuming and expensive, especially if the cohort needs to be followed for a prolonged length of time. Diseases that are rare or that take many years to develop may be better suited for a case-control study as it can be difficult to follow participants for many years, especially if the outcome of interest is rare. The longer the time period, the more likely participants will be lost to follow-up, and multiple exposures can potentially confound the relationship.

A cohort study was carried out in Norway to ascertain characteristics that would predict the risk of fibromyalgia (FM). The authors examined the association among leisure time, physical exercise, BMI, and risk of FM (Mork, Vasseljen, & Nilsen, 2010). A longitudinal study followed 15,900 women without FM or physical impairment at baseline for 11 years. At the end of the study period, there were 380 reported cases of FM, and RRs were calculated for each of the study variables (exposures). Women who reported the highest exercise level had an RR of 0.77 (95% confidence interval [CI], 0.55–1.07). In looking at exercise, the authors controlled for the potential confounding factor of BMI. Overweight or obese women (BMI > 25.0 kg/m²) had a 60% to 70% higher risk of FM compared with women of normal weight (BMI = 18.5 to 24.9 kg/m²).

Overweight or obese women who exercised more than 1 hour/week had an RR of 1.72 (95% CI, 1.07–2.76), compared with normal-weight women with a similar activity level. The risk for overweight or obese women who were inactive (RR, 2.09; 95% CI, 1.36–3.21) or exercised less than 1 hour/week (RR, 2.19; 95% CI, 1.39–3.46) showed a positive association between risk of developing FM and low levels of exercise. The authors concluded that being overweight or obese was associated with an increased risk of FM, especially among women who also reported low levels of physical exercise. On the basis of these findings, they recommended that community-based measures aimed at reducing the incidence of FM should emphasize maintaining a normal weight and regular exercise.

Case-Control Studies

In a *case-control* study, the APRN must first identify a group of individuals with the outcome of interest (cases). A second group is identified without the outcome of interest (controls). The proportion of those cases that have a history of exposures is then compared to the proportion of the cases that were not exposed, and the proportion of the controls who were exposed is compared to the proportion of the controls who were not exposed. The measure of the effect of exposure is expressed as an odds ratio (OR), which is the ratio of the odds of having been exposed if you are a case to the odds of having been exposed if you are a not a case. If the exposure is not related to the disease or outcome, the OR = 1. If the exposure is related to the disease or outcome, the OR >1, and if the OR <1, the exposure is considered protective. To calculate the OR, construct a 2×2 table in which the columns represent the cases and controls and the rows represent the exposed and nonexposed populations. It is important to set up the table correctly. If it is not set up correctly, it will affect the interpretation and conclusions. Once the table is complete, multiply the cross products to obtain the result (see Table 3.3).

In a case-control study, if there is an association between an exposure and disease, the history of exposure should be higher in persons who have the disease (cases) compared to those who do not have disease (controls). It is important to keep in mind that the OR is not a calculation of risk and cannot predict which exposures/risk factors will develop into a case or disease. The fact that a person is obese may put that person at risk for diabetes, but it does not mean

TABLE 3.3 • Calculation of Odds Ratio in a Case-Control Study

	Cases	Controls
Exposure History	a	b
No Exposure History	c	d
Totals	a + c	b + d
	Proportion of cases exposed = a/a + c	Proportion of controls exposed = b/b + d
Odds ratio = ad/bc		

that that person will get diabetes. In case-control studies, one cannot calculate RR; therefore, we cannot conclude that if you are obese you will develop diabetes, but rather, if your OR is greater than 1, you could conclude that those with diabetes (outcome) are more likely to be obese (risk factor/exposure).

Selection of cases and controls is an important step in case-control studies. Definite criteria should be used so that there is no ambiguity about how to distinguish between a case and a control. Exposure is not always all or nothing. Controls should resemble the cases as closely as possible except for the exposure to the factor under study. If the cases are drawn from a particular clinic, then ideally the controls should be drawn from the same clinic population. Matching is one method that can be used to select a sample so that potential confounders are distributed equally between the cases and controls. For example, if an APRN plans to evaluate an intervention to reduce burden among caregivers of dependent elderly in the home, it would be important to recognize the characteristics of the population studied prior to implementing the intervention. It is known that men and women have differing characteristics that affect their role as caregiver (e.g., women find the physical demands of caregiving more burdensome than do men; Curley, 1997). By matching for gender in the study, the APRN can eliminate this potentially confounding factor (gender). The problem with matching is that the investigator is not always aware of all of the potential confounding factors. It can be difficult to match each subject in a study, and in some cases, investigators can overmatch. When an investigator overmatches, one loses the ability to look at the matched variables as risk factors.

In case-control studies, the investigator begins with cases and controls and goes back retrospectively to look for exposures. In cohort studies, the investigator begins with exposed and nonexposed individuals and follows individuals over time to see who develops or does not develop an outcome or disease. Case-control studies allow the APRN to look at cases and the probability of having an exposure or risk factor. Cohort studies allow an APRN to follow a cohort over time to determine whether being exposed to a risk factor impacts the likelihood of developing a disease or diseases, or improves outcomes (as in an intervention). If associations are found, further studies are necessary to determine causal links and to prevent ecologic fallacy. When examining the results of case-control and cohort studies, it is important for the APRN to consider whether or not all other explanations for an identified association have been eliminated. No single epidemiological study can satisfy all criteria for causality. The APRN needs to look at the accumulation of evidence, as well as the strength of individual studies.

Randomized Controlled Trials

Randomized controlled trials (RCTs) or clinical trials are useful for evaluating treatments (including technology) and for assessing new ways of organizing and delivering health services. In population-based studies, the issue is often health promotion and disease prevention rather than treatment of an existing disease. Interventions can also be studied in RCTs, with the target involving defined populations rather than individuals and often involving educational, program, or policy interventions. When carefully designed, RCTs can provide the strongest evidence for evaluating treatments and interventions.

The basic design of an RCT is to assign patients randomly to either receive the new treatment/intervention or not receive the new treatment/intervention. Inclusion and exclusion criteria for the participants must be precise and written in advance to eliminate any errors within the study or any future comparison studies. As with cohort studies, RCTs can compare more than two groups. Analysis is carried out to compare outcomes between the randomized groups. As mentioned earlier, comparisons can be made between different interventions, different treatments, or to a control group that has received no intervention or treatment.

A randomized trial of a fall prevention strategy was carried out by Dykes et al. (2010). The objective of the study was "[t]o investigate whether a fall prevention tool kit (FPTK) using health information technology (HIT) decreases patient falls in hospitals" (p. 1912). The design was a cluster randomized study. In a clustered design, study groups of subjects (instead of individuals) are randomized to each intervention. In this case, medical units that met the inclusion criteria for the study were matched for unit census, length of stay, and fall rates. Matched units were then randomly assigned to either the intervention group or the control group. Eight units in four hospitals met the inclusion criteria and were entered into the study. The four units in the control group received an educational program on fall risk assessment and prevention and were provided usual care. The four units in the intervention group received the FPTK software integrated into an existing health information technology application. The FPTK tailors fall prevention interventions to the identified risk factors of each patient. The software also produces alerts such as bed posters, educational handouts for patients, and individualized plans of care. The primary outcome measure was falls per 1,000 patient days. As part of the data analysis, the researchers adjusted for possible confounders such as age and fall risk scores. The intervention and control groups had similar lengths of stay and no differences in gender composition. The researchers also monitored adherence to the protocol. Analysis revealed that the intervention group had a significantly lower adjusted fall rate (3.15; 95% CI, 2.54–3.90) per 1,000 patient wdays as compared to the control group (4.18; 95% CI, 3.45–5.06). The researchers hypothesized, after completion of the study, that the intervention effect was greater in older patients than in younger patients.

This study illustrates how useful the randomized trial design is for testing a new intervention. An advantage of the cluster randomized design is the ability to study interventions that cannot be directed toward selected individuals. In this case, the design simplified the ability of the researchers to control confounders and to prevent *contamination bias* (discussed further in Chapter 4), which occurs when patients in the control group inadvertently receive the intervention (see in Chapter 4).

Sample Size

Sample selection and sample size determination are critical steps in the research process. Sample size determination is necessary to identify the minimum number of subjects needed to enroll in a study to identify true differences and associations between groups, and thus has implications for the investigators as they need to allocate ample resources based on sample size to carry out the study.

Power analysis is used to determine sample size. There are several factors that influence the size of the sample: variance, significance, power, and effect size.

Variance

Variance is the variation about the mean. For example, if you are looking at a continuous variable such as blood pressure, the variance away from the mean is defined as s^2. Variance (s^2) is the square of the standard deviation (s). The standard deviation takes into account all blood pressure measurements and essentially sums the difference of each blood pressure measurement away from the mean (see a statistic textbook for more details). If you do not have data with which to calculate the standard deviation, you can review the literature or look at a pilot data set to determine this number. A study that has very little variance (i.e., most of the values fall close to the mean) would require a smaller sample size than a study in which the blood pressure measurements have a very large range and a wider sigmoid curve.

Significance and Power

Significance is the probability that an observed difference or relationship exists and usually is defined as a *p*-value ($p < .05$). The smaller the *p*-value (e.g., $p < .01$), the larger the required sample size. *Power* (1-β) is the capacity of the study to detect differences or relationships that actually exist in the population or the capacity to correctly reject a null hypothesis, that is, prevent a type II error. The larger the power required, the less likelihood of committing a type II error. Most studies use a power of 80% or 0.80, or if a more rigorous power is necessary (e.g., 90%), a larger sample size is required.

Effect Size

Effect size is the actual difference between groups and treatments that you hope to see in your study. One way to identify effect size is to review previous studies or another method is to conduct a pilot study. For example, if you are designing an educational intervention and want to see a 20% improvement of knowledge after the intervention, 20% is your effect size. If you want to see a smaller change in knowledge (e.g., 10%), then a larger sample will be required to detect a smaller effect or difference. In summary, effect sizes occur along a range of values. For example, if you want to see a 5% change in results of an outcome, you will need many more participants than if you want to see a 30% change.

Understanding what goes into power analysis is an important step in designing a study. Power analysis can be calculated using computer programs. There are many free software programs available on the Internet to assist with power analysis. Typing "sample size calculation" in a search engine such as Yahoo or Google will lead an APRN to many sites (Burns, 2000; Duffy, 2006).

Screening

Screening is a tool used to detect disease in groups of asymptomatic individuals with the goal of reducing and/or preventing morbidity and mortality.

Screening tests can be applied to groups of individuals or to high-risk populations. There are multiple examples of screening tests, including the Pap smear, the tuberculosis skin test (PPD test), the mammogram, and so on.

Determining whether a screening test is appropriate requires the APRN to address several aspects of the disease of interest. Screening is neither available nor appropriate for all diseases. In order for a screening program to be effective, certain criteria should be met. The target population needs to be identifiable and accessible and the disease should affect a sufficient number of people to make screening cost-effective. The preclinical period should be sufficient to allow treatment before symptoms appear so that early diagnosis and treatment make a difference in terms of outcome.

Finally, it is necessary for the screening test to be sensitive enough to detect most cases of the disease and to be specific enough to limit the number of false-positive tests. Screening tests should also be relatively inexpensive, easy to administer, and have minimal side effects.

The validity of a screening test refers to its ability to accurately identify those who have the disease. Sensitivity and specificity are measures of a screening test's validity. Sensitivity is a measure of a screening test's ability to accurately identify disease when it is present. Specificity is a measure of a screening test's ability to correctly identify a person without disease with a negative test. The positive predictive value (PPV) is a measure of the probability of a positive test result when the disease is present. The negative predictive value (NPV) of a test is a measure of the probability that the disease is absent when there is a negative test (see Table 3.4).

Directing screening tests toward high-risk populations has many advantages. By screening populations with a higher disease prevalence, we can actually increase the positive predictive value of that test. Screening low-prevalence populations can lead to more false positives, which can be costly and harmful to patients. Thus, selection of the disease to be tested and the patient population to be screened are both important to consider when designing a new test.

The APRN can evaluate the success of screening programs by looking at a variety of outcomes. For example, some of the outcomes that can be followed include the reduction in overall mortality in screened individuals, a reduction in the case fatality rate in screened individuals, an increase in the percentage of cases detected at earlier stages, a reduction in complications, and improvement of quality of life in screened individuals.

TABLE 3.4 • Computing Sensitivity, Specificity, and Predictive Values in Screening Tests

	Disease	No Disease	Totals	
+ Test	a	b	a + b	PPV = a/a + b
− Test	c	d	c + d	NPV = d/c + d
Totals	a + c	b + d		
	Sensitivity = a/a + c	Specificity = d/b + d		

In 2009, the U.S. Preventive Services Task Force (USPSTF) released their recommendations for breast cancer screening (U.S. Preventive Services Task Force [USPSTF], 2009). Currently, a new update is in the process of development and can be found on the USPSTF website (www.uspreventiveservicestaskforce .org/Page/Document/UpdateSummaryDraft/breast-cancer-screening1). If you visit this website, you can add yourself to their e-mail list and receive the latest updates on breast cancer screening. There are also screening guidelines on a variety of disease states with recommendations (e.g., colorectal, prostate, and cervical cancers). One of the recommendations for breast cancer is that biennial screening with mammography should begin at age 50 for most women. The recommendation is based on the findings that the highest false-positive test rate and the most unnecessary biopsies occur in the 40- to 50-year age group. The recommendation also takes into consideration the belief that the cumulative effect of exposure to multiple mammographies over time is not benign. There is ample evidence that the most benefit for breast screening using mammography is derived from screening women aged 50 to 74 every 2 years (Lefevre, Calonge, Dietrich, & Melnikow, 2010; USPSTF, 2009). These guidelines provide an example of how evidence on the specificity and sensitivity of a screening test can be used to create more evidence-based clinical guidelines. Therefore, screening tests need to be tailored to the disease under investigation, and many factors need to be taken into consideration (e.g., How many false negatives can be missed? How many false positives are acceptable? Can screening and early detection really make a difference in the outcome of the disease?). Understanding these factors and balancing them with targeted screening in high-risk populations are important considerations in screening implementation.

SUMMARY

The natural history of disease refers to the progression of a disease from its preclinical state to its clinical state, and knowledge of these stages provides a framework for understanding approaches to the prevention and control of disease. Primary prevention refers to the process of altering susceptibility or reducing exposure to susceptible individuals and includes general health promotion and specific measures designed to prevent disease prior to a person getting a disease. Primary prevention measures are generally carried out during the stage of susceptibility. With secondary prevention, it is sometimes possible to either cure a disease at a very early stage or slow its progression to prevent complications and limit disability. Secondary prevention measures are carried out during the preclinical or presymptomatic stage of disease. Tertiary prevention takes place during the middle or later stages of a disease (the clinical stage of disease) and refers to measures taken to alleviate disability and restore effective functioning.

The dynamic nature of disease calls for a sophisticated model for explaining causation. When designing interventions for populations, the APRN needs to keep in mind that disease develops as the result of many antecedent factors and not as a result of a single, isolated cause.

Descriptive epidemiology is used to describe the distribution of disease and other health-related states and events in terms of personal characteristics, geographical distribution, and time. It also helps APRNs design studies and measure mortality and prognosis. Analytic epidemiology looks at the origins and causal factors of diseases and other health-related events. Epidemiologic methods can be used to identify populations at risk and to evaluate interventions provided to patient populations. Population-based evaluation and planning depend on understanding the many and varied factors that influence health and disease. APRNs can use their understanding of epidemiological methods in concert with their clinical expertise to develop policies and implement and evaluate new programs and interventions to improve population outcomes.

EXHIBIT 3.1 • List of Useful Formulae

<u>**Calculating Rates**</u>

Incidence rates describe the occurrence of *new* disease cases in a community over a period of time relative to the size of the population at risk.

$$\text{Incidence rate} = \frac{\text{Number of } new \text{ cases during a specified period}}{\text{Population at risk during the same specified period}} \times \text{Constant multiplier}$$

Prevalence rates are the number of *all* existing cases of a specific disease in a population *at a given point in time* relative to the population at risk.

$$\text{Prevalence rate} = \frac{\text{Number of } existing \text{ cases at a specified period}}{\text{Population at risk at the same specified period}} \times \text{Constant multiplier}$$

Crude rates summarize the occurrence of births (crude birth rate) or deaths (crude death rate). The numerator is the number of events and the denominator is the average population size (usually estimated as a midyear population).

$$\text{Crude death rate} = \frac{\text{Number of deaths in a population during a specified period}}{\text{Population estimate during same specified time}} \times \text{Constant multiplier}$$

Specific rates are used to overcome some of the biases seen with crude rates. They are used to control for variables such as age, race, gender, and disease.

$$\frac{\text{Age-specific}}{\text{death rate}} = \frac{\text{Number of deaths for a specified age group during a specified time}}{\text{Population estimate for the specified age group during the same specified time}} \times \frac{\text{Constant}}{\text{multiplier}}$$

(continued)

EXHIBIT 3.1 • List of Useful Formulae (*continued*)

Case fatality rate is used to measure the percentage of people who die from a certain disease. This rate tells you how fatal or severe a disease is compared to other diseases.

$$\text{Case fatality rate} = \frac{\text{Number of individuals dying after disease onset or diagnosis}}{\text{Number of individuals with the specified disease}} \times 100$$

Proportionate mortality ratio is useful for determining the leading causes of death.

$$\text{Proportionate mortality ratio} = \frac{\text{Number of deaths from a specified cause during specified time period}}{\text{Total deaths during the same period}} \times 100$$

Calculations Used in Health Impact Assessment

Number needed to treat (NNT) is the number of patients needed to receive a treatment to prevent one bad outcome. The NNT calculated should be rounded up to the next highest number. Before the NNT can be calculated, the absolute risk reduction (ARR) must be identified.

$$\text{ARR} = \text{Incidence in exposed} - \text{Incidence in nonexposed}$$
$$\text{NNT} = 1/\text{ARR}$$

The NNT can also be calculated in randomized trials using mortality rates:

$$\text{NNT} = 1/(\text{Mortality rate in untreated group} - \text{Mortality rate in treated group})$$

Disease impact number (DIN) is the number of those with the disease in question among whom one event will be prevented by the intervention.

$$\frac{1}{\left(\text{ARR} \times \dfrac{\text{Proportion of people with the disease}}{\text{who are exposed to the intervention}} \right)}$$

Population impact number (PIN) is the number of those in the whole population among whom one event will be prevented by the intervention.

$$\frac{1}{\left(\text{ARR} \times \dfrac{\text{Proportion of people with the disease who are exposed to the intervention}}{} \times \dfrac{\text{Proportion of the total population with the disease of interest}}{} \right)}$$

Years of potential life lost (YPLL) is used for setting heath priorities. Predetermined standard age at death in the United States is 75 years.

$$\text{YPLL (75)} = 75 - \text{Age at death from a specific cause}$$

Add the years of life lost for each individual for specific cause of death = YPLL

(continued)

EXHIBIT 3.1 • List of Useful Formulae (*continued*)

<u>Calculations Used in Screening Programs</u>
Sensitivity: the ability of a screening test to identify accurately those persons with the disease

$$\text{Sensitivity} = TP/(TP + FN)$$

Specificity: reflects the extent to which it excludes the persons who do not have the disease

$$\text{Specificity} = TN/(TN + FP)$$

	Disease	No Disease
+ Test	True positive (TP)	False positive (FP)
− Test	False negative (FN)	True negative (TN)

Adapted from Fulton, Lyon, and Goudreau (2010).

EXERCISES AND DISCUSSION QUESTIONS

Exercise 3.1 A study was conducted surveying men and women for high blood pressure (HTN). The results showed that there were 50 men and 75 women per 100,000 who had HTN. The male and female population totals were 230,000 and 189,000, respectively.
- What is the absolute number of men and women affected (i.e., how many men and women were identified with HTN in this study)?
- Is this incidence or prevalence? Why?

Exercise 3.2 You are working in a community hospital in a small town in Tennessee. The town's population is 23,000. There were six new cases of Rocky Mountain spotted fever diagnosed in the past year.
- Calculate the incidence of Rocky Mountain spotted fever per 1,000 and per 100,000.

Exercise 3.3 A rapid screening test for women with HPV (human papillomavirus) is being evaluated for its effectiveness and sensitivity as a screening test in college healthcare clinics. In order to determine the effectiveness of the HPV test, it was administered to 2,000 female college students. Tests were confirmed by comparisons to the gold standard test (Pap smears). Prevalence of HPV was 12% in the female college population; 352 students tested positive for HPV. The HPV test was found to be 92% specific. Create a 2 × 2 table that accurately describes this test and use this information to answer the following questions.

	HPV	No HPV	Totals
+ Test			
− Test			
Totals			

- What is the sensitivity of this test?
- What is the positive predictive value of this test?
- What is the negative predictive value of this test?
- If everything else remained the same, what would happen to the predictive value of a positive test if the disease prevalence increased in the population?
- How many false negatives are there with this test?
- How many false positives are there with this test?
- Explain how false positives and false negatives can affect your patient population.
- If the gold standard test (Pap smear) has a sensitivity of 94% and a specificity of 88%, which test (the new HPV test or Pap test) would you prefer to use in your healthcare clinic if you want to reduce the number of false-negative test results in your clinic? Which test would you prefer if you want to reduce the number of false-positive test results? Explain your answer using results from previous calculations.

Exercise 3.4 An investigator samples a group of clients from a clinic based on their disease status—in particular, whether or not they have HTN. Of the 250 people sampled, 40% were found to have HTN. Knowing their disease status, a questionnaire is administered to the people in the study to determine how many have a family history (FHx) of stroke (in a first-degree relative). Of the people without HTN, 8% had a FHx of stroke. Of the people with HTN, 37% had a FHx of stroke. Create a 2 × 2 table using this information and answer the following questions.

	HTN	No HTN	Totals
+ FHx stroke			
− FHx stroke			
Totals			

- What type of study design is this?
- Can you calculate RR (relative risk) using these data? Why or why not?
- Can you calculate OR (odds ratio) using these data?
- Calculate the correct descriptive statistic for this study (either RR or OR).
- What is the correct interpretation of the statistic used?
  a. Patients with a FHx of stroke are 6.75 times more likely to develop HTN than patients with no FHx of stroke.
  b. Patients with HTN are 6.75 times more likely to have a FHx of stroke than those with normal blood pressure.
- What are possible errors that could be made in this type of study?

Exercise 3.5 A study is conducted at your hospital to learn about the relationship between HIV and intravenous (IV) drug usage. You identify patients from your emergency department who are IV drug users and those who are not and follow them for 1 year. During that year, you identify 69 new cases of HIV out of 253 who are IV drug users, and there are 17 new cases of HIV out of 450 who are not IV drug users. (The overall rate in both groups combined = 86 cases of HIV out of 703.) You are interested in developing an intervention to reduce the incidence of HIV and you would like to target a prevention program addressing risk factors. Create a 2 × 2 table using this information and answer the following questions.

	+HIV	–HIV
+ IV drug use		
– IV drug use		
Totals		

- Calculate the incidence rate of HIV in the IV drug users ($Iexp$), in the non-IV drug users ($Inonexp$), and overall (I). Express all rates as "per 1,000."
- What type of study design is this?
- Calculate the relative risk (RR) for this exposure.
- Calculate the attributable risk (AR) for this exposure. Interpret this result.
- Calculate the AR proportion for this exposure. Interpret this result.
- What are some problems that may be associated with this kind of study design?
- What are possible confounders?

Exercise 3.6 For the following scenarios, describe the type of study design: Answer a, b, c, or d.
   a. Cross-sectional study
   b. Case-control study
   c. Cohort study
   d. Correlation study

   _____ A study was done to look at melanoma and sun exposure in a population in Arizona. Prevalence rates in Arizona were compared to prevalence rates of melanoma and sun exposure in Alaska. The researchers found people in Arizona had a higher prevalence of melanoma and sun exposure than those in Alaska.

   _____ Over a 3-month period, 12,000 patients with hepatitis will be categorized as alcoholic or nonalcoholic. Then over the next 20 years, new cases of liver cancer will be classified out of the 12,000.

   _____ Over a 6-month period, all incoming residents into a nursing home over 55 years of age were asked whether they currently have diabetes and whether they have a history of skin infections.

   _____ Over a 1-year period, 100 cases of hepatitis were identified and a similar number of persons without hepatitis were recruited to participate in a statewide study looking at prior history of alcohol usage.

   _____ All school children in five schools are given a physical fitness test during May and June 2015. At the time the test results are collected, current risk factors for obesity were ascertained.

Exercise 3.7 During the course of the spring semester at the School of Nursing (SON), 13 students developed colds. There are 22 students who enrolled in the SON for the first time at the start of the spring semester (new to school), and 88 students are continuing at the school from the previous fall semester. Thirty-two students had a cold at some point during the spring semester. According to a survey done by students at the SON on the last day of the spring semester, three students claimed to have a cold at the time of the survey.
- What was the point prevalence per 1,000 of colds at the time of the survey?
- What was the incidence per 1,000 of colds during the spring semester?
- What was the period prevalence per 1,000 of colds during the spring semester?

Exercise 3.8 You are asked to assess the state of health of a population after an outbreak of *Escherichia coli* that occurred in January 2014. Your community midyear population in 2014 was 90,150. You have obtained some statistics 1 year after the outbreak, and your hospital administrator would like you to assess the impact of the outbreak on the community. You are asked to look at illnesses due to *E. coli*, which have peaked since the disaster. You determined there were 2,905 total deaths in your community in 2014. This includes 128 deaths from *E. coli*; 274 people were sick with *E. coli* during 2014. Use this information to answer the following questions.
- What was the cause-specific mortality rate per 100,000 for *E. coli* in 2014?
- What was the case-fatality rate for *E. coli* in 2014?
- What is the crude mortality rate per 100,000 in this community?
- What was the proportionate mortality rate for *E. coli* in 2014?

Exercise 3.9 You are reviewing the survival statistics from your hospital using a new treatment (Treatment A) compared to the old treatment (Treatment B) for breast cancer. The following table lists the number of survivors after each year of treatment for both treatments A and B. Answer the following questions using the table. Assume no patients were lost to follow-up.

Treatment A	Number Survived				
	At 1 Year	At 2 Years	At 3 Years	At 4 Years	At 5 Years
Cohort (N = 1,229)	1,102	987	835	725	633

Treatment B	Number Survived				
	At 1 Year	At 2 Years	At 3 Years	At 4 Years	At 5 Years
Cohort (N = 1,179)	1,084	886	755	602	544

- Calculate the survival rates for treatments A and B for each year after treatment: P1, P2, P3, P4, and P5.
- Calculate the probability of surviving for 1, 2, 3, 4, and 5 years cumulatively for each of the treatments.
- Your administrator would like to know how the treatments compare to each other. You are asked for the following information:
  - What is the likelihood of surviving 5 years if you made it to 4 years of treatment for each of the treatments?
  - How does treatment A compare to treatment B for each year of survival after treatment?
  - Which treatment has the best 5-year survival rate?
- Plot the survival curve for both treatments on the same graph.
- Why might there be differences between these two treatments?
- What are some potential confounders that may contribute to one treatment working better than the other?
- Explain the advantages and disadvantages of screening tests.
- What are the limitations to performing survival analysis?
- How might patients lost to follow-up affect the validity of survival analysis?
- What are the differences between the actuarial method of survival analysis and the Kaplan–Meier method?

Exercise 3.10

- Perform a search to determine the incidence, prevalence, and survival rates for one of the following cancers in your state (lung cancer, breast cancer, colon cancer, prostate cancer)
  - Perform a search and describe the screening recommendations for the cancer you selected.
  - Describe the advantages and disadvantages of cancer screening for the cancer you selected.
  - How does the incidence, prevalence, and survival rates in your state compare to the national rates.
  - What are potential confounders for the cancer you selected?
  - What disparities in cancer incidence, mortality, and survival were you able to determine from your search?

Exercise 3.11

- What are the factors that contribute to sample size calculation?
- For each of these factors, describe how they impact sample size.

REFERENCES

Burns, K. (2000). Power and effect size: Research considerations for the clinical nurse specialist. *Clinical Nurse Specialist, 14*(2), 61–68.

Centers for Disease Control and Prevention. (2010, August 3). Vital signs: State specific obesity pre-valence among adults—United States, 2009 (Early release). *Morbidity and Mortality Weekly Report (MMWR), 59*, 1–5. Retrieved from http://www.cdc.gov/mmwr/preview/mmwrhtml/mm59e0803a1.htm

Centers for Disease Control and Prevention. (2011). Decrease in smoking prevalence—Minnesota, 1999–2010. *Morbidity and Mortality Weekly Report (MMWR), 60*(5), 138–141. Retrieved from http://www.ncbi.nlm.nih.gov/pubmed/21307824

Centers for Disease Control and Prevention. (2014a). *Fast facts: Smoking and tobacco use.* Retrieved from http://www.cdc.gov/tobacco/data_statistics/fact_sheets/fast_facts/index.htm#use

Centers for Disease Control and Prevention. (2014b). *About the Morbidity and Mortality Weekly Report (MMWR) series.* Retrieved from http://www.cdc.gov/mmwr/about.html

Centers for Disease Control and Prevention. (2014c). *Overweight prevalence maps.* Retrieved from http://www.cdc.gov/obesity/data/prevalence-maps.html

Curley, A. L. (1997). *An investigation of burden, control, and professional support of abused elderly* (Unpublished doctoral dissertation). Rutgers, The State University of New Jersey, New Brunswick, NJ.

Duffy, M. (2006). Resources for determining or evaluating sample size in quantitative research reports. *Clinical Nurse Specialist, 20*(1), 9–12.

Dykes, P., Carroll, D., Hurley, A., Lipsatz, S., Benoit, A., Chang, F., . . . Middleton, B. (2010). Fall prevention in acute care hospitals: A randomized trial. *JAMA, 304*(17), 1912–1918.

Fontaine, K., Redden, D., Wang, C., Westfall, A., & Allison, D. (2003). Years of life lost due to obesity. *JAMA, 289*(2), 187–193.

Fulton, J. S., Lyon, B. L., & Goudreau, K. A., (2010). *Foundations of clinical nurse specialist practice.* New York, NY: Springer Publishing Company.

Gillespie, C. D., & Hurvitz, K. A. (2013). Prevalence of hypertension and controlled hypertension—United States, 2007–2010. Retrieved from http://www.cdc.gov/mmwr/preview/mmwrhtml/su6203a24.htm?s_cid=su6203a24_w

Gordis, L. (2014). *Epidemiology* (5th ed.). Canada: Elsevier Saunders.

Harkness, G. (1995). *Epidemiology in nursing practice.* New York, NY: Mosby.

Heller, R. F., & Dobson, A. J. (2000). Disease impact number and population impact number: Population perspectives to measures of risk and benefit. *British Medical Journal, 321*(7266), 950–953.

Heller, R. F., & Page, J. (2002). A population perspective to evidence based medicine: "Evidence for population health." *Journal of Epidemiology and Community Health, 56,* 45–47.

Jekel, J. F., Katz, D. L., Elmore, J. G., & Wild, D. M. J. (2007). *Epidemiology, Biostatistics, and Preventative Medicine* (3rd ed.). Philadelphia, PA: Saunders Elsevier.

Lefevre, M., Calonge, N., Dietrich, A., & Melnikow, J. (2010). Mammography screening for breast cancer: Recommendation of the U.S. Preventative Services Task Force [Editorial]. *American Academy of Family Physicians, 304*(17). Retrieved from www.aafp .org/afp

Mork, P. J., Vasseljen, O., & Nilsen, T. I. L. (2010). Association between physical exercise, body mass index, and risk of fibromyalgia: Longitudinal data from the Norwegian Nord-Trøndelag Health Study. *Arthritis Care & Research, 62,* 611–617. doi:10.1002/ acr.20118

National Heart, Lung, and Blood Institute and Boston University. (2010). *The Framingham study.* Retrieved November 20, 2010, from http://www.framinghamheartstudy.org/ about-fhs/history.php

Spoelstra, S., Given, B., von Eye, A., & Given, C. (2010). Falls in the community-dwelling elderly with a history of cancer. *Cancer Nursing, 33*(2), 149–155.

Tresserras, R., Canela, J., Alvarez, J., Sentis, J., & Salleras, L. (1992). Infant mortality, per capita income, and adult illiteracy: An ecological approach. *American Journal of Public Health, 82*(3), 435–438.

U.S. Preventative Services Task Force. (2009). *Screening for breast cancer.* Retrieved from http://www.uspreventiveservicestaskforce.org/uspstf/uspsbrca.htm

Epidemiological Methods and Measurements in Population-Based Nursing Practice: Part II

Patty A. Vitale and Ann L. Cupp Curley

In order to provide leadership in evidence-based practice, advanced practice registered nurses (APRNs) require skills in the analytic methods that are used to identify population trends and evaluate outcomes and systems of care (American Association of Colleges of Nursing [AACN], 2006). APRNs need to be able to carry out studies with strong designs and solid methodology, taking into account the factors that can affect study results. This chapter discusses the complexities of data collection and the strengths and weaknesses of study designs used in population research. Critical components of data analysis are discussed, including bias, causality, confounding, and interaction.

ERRORS IN MEASUREMENT

A dilemma that may occur with population research is the difficulty of controlling for variables that are not being studied but that may have an impact on the results. Finding a statistical association between an intervention and an outcome or an exposure and a particular disease is meaningful only if variables are correctly controlled, tested, and measured. The purpose of a well-designed study is to properly identify the impact of the variable (or variables) under study and to avoid bias and/or design flaws caused by another, unmeasured variable.

Statistics are used to analyze population characteristics by inference from sampling (Statistics, 2002, p. 1695). They help us to translate and understand data. Before we can begin to understand a measured difference between groups, we have to identify the variation. But statistical analysis cannot overcome problems caused by a flawed study. When a researcher draws the wrong conclusion because of a problem with the research methodology, the result is a type I or type II error, also referred to as *errors of inference*. A *type I error* occurs when a null hypothesis is rejected when in fact it is true. A *type II error* occurs when one fails to reject a null hypothesis when in fact it is false.

Take, for example, an APRN who carries out a study to determine whether a particular intervention improves medication compliance in hypertensive patients. To keep the example simple, the intervention will simply be referred to as "Intervention A." A null hypothesis proposes no difference or relationship between interventions or treatments. In this case, the null hypothesis is: There is no difference in medication compliance between hypertensive patients who receive Intervention A and those who receive no intervention. Let us assume that the APRN completes the study and carries out the statistical analysis of the data. The following conclusions are possible:

1. There is no significant difference in medication compliance between the two groups.
2. There is a significant difference in medication compliance between the two groups.

Now let us assume that the correct conclusion is number 1, but the APRN concludes that there is a difference in medication compliance between the two groups (rejects the null hypothesis when it is true). The APRN has committed a type I error. If the correct conclusion is number 2, but the APRN concludes that there is no difference in medication compliance between the two groups (fails to reject the null hypothesis when it is false), then a type II error has occurred (Table 4.1).

When using data or working with data sets, it is critical to understand that mistakes can occur where measurements are involved. There are two basic forms of error of measurement: *random error* (also known as nondifferential error) and *systematic error* (also known as bias). Random errors occur as the result of the usual, everyday variations that are expected and that can be anticipated during certain situations. The result is a fluctuation in the measurement of a variable around a true value. Systematic errors occur not as the result of chance but because of inherent inaccuracies in measurement. They are typically constant or proportional to the true value. Systematic error is generally considered the more critical of the two. It can be the result of either a weak study design or a deliberate distortion of the truth.

Random Error

Random error measurements tend to be either too high or too low in about equal amounts because of random factors. Although all errors in measurement

TABLE 4.1 • Type I and Type II Errors

	Relationship Does Not Exist	Relationship Exists
Conclude Relationship Does Not Exist (Fail to reject Null Hypothesis)	Correct Decision	Type II Error (β)
Conclude Relationship Exists (Reject Null Hypothesis)	Type I Error (α)	Correct Decision Power ($1 - \beta$)

are serious, random errors are considered to be less serious than bias because they are less likely to distort findings. Random errors do, however, reduce the statistical power of a study and can occur because of unpredictable changes in an instrument used for collecting data or because of changes in the environment. For example, if one of three rooms being used to interview subjects became overheated occasionally during data collection, making the subjects uncomfortable, it could affect some of their responses. This effect in their responses is an example of a random error of measurement.

Systematic Error

There are several types of systematic error or bias and all of them can impact the validity of study results. Bias can occur in many ways and is commonly broken down into 2 categories: selection and information bias. Such things as how the study design is selected, how subjects are selected, how information is collected, how the study is carried out (the conduct), or how the study is interpreted by investigators are all forms of potential bias. These problems can result in a deviation from the truth, which can lead to false conclusions.

Selection Bias

Selection bias occurs when the selected subjects in a sample are not representative of the population of interest or representative of the comparison group, and as a result, this selection of subjects can make it appear (falsely) that there is or is not an association between an exposure and an outcome. Selection bias is not simply an error in the selection of subjects for a study, but rather the systematic error that occurs with "selecting a study group or groups within the study" (Gordis, 2014, p. 263). Nonprobability sampling (nonrandom sampling) is strongly associated with selection bias. In nonprobability sampling, members of a target population do not share equal chances of being selected for the study or intervention/treatment group. This can occur with studies using convenience samples or volunteers. People who volunteer to participate in a study may have characteristics that are different from people who do not volunteer, and this can impact the outcome of the results and is simply referred to as *volunteer bias.* Similarly, people who do not respond to surveys may possess characteristics different from those who do respond to surveys. Thus, it is important to characterize nonresponders as much as possible, as the characteristics of responders may be very different from those of nonresponders and can lead to errors in survey interpretation. The best way to avoid this type of bias is to keep it at a minimum unless the characteristics of nonresponders can be identified and addressed. Another form of selection bias is *exclusion bias,* and this can occur when one applies different eligibility criteria to the cases and controls (Gordis, 2014). *Withdrawal bias* can occur when people of certain characteristics drop out of a group at a different rate than they do in another group or are lost to follow-up at a different rate. This can also lead to systematic error in the interpretation of data. APRNs must be aware of these types of error early in their study design. All of these types of systematic error can have an impact on how data are interpreted; therefore, minimizing these types of error through careful assessment of subject selection and eligibility criteria, and monitoring of characteristics in the populations of interest are critical for successful research and program implementation. Finally, probability sampling methods (random sampling) can be used to ensure that all members of a target population have an equal chance of being selected into a study, thereby eliminating the chance of selection bias (Shorten & Moorley, 2014).

Information Bias

Information bias deals with how information or data are collected for a study. This includes the source of data that are collected, such as hospital records, outpatient charts, or national databases. Many of these types of data are not collected for research purposes; so they may be incomplete, inaccurate, or contain information that is misleading. This can complicate data analysis as the information abstracted from these sources may be incorrect and can lead to invalid conclusions. *Measurement bias* is a form of information bias and occurs during data collection. It can be caused by an error in collecting information for an exposure or an outcome. Calibration errors can occur when using instruments to measure outcomes. This type of bias can also occur when an instrument is not sensitive enough to measure small differences between groups or when interventions are not applied equally (e.g., blood pressure measurements taken using the wrong cuff size). Information bias also includes how the data are recorded and classified. This can lead to *misclassification bias,* in which a control may be recorded as a case or a case is classified as having an exposure or exposures that he or she did not actually have. Misclassification bias can be subdivided into differential and nondifferential. For example, *differential misclassification* occurs when a case is misclassified into exposure groups more often than controls. In this case, this type of bias usually leads to the appearance of a greater association between exposure and the cases than one would find if this bias was not present (Gordis, 2014). In *nondifferential misclassification,* the misclassification occurs as a result of the data-collection methods such that a case is entered as a control or vice versa. In this situation, the association between exposure and outcome may be "diluted," and one may conclude there is not an association when one really exists (Gordis, 2014). Another example of misclassification bias occurs when members of a control group are exposed to an intervention. This results in *contamination bias.* An example would be a nurse who floats from the floor where hourly rounding is being carried out to a control floor where no rounding is supposed to occur, but the nurse carries out hourly rounding on the control floor. In this case, contamination bias minimizes the true differences that would have been seen between groups. However, these cases should not be reassigned; in fact, any unexpected or unplanned crossover that occurs should be analyzed in the original group to which it was assigned by the investigator. This is known as the *intent-to-treat principle.* For example, patients who are assigned to one group or another and crossover intentionally or accidentally to the other group should be analyzed according to their original assignment. *Intent to treat* simply means that you assign patients to the original group you intended to treat them in from the start of the study regardless of the treatment they received.

If information is obtained from interviews, there can be bias introduced based on how the questions are asked or there may be variance between interviewers in how the questions are prompted to the subject. *Recall bias* happens when subjects are asked to remember or recall events from the past. For example, people who experience a traumatic event in their lives may recall events of that day more accurately and with more detail than someone asked to recall events from a day without significance. *Reporting bias* occurs when a subject may not report a certain exposure as he or she may be embarrassed or not want to disclose certain personal information, or the subject may report certain things to gain approval from the investigator (Gordis, 2014). The effects of bias can impact a study in two ways. It can make it appear that there is a significant effect when one does not exist (type I error), or there is an effect but the results suggest there is no effect (type II error) (see Table 4.1).

Finally, an APRN needs to be aware of *publication bias* (another type of *information bias*), particularly when carrying out systematic reviews or meta-analyses. Publication bias refers to the tendency of peer-reviewed journals to publish a higher percentage of studies with significant results than those studies with nonsignificant or negative statistical results. This problem has been identified and studied for decades, and there is evidence that the incidence of publication bias is on the increase (Joober, Schmitz, Annable, & Boksa, 2012). Song et al. (2009) completed a meta-analysis to determine the odds of publication by study results. Although they identified many problems that were inherent in studying publication bias (e.g., they pointed out that studies of publication bias may be as vulnerable as other studies to selective publication), they concluded that "[t]here is consistent empirical evidence that the publication of a study that exhibits significant or 'important' results is more likely to occur than the publication of a study that does not show such results" (p. 11). Among their recommendations was that all funded or approved studies should be registered and the results publicly available.

There are several issues related to publication bias. It can give readers a false impression about the impact of an intervention, it can lead to costly and futile research, it can distort the literature on a topic, and can be unethical. People who participate in research studies (subjects) are often told that their participation will lead to a greater understanding of a problem. There is a breach of faith when the results of these studies are not published and shared in the scientific community (Joober et al., 2012; Siddiqi, 2011). The publication of both categories of research is ethical and provides a more balanced and objective view of current evidence.

In summary, bias must be recognized and addressed early in the study design. Ultimately, bias should be avoided when possible, but if it is recognized, it should be acknowledged in the interpretation of results and addressed in the study discussion.

CONFOUNDING

Confounding occurs when it appears that a true association exists between an exposure and an outcome, but in reality, this association is confounded by another variable or exposure. An interesting study by Matsumoto, Ishikawa, and

Kajii (2010) raised questions about the potential confounding effect of weather on differences found among communities in Japan. They investigated the rural–urban gap in stroke incidence and mortality by conducting a cohort study that included 4,849 men and 7,529 women in 12 communities. On average, subjects were followed for 10.7 years. Information on geographic characteristics (such as population density and altitude), demographic characteristics (including risk factors for stroke), and weather information (such as rainfall and temperature) were obtained and analyzed using logistic regression. The researchers discovered a significant association between living in a rural community and stroke, independent of risk factors. However, further analyses revealed that the actual link may be between the weather and stroke. They proposed that the difference seen in the incidence of stroke in these communities may be related not to living in a rural versus an urban community, but by the weather differences between communities. Low temperatures are known to cause an increase in coagulation factors and plasma lipids, and therefore, differences in weather could have an impact on the incidence of stroke. They cite the small number of communities as a limitation of the study, and for this reason they did not generalize their findings. But they did raise an important point: It is important to be aware of the many variables (e.g., biologic, environmental, etc.) that may confound a relationship in population studies (Matsumoto et al., 2010).

Identification of confounding or other causes of spurious associations are important in population studies. A confounder is a variable that is linked to both a causative factor or an exposure and the outcome. There are many examples of confounders, such as age, gender, and socioeconomic status. Confounding occurs when a study is performed, and it appears from the study results that an association exists between an exposure and an outcome, when, in fact, the association is actually between the confounder and the outcome. Another example of confounding might occur if an APRN carried out a study to determine whether there is a relationship between age and medication compliance without controlling for income. Younger, working patients might be more compliant not because of the age factor, but because they have the resources to buy their medications. If confounding is ignored, there can be long-term implications as the APRN may implement interventions for medication compliance with education programs aimed at older patients without considering problems related to income. The intervention would ultimately not succeed because the relationship is false or not causal due to confounding. By definition, confounders must be known risk factors for the outcome and must not be affected by the exposure or the outcome (Gordis, 2014). Confounding, although difficult to avoid, must be recognized and accounted for in studies.

There are some techniques that an APRN can use to reduce the effects of confounding variables. Random assignment to treatment and nontreatment groups can reduce confounding by ensuring each group has similar shared characteristics that otherwise might lead to spurious associations. In the earlier example, if you were concerned about the socioeconomic status and education level, you may stratify early on for those characteristics and randomly assign from each of those groups so that they are equally represented in your intervention and nonintervention groups. When random assignment is not possible, the matching of cases and controls for possible confounding variables can improve equal representation of subjects and can minimize the effect of confounding.

Investigators can match groups or individuals. Group matching allows groups with similar characteristics of interest to be matched to each other. Each group should share a similar proportion of the characteristics of interest. Usually, cases should be selected first, and the control group should be selected with similar proportions of the characteristics of interest (Gordis, 2014).

In individual matching, each individual case is matched to a control with similar characteristics of interest. This is referred to as matched pairs. One has to be careful not to match cases and controls for too many characteristics, as it can be difficult to find a control or the control may be too similar to the case and true differences may not be able to be demonstrated in the analysis phase. Using strict inclusion and exclusion criteria also can be helpful and should be applied similarly for comparison groups. There are limitations to the latter two methods.

Although it is possible to match for known confounding variables, there may be other unknown confounding variables that cannot be controlled for and, if not recognized, can impact study conclusions. If the study groups are matched for gender, then gender cannot be evaluated in the final analysis. Additionally, if the study is matched for too many variables, this can also limit the study as all of the matched variables cannot be studied, and this may limit the ability to make valid conclusions. There is a similar problem with inclusion and exclusion criteria as both criteria should be applied the same to each of the study groups. The method for analyzing data can also help reduce problems related to confounding.

Multivariable regression, for example, can measure the effects of multiple confounding variables. This method is useful only when the variables are recognized and acknowledged. Recognition of confounders requires a basic understanding of the relationship between an exposure and a disease or an outcome, and can also be identified by performing a stratified analysis first. Once confounders are determined, then these variables can be added in and removed from the model one at a time. Interaction needs to be assessed, and the exposure–disease relationship is determined. These inferential methods estimate the contribution of each variable to the outcome while holding all other variables constant in the model. The objective is to include a set of variables that are theoretically or actually correlated with both the intervention and the outcome to reduce the bias of treatment effect. Therefore, the goal of regression analysis is to identify causal relationships by recognizing the confounders to ensure found relationships are real and not spurious (Kellar & Kelvin, 2013; Starks, Diehr, & Curtis, 2009).

INTERACTION

Whenever two or more factors or exposures are being studied simultaneously, the possibility of *interaction* exists. Interaction occurs when one factor impacts another such that one sees a greater or lesser effect than would be expected by one factor alone. *Synergism* occurs when the combined effect of two or more factors is greater than the sum of the individual effects of each factor. And conversely, the opposite or negative impact can be seen with *antagonism* of factors. One example of antagonism is seen with the interaction of exercise and diet. The combination of these two factors can actually reduce the risk of heart disease more than each factor alone. Synergistic models can have an additive effect in which the effect of one factor or exposure is added to another or can have a multiplicative effect in which the effect of one factor multiples the effect of another factor. For example, epidemiologists identified an interactive effect between cigarettes and alcohol; these two factors together have a multiplicative effect on the risk of developing digestive cancers (Sjödahl et al., 2007). There are many synergistic effects that can be found in clinical practice, especially as they pertain to drugs. First-generation antihistamines, such as chlorpheniramine, have a synergistic effect on opioids such as codeine. Patients are warned not to take them in combination as the sedative effects are more significant when taken together. APRNs who carry out investigations need to be aware of the potential interactions when examining the effects of multiple exposures on an outcome. A discussion on how to determine whether a model is multiplicative or additive can be found in more detail in an advanced epidemiologic textbook, but a basic understanding is necessary for interpreting the different outcomes that can occur from multiple exposures.

There are clearly many sources of error that can occur while conducting a study. The informed APRN needs to identify and acknowledge these types of errors and work to minimize them. Therefore, it is essential that APRNs recognize when errors occur and how they can impact a study, and should be familiar with measures that can be taken to avoid or minimize errors.

RANDOMIZATION

Randomized controlled trials (RCTs) are considered inherently strong because of their rigorous design. Random selection of a sample and random assignment to groups are objective methods that can be used to prevent bias and produce comparable groups. Random assignment helps to minimize bias by ensuring that every subject has an equal chance of being selected and that results are more likely to be attributed to the intervention being tested and not to some other extraneous factor such as how subjects were assigned to the treatment or control group. It is impossible to know all of the characteristics that could influence results. The random assignment of subjects to different treatment groups helps to ensure that study groups are similar in the characteristics that might affect results (e.g., age, gender, ethnicity, and general health). As a general rule, the greater the number of subjects that are chosen and assigned into the treatment or nontreatment groups, the more likely that the groups will be similar for important characteristics (Shott, 1990).

Blinding

Another problem encountered in research occurs when investigators or subjects themselves have an effect on study results. This can happen when a researcher's personal beliefs or expectations of subjects can influence his or her interpretation of the outcome. Sometimes observers can err in measuring data toward what is expected. If subjects know or believe that they are given a placebo or the nonexperimental treatment, it may cause them to exaggerate symptoms that they would dismiss if given the experimental treatment. These actions by both investigators and subjects are not necessarily intentional; they can occur subconsciously.

The best way to eliminate or minimize this type of bias is to use a *single-blind* or a *double-blind* study design. In a double-blind study, both the subjects and the investigators are blinded, that is, unaware of which group is receiving the experimental treatment or intervention. Sometimes it is impossible to blind the investigator because of the nature of the treatment, in which case a single-blind design, in which the subjects are unaware of which group they are in, can be used. If blinding cannot be used, measures need to be taken that ensure that study groups are followed with strict objectivity.

DATA COLLECTION

As mentioned earlier, how data are collected and analyzed can lead to bias when conducting a study. The training of investigators to ensure that data are collected uniformly from all subjects and the use of a strict methodology for data collection and analysis contribute to a strong study design. Objective criteria should be used for the collection of all data. Strict inclusion and exclusion criteria should be developed in writing so that there are no questions as to what criteria are to be applied to the study. Avoiding subjective criteria is important as it can lead to inconsistent application of criteria. For example, if you chose "ill appearance" as an exclusion criterion, it may be difficult to apply this criterion uniformly as each APRN may have different levels of experience making this assessment. Objective criteria, such as heart rate greater than 120 beats per minute, respiratory rate greater than 24 breaths per minute, or oxygen saturations less than 90%, are easy to apply uniformly. Of course, even those criteria can be incorrectly assessed by someone who is inexperienced; however, one can see that these types of data are more easily reproducible within and between studies. One way to assess reliability between raters in a study is by using the *kappa statistic*. This statistic tests how reliable different investigators or data collectors are in their assessment or interpretation of data beyond what one would expect by chance alone.

$$Kappa = \frac{(\text{Percent agreement observed}) - (\text{Percent agreement expected by chance alone})}{100\% - (\text{Percent agreement expected by chance alone})}$$

If you were to evaluate two observers without any training, you would expect them to agree a certain percentage of the time and that percentage represents the chance of agreement, usually around 50%. Using the kappa statistic, you can estimate how reliable this agreement is by subtracting out the percentage expected by chance alone. Kappa values that are greater than 0.75 represent excellent agreement, and those values less than 0.40 represent poor agreement. These values, although not perfect, can give an investigator an assessment of how well her or his observers are agreeing with each other in their data interpretation (Landis & Koch, 1977). The kappa statistic appears frequently in the literature, and the APRN should be familiar with its use and limitations (Maclure & Willett, 1987).

One of the first steps in data analysis is to compare the demographic information of each of the groups studied to ensure that they are matched for important characteristics and that they represent the population of interest. Frequencies of data can be generated and compared for similarities and differences. This should be done early on so that any imbalance between groups is addressed before it becomes a problem in the analysis stage. This reiterates the importance of generating strict inclusion and exclusion criteria that can be followed with minimal error.

CAUSALITY

Ernst Mach, an Austrian professor of physics and mathematics and a philosopher, argued that all knowledge is based on sensation and that all scientific measurements are dependent on the observer's perception. He proposed that "in nature there is no cause and effect" (Hutteman, 2013, p. 102). This is a relevant quote to begin a discussion of causality, because causality is a complex issue faced by all investigators. A single clinical disease can have many different "causes," and one cause can have several clinical consequences. Causality becomes even more complex when we begin to look at chronic diseases. Chronic diseases can have multiple etiologies. Cardiac disease, for example, has multiple causes such as genetic predisposition, obesity, smoking, lack of exercise, poor diet, or any combination of these factors.

A useful definition of causation for population research is that an increase in the causal factor or exposure causes an increase in the outcome of interest (e.g., disease). With that said, if an association is found between an exposure and an outcome, then the next question is: Is it causal? There are many theories of causation, some of which have been addressed in Chapter 3, but no one theory can explain entirely the complex interactions of an exposure with the development of disease or an outcome.

There are multiple criteria that can help determine causality. No one criterion in and of itself determines causality, but each one may help strengthen the argument for or against causality. One important criterion is the determination of a statistical *strength of association*. Statistics are used to test hypotheses: Is an exposure or risk factor present significantly more often in a population with the disease than without? If a new intervention is put into place, is there a significant improvement in the targeted outcome? The strength of association is measured by such things as relative risk and attributable risk. Another criterion is the confirmation of a *temporal relationship*: The suspected exposure or risk factor needs to occur before the disease or outcome. For example, a person needs to smoke before he or she develops lung cancer in order to attribute lung cancer to smoking as a potential causal agent. To show a causal relationship requires the elimination of all known *alternative explanations* and an experienced investigator will seek out other potential explanations to explain why such a relationship may not exist (Katz, Elmore, Wild, & Lucan, 2013).

Two additional important considerations are scientific plausibility and the ability to replicate findings. *Scientific plausibility* refers to coherence with our current body of knowledge as it relates to the phenomenon under study. That is, do the results make sense based on what we know about the phenomenon? For example, is it biologically plausible that exposure to cigarette smoke (e.g., benzene, nicotine, tar) could convert normal cells into cancer cells?

Additionally, the ability to *replicate findings* in different studies and in different populations provides strong evidence that a causal association exists. Other criteria for causation include the *dose–response* relationship. For example, with increasing exposure (e.g., smoking), one can see increasing risk of disease (e.g., lung cancer). Similarly, if one has a *cessation of exposure*, one would expect a cessation or reduction of disease. Finally, another criterion worth mentioning is consistency with other knowledge. This criterion takes into consideration knowledge of other known factors (e.g., environmental changes, product sales, behavioral changes) that may indicate a causal relationship. For example, if a law is passed that prohibits smoking in public places, it may result in fewer cases of smoking-related diseases reported in area hospitals. These criteria, in concert with a strong study design and methodology, can assist an APRN in determining the likelihood of causality when an association is found between an exposure and an outcome (Gordis, 2014).

Causes can be both direct and indirect. An example of a direct cause would be an infectious agent that causes a disease. Pertussis (whooping cough, a bacterial infection) is caused by *Bordetella pertussis*. The disease is a direct cause of the organism. Toxic shock syndrome is an example of an indirect cause. Although the staphylococcal organism and its toxins are the direct cause of the syndrome, the indirect cause (and the first factor that was identified) is tampons.

Even the infectious disease process is not simple. Both the host and the environment can have an impact on the infectious disease process. Characteristics of the host (e.g., age, previous exposures, general health, and immune status) can influence the development of the disease. Environmental conditions also play a role. A good example is influenza, which is most prevalent during certain times of the year. Infectious disease departments document these seasonal trends during the year, and they are available for hospitals to review. Such information can assist in antibiotic selection, hospital staffing, and educational campaigns to ensure immunizations or prevention programs are put into place. Awareness of seasonal fluctuations in certain diseases, trends in drug resistance, or changes in the community that affect the overall management of a patient are important in an APRN's practice. By following these trends, the APRN can better assess the needs of the community and ensure that appropriate resources are available to address the fluctuations that occur naturally in all communities.

SCIENTIFIC MISCONDUCT (FRAUD)

Scientific misconduct includes (but is not limited to) gift authorship, data fabrication and falsification, plagiarism, and conflict of interest. It can have an impact on researchers, patients, and populations (Karcz & Papadakos, 2011). No one wants to believe that there are investigators who commit fraud by deliberately distorting research findings, but it does happen. Unfortunately, in some cases, the fraud is intentional; in other cases it occurs via a series of missteps from methodology to analysis. As mentioned earlier, multiple forms of bias or confounding can be introduced into a study, and these, if ignored, can lead to spurious results. Intentionally ignoring these issues, especially without addressing them as a limitation, can be fraudulent. Acceptance for publication in a prominent peer-reviewed journal and/or evidence that the protocol was approved by an institutional review board (IRB) does not ensure the accuracy and/or ethical conduct of that research.

Perhaps one of the most infamous cases of fraud involved a well-respected peer-reviewed journal. In 1998, *The Lancet* published an article written by Andrew Wakefield and 12 others that implied a link between the measles–mumps–rubella (MMR) vaccine and autism and Crohn's disease. Although epidemiologists pointed out several study weaknesses, including a small number of cases, no controls, and reliance on parental recall, it received wide notice in the popular press. It was 7 years before a journalist uncovered the fact that Wakefield altered facts to support his claim and exploited the MMR scare for financial gain. *The Lancet* retracted the paper in 2010 (Godlee, Smith, & Marcovitch, 2011). A series of articles in the *British Medical Journal* (Deer, 2011) revealed how Wakefield and his associates distorted data for financial gain. Before this article was retracted, it caused widespread fear among parents and accelerated an antivaccine movement that many blame for the resurgence of infectious diseases among children.

In 2006, a writer for *The New York Times* (Interlandi, 2006) wrote an article that described a case of fraud that involved a formerly tenured professor at the University of Vermont. Dr. Eric Poehlman was tried in a federal court and found guilty. He was sentenced to 1 year and 1 day in jail for fraudulent actions that spanned 10 years. His misconduct included using fraudulent data in lectures and in published papers, and using these data to obtain millions of dollars in federal grants from the National Institutes of Health (NIH). He pleaded guilty to fabricating data on obesity, menopause, and aging. Interlandi's article, which includes a very detailed account of Dr. Poehlman's actions and his downfall, documents how a "committed cheater can elude detection for years by playing on the trust—and self-interest—of his or her junior colleagues" (p. 3).

It is safe to say that the majority of researchers carry out their research with scrupulous attention to detail and with integrity, but APRNs need to be aware that instances such as those mentioned earlier do happen. As stated in Chapter 3, it is important that when an APRN is making decisions related to population-based evaluation, the decisions need to be based on a sound methodological framework that includes ethical considerations of the effect of the research on the population as a whole. It is also important that APRNs are aware that fraud occurs in research and that they should be vigilant not only in how they carry out research but also in how they critically review the results of studies by other investigators.

STUDY DESIGNS

There is no perfect study design; however, there are strategies that can be used to decrease the threat of bias and increase the likelihood that hypotheses are answered accurately. The awareness that bias and confounding can cause a threat to the validity of study results is important and may be unavoidable; however, recognizing these limitations and addressing them within your study is even more critical. The design of high-quality and transparent studies creates a good foundation for evidence-based practice. Table 4.2 outlines the strengths and weaknesses of study designs used in population research.

Randomized Controlled Trials

When carefully designed, RCTs can provide the strongest evidence for the effectiveness of a treatment or intervention. Subjects are randomly assigned to either the intervention group (which will receive the experimental treatment or intervention) or the control group (which will receive the nonexperimental treatment or no intervention). Inclusion and exclusion criteria for the participants must be precise and spelled out in advance.

RCTs are considered strong designs because of their ability to minimize bias; however, if the randomization is not executed in a truly random manner, then the design can be flawed, or if the data are not reported consistently,

TABLE 4.2 • Strengths and Weaknesses of Study Designs

Type of Study	Strengths	Weaknesses
Randomized controlled trials	• Lower likelihood of confounding variables • Minimize bias in treatment assignment • Able to control intervention or treatment	• Labor intensive • Costly • Lengthy • Sometimes impractical or unethical to conduct
Cohort designs	• Able to identify confounding and address in the study • Able to control exposure • Able to calculate relative risk and incidence rates • Can study multiple outcomes	• Labor intensive • Costly • Lengthy
Case-control	• Inexpensive • Shorter time to completion • Able to study variables with long latency or impact periods • Provides a means to compare groups • Able to calculate odds ratios • Able to study rare or fatal diseases • Can study multiple exposures	• Risk of bias and confounding variables • Sometimes unable to measure or determine exposure • Selection bias • Measurement error • Recall bias • Cannot assess risk
Cross-sectional	• Able to calculate prevalence of population studied • Assesses exposures and outcomes at one time • Provides a snapshot of study population • Inexpensive	• Risk of confounding variables • Selection bias • Cannot control for or identify the significance of potentially important variables • Cannot assess risk

then errors can lead to invalid conclusions. Consolidated Standards of Reporting Trials (CONSORT) is a method that has been developed to improve the quality and reporting of RCTs. It offers a standard way for authors to prepare reports of trial findings, facilitate their complete and transparent reporting, and aid their critical appraisal and interpretation (CONSORT Group, 2014). The CONSORT checklist items focus on reporting how the trial was designed, analyzed, and interpreted; the flow diagram displays the progress of all participants through the trial (CONSORT Group, 2014). The CONSORT guidelines are endorsed by many professional journals and editorial organizations. They are part of an effort to improve the quality and reporting of research that is conducted to make better clinical decisions. Both the CONSORT checklist and the CONSORT flow diagram can be accessed at www.consort-statement.org/consort-2010.

RCTs are believed to provide the most reliable scientific evidence, but they can be expensive, time-consuming, and sometimes difficult to conduct for ethical reasons. There are general guidelines that APRNs can follow when conducting a study to provide a framework for a quality design. They are as follows:

- Formulate an answerable research question (see Chapter 5).
- Complete an extensive review of the literature to determine what is currently known about the problem and to provide a sound theoretical background (see Chapter 5).
- Select a study design that will best answer the research question.
- Choose a study design that is feasible in terms of both time and money.
- Once a design is chosen, plan every step of the research process before beginning the study (e.g., determination of inclusion and exclusion criteria, selection of primary and secondary outcomes of interest).
- Ensure that comparison groups are as similar as possible; stratify for possible confounders early on to avoid making false conclusions.
- Determine sufficient sample size to ensure the study has adequate power for result interpretation.
- Use objective criteria for the collection of all data.
- Train all investigators to ensure that data are collected uniformly.
- Choose the appropriate methods for data analysis.
- Provide sufficient and clear details of the study in papers and presentations to allow others to understand how the study was carried out and to allow them to assess for possible biases (e.g., provide an audit trail).

Cohort Studies

Cohort designs can be either prospective or retrospective. In a prospective cohort design, the investigator selects a group of individuals who were exposed to a factor of interest and compares it to a group of nonexposed individuals and follows both groups to determine the incidence of an outcome (e.g., disease). This type of design should be carried out when the APRN has good evidence (a sound theoretical base) that links an exposure to an outcome. A well-designed, prospective cohort study has the potential to provide better evidence than a poorly designed RCT. One of the major problems with cohort studies is that they can be time-consuming and expensive if the cohort needs to be followed for a prolonged period of time, and the longer the time period involved, the more likely that participants can and will be lost to follow-up. This potential loss of subjects can result in withdrawal bias, particularly when people with certain characteristics drop out of one group at a different rate than that of another group or are lost to follow-up at different rates. Both of these occurrences can lead to spurious results or results that are difficult to generalize. For example, subjects who participate for the duration of a study may be healthier than those who drop out, leading to potential characteristic differences between groups that may affect the final analysis. These types of differences can falsely dilute observed differences between groups or falsely strengthen results and should be avoided when possible.

When conducting a cohort study, investigators should provide detailed information on the following: subjects' data that are lost or incomplete, subjects' rates of withdrawal or loss to follow-up, characteristics of subjects that are lost to follow-up or who have withdrawn from the study, and, when possible, reasons for the dropouts. They should also include detailed descriptions of the groups that are included in the analysis of outcomes (e.g., age, gender, family history, and severity of disease).

Des Jarlais, Lyles, Crepaz, and the TREND Group (2004) first presented the Transparent Reporting of Evaluations with Nonrandomized Designs (TREND) in the *American Journal of Public Health*. These guidelines provide a framework for the design and reporting of nonrandomized studies in order to facilitate research synthesis. The TREND checklist has 22 steps and was designed for use as an evaluation tool of nonrandomized behavioral or public health intervention studies. The TREND statement and checklist are available through the Centers for Disease Control and Prevention website, www.cdc.gov/trendstatement. These types of studies should include a defined intervention and research design that provides for an assessment of the efficacy or effectiveness of the intervention. The authors place emphasis on "description of the intervention, including the theoretical base, description of the comparison condition, full reporting of outcomes, and inclusion of information related to the design needed to assess possible biases in the outcome data" (Des Jarlais et al., 2004, p. 362). These guidelines provide APRNs with a comprehensive checklist for designing studies and writing research reports.

Case-Control Studies

In a *case-control* study, the investigator first identifies a group of individuals with the attribute of interest (cases), and a second group is identified without the attribute of interest (controls). Cases and controls can be matched individually or as a group for variables that might cause confounding (e.g., age, gender, and ethnicity), or they can be unmatched. If unmatched, then each group should have similar characteristics. As mentioned earlier, matching can be on an individual level or group level. In Chapter 3, we defined the odds ratio (OR) in case-control studies as the odds of being an exposed case compared to the odds of being an exposed control (ad/bc). This is the calculation for an unmatched study. However, when we calculate the OR for a matched

TABLE 4.3a • 2 × 2 Table for Calculating Odds Ratio in an Unmatched Case-Control Study

	Cases	Controls
Exposed	a	b
Nonexposed	c	d
OR = ad/bc (unmatched pairs)		

TABLE 4.3b • 2 × 2 Table for Calculating Odds Ratio in a Matched Pairs Case-Control Study

	Exposed Controls	Nonexposed Controls
Exposed Cases	a	b
Nonexposed Cases	c	d
OR = b/c (matched pairs)		

pairs study (e.g., matching of individual pairs for a variety of characteristics), we need to take into consideration only those situations in which cases have different exposures. We are not interested in comparing cases with controls if both are exposed (as in "a") or both are unexposed (as in "d"). Therefore the OR for a matched case-control study is calculated as b/c. Also, of note in a matched case-control study, the 2 × 2 table is set up differently as individual cases are matched to individual controls (Tables 4.3a and b).

Case-control studies tend to be inexpensive and relatively quick to complete, but they have several weaknesses. Because subjects in the groups are not randomly assigned, associations found in the analysis may be the result of exposure to another, unknown variable. To decrease the likelihood of bias, definite criteria should be used so that there is no ambiguity about how to distinguish between a case and a control. Controls should resemble the cases as closely as possible except for exposure to the factor under study. If the cases are drawn from a medical surgical unit in an acute care hospital, then ideally the controls should be drawn from the same population. Matching, as previously described, is one method that can be used so that potential confounders are distributed equally between the cases and controls. A problem with case-control studies is that data are usually abstracted from medical records that are not designed for collection of research material; so data obtained from medical records may be limited and may not provide adequate or accurate information on exposures. For example, data collected from medical records may be incomplete (e.g., missing diagnoses), may use old diagnostic criteria, or may be coded or entered incorrectly. Additionally, if abstracting data from interviews, biases, such as recall bias or reporting bias, may play a role in how data are recorded and ultimately can affect the interpretation and final conclusions of a study.

DATABASES

Databases have become ubiquitous in the healthcare field, and their use is growing. Many of the larger and better known databases are discussed throughout this text. There is a good reason for their frequent mention. Nurses in all fields and in all positions enter data electronically into databases of some kind. Managers use databases to assess the level of satisfaction of their patient population and nursing staff. Direct care nurses use data to assess the performance of their units on important patient care indicators (such as falls) and record patient information into electronic health records that may be linked with larger databases or registries. Departments dedicated to quality improvement track infection rates, readmission rates, and other identified indicators of quality of care.

Some databases are for a single site (e.g., one acute care hospital or one community), but it is becoming increasingly common for databases to be linked or for databases to include information at the state, regional, and national level (e.g., trauma registries that log all incoming trauma data from all trauma centers in the state). State and federal regulatory agencies, such as the Agency for Healthcare Research and Quality (AHRQ) and the Centers for Medicare & Medicaid Services (CMS), are requiring healthcare providers to report specific patient safety indicators. Some of these data, such as those compiled by CMS, are being posted for public view. Other organizations, such as the American Nurses Credentialing Center (ANCC), are requiring data entry for accreditation by programs, such as Magnet, and setting performance standards using benchmarks.

Databases are being developed to meet the needs of specific populations. One such database was developed for quality-improvement and service planning for palliative care and hospice facilities in North Carolina. The system was developed and implemented over a 2-year period and grew from one community-based site to four. The patient data are entered at the point of care (e.g., hospital, nursing home, and hospice). The information captured by the database has strengthened the ability of providers to identify areas for improvement in quality of care and the service needs of the palliative care population (Bull et al., 2010).

Nursing care data that are captured using technology can be aggregated, analyzed, and benchmarked. The information can provide APRNs with a clear picture of the population that they serve and help to guide decisions for the provision of services. Patrician, Loan, McCarthy, Brosch, and Davey (2010) described the creation of the nurse-sensitive indicators for military nursing outcomes database (MilNOD; www.usuhs.edu/tsnrp/index.php). Prospective data are collected and entered into the database each shift by nurses. Information is collected on direct staff hours by levels (RN, LPN), patient census and acuity, falls, medication errors, and other identified indicators for 56 units in 13 military hospitals. The information allows nurse leaders to track nursing and patient quality indicators and to target areas for managerial and clinical performance improvement.

There are many issues that the APRN needs to be aware of when using or developing databases. Databases require a high level of technological expertise to create, maintain, and use. Trained technicians and specialized equipment are required. Unanticipated technology-related problems can occur. In North Carolina, the mountains created a barrier for wireless communication of data and another system had to be installed to be able to communicate among sites. MilNOD designers identified the need to focus on a standardized approach for data collection. To minimize bias in their data set, the designers also created standardized definitions and specific and detailed protocols to ensure data are entered accurately and consistently.

Roberts and Sewell (2011) have outlined important requirements for the development and use of databases. Among the important points that they make is that nurses must understand the basics of entering data into databases and how data must be structured. Computer systems must be able to communicate with each other. This includes systems located within one site as well as systems in other sites if it is a multisite system. They also emphasize the need to be consistent in how data are coded.

Successful databases are created collaboratively. Members of the healthcare team who will be entering and using the data need to work together with technicians who understand systems. And the creation of a workable database is just a beginning. Once the data are entered, they need to be analyzed and checked for accuracy (*data editing*). Posting data that are summarized and benchmarked using graphs and trend lines on shared drives that are accessible to direct care nurses as well as nurse leaders brings the information to people who directly impact care and helps nurses to identify areas for improvement. Nurses at all levels should be involved in data management and analysis.

SUMMARY

APRNs need to carry out studies with strong methodology and designs and understand the factors that can influence study results. One problem with population research is that it is difficult to identify and control for variables that are not part of the study but that may have an effect on the results. When a researcher analyzes data in a study and draws the wrong conclusion, the result is a type I or type II error, also referred to as errors of inference. A type I error occurs when a null hypothesis is rejected when in fact it is true. A type II error occurs when a null hypothesis is not rejected when in fact it is false. There are two kinds of error of measurement—random error and systematic error, and it is essential that APRNs are aware how these errors can occur, how they can impact a study, and what measures can be taken to avoid or minimize them. RCTs are considered the gold standard in population research and offer the best protection for preventing bias, but they are not always feasible. Well-designed cohort and case-control studies are acceptable alternatives when RCTs are not an option.

Databases are increasingly used in healthcare. Aggregated data provide valuable information about population groups that can be used to direct care and establish evidence for clinical guidelines. APRNs should work closely with technology experts in the planning, implementation, and use of databases in order to maximize their ability to analyze data in an accurate and systematic manner. Strong methodology and data collection with a sound research design are the foundation for an excellent study/intervention that ultimately can contribute to evidence-based practice.

EXERCISES AND DISCUSSION QUESTIONS

Exercise 4.1 Over a period of several months, you notice a significant increase in the number of pediatric patients (less than 1 year of age) who present to the emergency department (ED) with traumatic injuries. You are concerned because many of these injuries could have been prevented and some of them appear nonaccidental. You decide to design an intervention to address risk factors for trauma in infants. There are many settings in which such an intervention can be implemented: the newborn nursery, outpatient clinics, and EDs. The target audience can be expectant parents, parents, healthcare providers, or any combination thereof.

- Where might you find data on traumatic injuries in your area? How can you use these data to help you design an intervention?
- Design an educational intervention to address the risk factors for traumatic injuries in infants. Decide on a site and a target audience. Identify an outcome.
- What type of study design might you use for your proposed intervention?
- What are the advantages and disadvantages of the design you have selected?
- What variables could be considered confounders?
- Describe some of the systematic errors that could occur in your study, and why.

Exercise 4.2 You are an administrator in an adolescent inpatient psychiatric hospital. You are concerned about a recent increase in the use of physical restraints in the hospital. You also notice an increased use of sedating medications. You have not had any recent changes in staffing or patient mix and acuity.

- How might you assess this situation?
- Where might you find the data in your hospital to support your concern?
- What type of study could you perform to identify the cause(s) for the increase in both physical and chemical restraint usage?
- How will you select your population of study?
- How will you select a control group or comparison group?
- What are potential errors in measurement that you may encounter?

Exercise 4.3 You are working in an ambulatory care clinic in an underserved community and are interested in improving the quality of healthcare that is provided in your area. You are concerned about an increase in the incidence of methicillin-resistant *Staphylococcus aureus* (MRSA) in the population that you serve. Before you launch an educational campaign aimed at both your staff and the community, you need to establish the severity of the problem.

- Identify a database at the local, state, or national level that can help you obtain the necessary information.
  - How can you determine the incidence and prevalence of MRSA in your community?
  - What are some of the potential errors that can occur in the reporting of MRSA to a local, state, or national database?

- How might this affect your interpretation of the data?
- What are some of the barriers to reporting in your community (i.e., hospital, outpatient clinic, nursing home)?
- You decide to begin collecting data on MRSA-related deaths for your local hospital.
  - What are some of the problems that may occur during data collection?
  - How might you avoid these problems?
- You determine from your investigation that there is a significant problem in your community.
  - Describe how you would address the increasing morbidity and mortality of MRSA in the population that you serve.
  - What type of study design would you use to evaluate the effectiveness of your intervention?
  - What are potential confounders?
  - Is there potential for interaction?

Exercise 4.4 Match the term with the correct definition.
  a. *Decision:* Conclude treatments are not different. *Reality:* Treatments are different.
  b. *Decision:* Conclude treatments are different. *Reality:* Treatments are different.
  c. *Decision:* Conclude treatments are not different. *Reality:* Treatments are not different.
  d. *Decision:* Conclude treatments are different. *Reality:* Treatments are not different.
  _____ Type I error
  _____ Type II error
  _____ Power

REFERENCES

American Association of Colleges of Nursing. (2006). *The essentials of doctoral education for advanced practice nursing.* Retrieved from http://www.aacn.nche.edu/publications/position/DNPEssentials.pdf

Bull, J., Zafar, Y., Wheeler, J., Harker, M., Gblokpor, A., Hanson, L., . . . Abernethy, A. (2010). Establishing a regional, multisite database for quality improvement and service planning in community-based palliative care and hospice. *Journal of Palliative Medicine, 13*(8), 1013–1020.

CONSORT Group. (2014). *CONSORT: Transparent reporting of trials.* Retrieved from http://www.consort-statement.org/

Deer, B. (2011). How the case against the MMR vaccine was fixed. *British Medical Journal, 342,* 77–82.

Des Jarlais, D., Lyles, C., Crepaz, N., & TREND Group. (2004). Improving the reporting quality of nonrandomized evaluations of behavioral and public health interventions: The TREND statement. *American Journal of Public Health, 94*(3), 361–366.

Godlee, F., Smith, J., & Marcovitch, H. (2011). Wakefield's article linking MMR vaccine and autism was fraudulent [Editorial]. *British Medical Journal, 342,* 64–66.

Gordis, L. (2014). *Epidemiology* (5th ed.). Canada: Elsevier Saunders.

Huttemann, A. (2013). A disposition-based process-theory of causation. In S. Mumford & M. Tugby (Eds.). *Metaphysics and science* (pp. 101 - 122). Oxford, U.K: Oxford University Press

Interlandi, J. (2006, October 22). An unwelcome discovery. *The New York Times.* Retrieved from http://www.nytimes.com/2006/10/22/magazine/22sciencefraud.html

Joober, R., Schmitz, N., Annable, L., & Boksa, P. (2012). Publication bias: What are the challenges and can they be overcome? *Journal of Psychiatry & Neuroscience, 37*(3), 149–152. doi:10.1503/jpn.120065

Karcz, M., & Papadakos, P. J. (2011). The consequences of fraud and deceit in medical research. *Canadian Journal of Respiratory Therapy, 47*(1), 18–27.

Katz, D., Elmore, J. G., Wild, D. M. G., & Lucan, S. C. (2013). *Jekel's epidemiology, biostatistics, preventive medicine, and public health* (4th ed.). Canada: Elsevier Saunders.

Kellar, S. P., & Kelvin, E. A. (2013). *Munro's statistical methods for health care research* (6th ed.). Philadelphia, PA: Wolters Kluwer/Lippincott Williams & Wilkins.

Landis, J. R., & Koch, G. G. (1977). The measurement of observer agreement for categorical data. *Biometrics, 33,* 159.

Maclure, M., & Willett, W. C. (1987). Misinterpretation and misuse of the kappa statistic. *American Journal of Epidemiology, 126*(2), 161–169.

Matsumoto, M., Ishikawa, S., & Kajii, E. (2010). Rurality of communities and incidence of stroke: A confounding effect of weather conditions? *Rural and Remote Health, 10,* 1493. Retrieved from http://www.rrh.org.au

Patrician, P., Loan, L., McCarthy, M., Brosch, L., & Davey, K. (2010). Towards evidence-based management: Creating an informative database of nursing-sensitive indicators. *Journal of Nursing Scholarship, 42*(4), 358–366.

Roberts, A., & Sewell, J. (2011). Data aggregation: A case study. CIN: *Computers, Informatics, Nursing, 29*(1), 3–7.

Shorten, A., & Moorley, C. (2014). Selecting the sample. *Evidence-Based Nursing, 17*(2), 32–33. doi:10.1136/eb-2014-101747

Shott, S. (1990). *Statistics for health care professionals.* New York, NY: W.B. Saunders.

Siddiqi, N. (2011). Publication bias in epidemiological studies. *Central European Journal of Public Health, 19*(2), 118–120. Retrieved from http://web.b.ebscohost.com/ehost/detail/detail?vid=14&sid=12f13f7c-adf3-40ee-8c3c-ed3d6d69996a%40sessionmgr115&hid=116&bdata=JnNpdGU9ZWhvc3QtbGl2ZQ%3d%3d#db=rzh&AN=2011210575

Sjödahl, K., Lu, Y., Nilsen, T., Ye, W., Hveem, K., Vatten, L., & Lagergren, J. (2007). Smoking and alcohol drinking in relation to risk of gastric cancer: A population-based, prospective cohort study. *International Journal of Cancer, 120*(1), 128–132.

Song, F., Parekh-Bhurke, S., Hooper, L., Loke, Y., Ryder, J., Sutton, A., . . . Harvey, I. (2009). Extent of publication bias in different categories of research cohorts: A meta-analysis of empirical studies. *BMC Medical Research Methodology, 9,* 79. Retrieved from http://web.ebscohost.com/ehost/pdfviewer/pdfviewer?hid=110&sid=01961f3d-cd2e-4770-86af-bc7107e2f85e%40sessionmgr113&vid=4

Starks, H., Diehr, P., & Curtis, J. R. (2009). The challenge of selection bias and confounding in palliative care research. *Journal of Palliative Medicine, 12*(2), 181–187.

Statistics. (2002). In *The American heritage dictionary of the English language* (4th ed., p. 1695). Boston, MA: Houghton Mifflin.

Applying Evidence at the Population Level

Ann L. Cupp Curley and Margaret M. Conrad

Nurses in advanced practice have an obligation to improve the health of the populations that they serve by providing evidence-based care. The American Association of Colleges of Nursing (AACN) has outlined eight essentials that represent the core competencies for the education of doctorally prepared advanced practice registered nurses (APRNs). The first essential listed is scientific underpinnings for practice (American Association of Colleges of Nursing, 2006). This competency stresses the integration of evidence-based practice into advanced nursing practice. APRNs are educated at the graduate level in research and critical appraisal skills and possess specialized clinical knowledge. These specialized abilities prepare the APRN to demonstrate the importance of evidence-based practice to others and to facilitate the incorporation of such evidence into practice (DeBourgh, 2001).

In this chapter, the APRN will learn how to integrate and synthesize information in order to design interventions that are based on evidence to improve population outcomes. Nurses need a sound knowledge of research methodology to support an evidence-based practice. They also require a wide array of knowledge gleaned from the sciences and the ability to translate that knowledge quickly and effectively to benefit patients (Porter-O'Grady, 2003). The goal of this chapter is to summarize the skills required for evidence-based practice and to provide specific examples of how APRNs use these skills to improve population outcomes.

The American Heritage Dictionary (2000) defines *evidence* as "[a] thing or things helpful in forming a conclusion or judgment" (p. 617). Melnyk and Fineout-Overholt (2010) define *evidence-based practice* as "a paradigm and life-long problem solving approach to clinical decision-making that involves the conscientious use of the best available evidence (including a systematic search for and critical appraisal of the most relevant evidence to answer a clinical question) with one's own clinical expertise and patient values and preferences to improve outcomes for individuals, groups, communities and systems" (p. 578). A related term is "best practices," which refers to providing care that has been improved in order to achieve superior outcomes (Lippencott Williams & Wilkins, 2007). Nurses require several skills to become practitioners of evidence-based care and to improve clinical outcomes. They must be able to identify clinical problems, recognize patient safety issues, compose clinical questions that provide a clear direction for study, conduct a search of the literature, appraise and synthesize the available evidence, and successfully integrate new knowledge into practice. The APRN plays an important role in this complex process of incorporating evidence-based practice into policies and standards of care to improve population outcomes. In population-based care, there is additional complexity in determining the values and needs of groups of people. Making decisions related to population-based health requires consideration of the effects of the intervention on the population as a whole. Balancing the overall needs of groups of people with the rights of individuals requires careful and thoughtful consideration. A sound evidence-based practice provides a foundation to better assess those needs based on evidence.

ASKING THE CLINICAL QUESTION

There are many situations that drive clinical questions. Clinical practice and observation, as well as information obtained by reading the professional literature, can lead nurses to ask questions such as "Why is this happening?" "Would this approach to care work in my clinical practice?" or "What can we do to improve this outcome?" An APRN who reads an article about an innovation in practice that leads to an improvement in a population outcome might wonder whether such an intervention would work in another setting. The observation that the readmission rates for a particular diagnosis are increasing, or that rates for a particular disease are higher in one population than in another, or that patient satisfaction scores for a particular group of patients are lower can all lead to a search of the literature for evidence to change and improve outcomes. It may also lead to further research to improve outcomes or the implementation of new interventions to change outcomes. But before the search can begin, it is important that clinical questions are defined clearly and in a way that can be answered and applied to practice.

Clinical questions need to be written in a format that provides a clear direction for examination. The PICO format provides a clear-cut method for developing clinical questions and is also one of the most popular methods used for this purpose. PICO is an acronym that stands for population studied (P), intervention (I), comparison (C), and outcome (O). Sometimes, practitioners use the PICOT format, in which the "T" stands for "time frame." For the purpose of this example, the PICO framework will be used. As you are formulating your PICO question, it is helpful to describe the type of question you are asking to better define your research method. Is this an intervention, diagnosis, etiology, or prognosis type of question? (Lansing Community College Library, 2014; Table 5.1). When constructing a PICO question, the first step is to select the type of question you wish to ask, and the next step is to describe the patient population to be studied. When retrieving background literature, it must be relevant to the

TABLE 5.1 • PICOT Questions > Types of Evidence > Databases

Type of Clinical Question	Primary Research	Synthesized Research (Secondary Literature)	Other Evidence (Secondary Literature)
	Use CINAHL and MEDLINE to find: • Randomized controlled trials (RCT) • Controlled trials • Case-control studies • Cohort studies • Descriptive studies • Qualitative studies • Instrument development research	Use Cochrane, CINAHL, and MEDLINE to find: • Systematic reviews • Meta-analyses	Use CINAHL, NGC, MEDLINE, Joanna Briggs Inst., nursing, healthcare, and government organizations to find: • Clinical practice guidelines Use published clinical articles (not research based), peer institution practices, expert clinician practices to find: • Expert opinion
Therapy "What is the best treatment or intervention?"	RCT, controlled trials	Systematic reviews	Clinical practice guidelines
Prevention "How can I prevent this problem?"	RCT, controlled trials	Systematic reviews	Clinical practice guidelines
Diagnosis / Assessment "What is the best way to assess or best diagnostic test for this patient?"	Instrument development research		**Evidence Pyramid** **Look for the highest level of evidence appropriate for your clinical question.** Level I Level II Level III Level IV Level V Level VI Level VII Level 1: Systematic reviews & meta-analysis of RCTs, evidence-based clinical practice guidelines Level 2: One or more RCTs Level 3: Controlled trials (no randomization) Level 4: Case-control or cohort study Level 5: Systematic review of descriptive and qualitative studies Level 6: Single descriptive or qualitative study Level 7: Expert opinion
Causation "What causes this problem?"	Cohort, case control, descriptive, or qualitative studies	Systematic reviews	
Prognosis "What are the long-term effects of this problem?"	Cohort or descriptive studies	Systematic reviews	
Meaning "What is the meaning of this experience for patients?"	Qualitative studies	Systematic reviews	

Source: Used with permission of Lansing Community College Library, Lansing, Michigan.

targeted population. Think about how to describe the population that you are interested in learning more about. What are its most important characteristics? For example, an APRN employed in a state correctional facility may observe both high rates of diabetes in the prison population and low rates of compliance with diabetes self-management. To accurately define the patient population, an APRN needs to identify any important characteristics of the population that need to be addressed or examined in the proposed study or intervention. Using the same example, prison populations are known to have high rates of mental illness, and the APRN decides to target this particular population for study. Therefore, the population studied would be described as follows:

- *Population:* Mentally ill inmates diagnosed with diabetes, housed in state prisons.

    The second step is to determine what intervention or process you want to study. As mentioned earlier, defining the method of study early on can help develop the PICO question more fully. In this particular example, the APRN hypothesized that increasing the self-efficacy of inmates with diabetes through a self-management course might help inmates manage their diabetes better. Having read in the professional literature about self-management courses for chronic illnesses used in other settings, the APRN postulates that a chronic disease self-management course might increase compliance rates with inmates through an increase in self-efficacy.

- *Intervention:* A chronic disease self-management program (CSMP).

    In this particular example, the APRN wants to measure self-efficacy and diabetes management before and after the CSMP. The comparison is, therefore, diabetes management before and after the intervention.

- *Comparison:* Diabetes management in mentally ill inmates housed in state prisons, diagnosed with diabetes before and after implementation of the CSMP.

    The last step is the outcome: What does the APRN want to see improved? What does the APRN expect to accomplish? The objective in this case was to increase self-efficacy and improve diabetes management in a targeted population of mentally ill inmates with diabetes after implementing a CSMP.

- *Outcome:* Self-efficacy (measured using a validated self-efficacy scale) and hemoglobin A_{1c} levels (as a measure of diabetes management).

    Using these steps, the APRN can compose the final PICO question: "Will a 6-week chronic disease self-management program increase the self-efficacy of insulin-dependent diabetic mentally ill inmates in a state prison setting?" (Conrad, 2008). Development of the PICO question provides the APRN with a better understanding of the clinical problem, allows for specific measures to be introduced, and provides the foundation for a well-designed study. The next step is to perform a thorough and comprehensive literature review.

THE LITERATURE REVIEW

The literature search should further define and clarify the clinical problem; summarize the current state of knowledge on the subject; identify relationships, contradictions, gaps, and inconsistencies in the literature; and finally, suggest the next step in solving the problem (American Psychological Association [APA], 2009). The search of the literature can be conducted by the APRN, or the APRN can engage the assistance of a research librarian if available. Librarians are educated to find and access information and are excellent resources for assisting with literature reviews. Navigating databases in order to find relevant information can be a complex process. The searcher needs to use the correct terms, search the correct databases, and use a well-designed and systematic search strategy. The searcher should also document each step of the process in order to provide an audit trail and avoid duplication of work (Hallyburton & St. John, 2010). An audit trail provides clarity to the method used to find the evidence and allows others to follow the decision-making process (Houde, 2009). In the absence of a librarian, there are steps that the APRN can take to increase the likelihood of a successful search.

In order to find the most relevant literature to inform decision making, the searcher should use key terms from the PICO question (i.e., population studied, intervention, comparison, and outcomes of interest). The first step is to search each key term separately and then to take steps to refine the search. The APRN should use at least two databases for the literature search. Access to some databases requires a subscription; others are free. The Cochrane Collaboration is an international organization that provides up-to-date systematic reviews (currently more than 8,000). It can be accessed through the Cochrane Collaboration website (www.cochrane.org) and requires a subscription in many countries, including the United States (with the exception of Wyoming). For a complete list of countries with free access, go to the Cochrane page at www.thecochranelibrary.com/view/0/FreeAccess.html. Some of the content is free. For example, access to summaries or older versions of the reviews can be accessed without a subscription, but for access to full systematic reviews, a paid subscription is required (The Cochrane Collaboration, 2014). PubMed is a free resource. It includes MEDLINE and is the United States National Library of Medicine (NLM) journal literature search system. It includes more than 20 million citations for biomedical literature from MEDLINE, journals, and online books, and includes citations from full-text content (U.S. National Library of Medicine, 2014). A free tutorial on how to use PubMed is available at www.nlm.nih.gov/bsd/pubmed_tutorial/ml001.html.

The Joanna Briggs Institute (JBI; http://joannabriggs.org) and the Cumulative Index to Nursing and Allied Health Literature (CINAHL) are excellent databases that both require a subscription. The JBI includes The JBI Library of Systematic Reviews, which is an international, not-for-profit, membership-based organization located within the University of Adelaide (Australia; The Joanna Briggs Institute, 2014). There are discounted rates for students to join. CINAHL is a comprehensive resource for nursing and allied health literature. It is owned and operated by EBSCO Publishing. EBSCO now sells five different versions (CINAHL, CINAHL Plus, CINAHL with Full Text, CINAHL Plus with Full Text, and CINAHL Complete). The main differences among them are the added content. CINAHL is the basic database (EBSCO Publishing, 2014).

Searches of a single keyword can result in a very large number of articles. For example, a CINAHL search for full-text articles using the keyword "diabetes" yielded a list of 81,693 articles. Including more than one concept in the search is more likely to provide relevant and useful articles. *Boolean logic* is the term used to describe certain logical operations that are used to combine search terms in many databases. Using the Boolean connector AND narrows a search by combining terms; it will retrieve documents that use two keywords. Combining words with a Boolean connector such as AND (e.g., *prisoners AND diabetes*) can narrow the search. In CINHAL, using *prisoners AND diabetes* yielded 33 articles. Using OR, on the other hand, broadens a search to include results that contain either of the words that are typed in the search. OR is a good tool to use when there are several common spellings or synonyms of a word. An example in this case would be *inmate OR prisoner*. Using NOT will narrow a search by excluding certain search terms. NOT retrieves documents that contain one but not the other of the search terms entered. It is appropriate to use when a word is used in different contexts. An example would be *prisoners NOT captives*. Parentheses indicate relationships between search terms. When they are used, the computer will process the search terms in a specified order and also combine them in the correct manner. For example, (*inmate OR prisoner*) AND diabetes combines inmate or prisoner and diabetes to get the most relevant results. A search conducted in the full-text database of CINAHL using these words and connectors yielded 232 articles.

There are other methods that can be used to make searches more relevant and useful. Specifying limits, such as English language only, peer-reviewed journals only, randomized controlled trials only, and a date range can narrow a search and increase the relevance of the information retrieved. Keep in mind that the more limits that are placed on the search, the fewer the results. A search using (*inmate OR prisoner*) AND diabetes, full text only, English only, limited to articles published in the past 5 years yielded 36 articles. However, it is recommended that the initial search should be broad and explored before restricting the search limits, as this could lead to information bias. For this PICO question, the following keywords were used both alone and in combinations: *chronic disease, chronic disease management program, diabetes, incarcerated, mentally ill, mental illness, prison, self-efficacy, and self-management.*

A search for the most current known evidence about a topic is not complete after the search of electronic databases. A hand search of current and relevant journals can reveal information that has not yet been entered into an electronic database. Studies can also appear in publications other than journals such as books, working papers, and unpublished doctoral dissertations. Projects and reports that are completed by specialized organizations, such as foundations and professional membership groups, may appear only on websites. Internet searching can help locate such resources and can scan organizational websites of professional and specialized organizations such as the American Diabetes Association, the American Public Health Association, the American Nurses Association, and the Robert Wood Johnson Foundation. The APRN should also consider contacting experts who may be aware of important findings and recent discoveries in a particular field. A technique known as snowballing (citation tracking using the citation databases such as Science Citation Index, Social Sciences Citation Index, and Arts and Humanities Citation Index) might also be helpful (Centre for Reviews and Dissemination [CRD], 2009). After reviewing the literature, many references can be found that may not have been discovered in an Internet search by simply reviewing the references of collected literature.

Finally, really simple syndication (RSS feeds) provides a convenient way for subscribers to obtain constantly updated information (see also Chapter 6). They function as a new version of a database. Rather than searching individual websites, nurses can browse content, summaries of content, headlines, and/ or links to information quickly and in one place from an aggregator that automatically downloads the new data to the user. Sites such as PubMed allow subscribers to customize the information for which they want alerts. For those who want to do the searching, Instant RSS Search (ctriq.org/RSS) provides a venue to find feeds for news, websites, podcasts, and more.

During the literature search, APRNs should keep in mind the difference between primary and secondary sources. Primary sources are those materials or documents created during the time under study and directly experienced by the writer. For example, an original article written by researchers that summarizes the methods and findings of a study carried out by them is an example of a primary source. Other examples of primary sources are letters, diaries, and speeches. Secondary sources interpret and analyze primary sources. An example is a news article announcing a new scientific discovery. A key here is that secondary sources generally analyze and interpret the findings in primary sources and this can lead to bias. It is always advisable to use primary sources when seeking evidence for a change in practice.

ASSESSING THE EVIDENCE

Once a list of articles is obtained, the next step is to assess and synthesize the evidence. Appraising evidence for its usefulness can be a challenge. While reviewing the evidence, the APRN needs to ask some fundamental questions that address the relevance of information such as "How confident am I that the relationships and knowledge in this particular study will apply to the situation in question?" Shapiro and Donaldson (2008) have identified some important questions related to evidence-based practice changes: "When is the evidence strong enough to use the results?" "Are the findings applicable to my setting?" "If I adopt the practice, what will it mean to the target population?" Another important question relates to the "efficacy" (evidence of an effect under ideal conditions, such as double-blind, randomized controlled trials) and "effectiveness" (evidence of what actually works in practice) of the findings and of the study. In summary, during the process of determining which studies to include in a synthesis, the APRN needs to ask not only "Does this intervention work?" and "For whom does this intervention work?" but also "When, why, and how does it work?"

All published evidence is not completed with equal rigor, and therefore, the value of published articles varies on a continuum from the lowest to the highest value. A search can potentially find an enormous number of articles, but not all articles may be useful. Because there is often a limited amount of time that is available to assess and synthesize the evidence, it is helpful to have a method that provides guidance as to which articles might be the most valid and useful. After conducting an extensive search of sources, the APRN must establish criteria for inclusion and exclusion of studies (Melnyk & Fineout-Overholt, 2005).

There are several organizations that provide guidelines for the conduct of systematic reviews and help healthcare professionals keep pace with the professional literature by providing completed systematic reviews. Information on five of them is listed in Table 5.2. Polit and Beck (2012) describe a systematic review as a summary of what is best evidence at the time the review

TABLE 5.2 • Online Resources for Evidence-Based Practice

Organization	Description	Web Link
The Cochrane Collaboration	The Cochrane Collaboration is an independent, not-for-profit organization	http://www .cochrane.org
	Systematic reviews are published in The Cochrane Library—summaries and abstracts are free of charge; a subscription is required for full use of the library resources	
	Publishes the Cochrane Handbook for Systematic Reviews	
The Joanna Briggs Institute (JBI), Australia	JBI is a professional, peer-review organization	http://connect .jbiconnectplus.org
	The JBI Library of Systematic Reviews is a refereed library that publishes systematic reviews of literature; subscription is required; student rates are available	
Centre for Reviews and Dissemination (CRD), University of York, UK	The CRD is part of the National Institute for Health Research (NIHR)	http://www.york .ac.uk/inst/crd
	The CRD makes available systematic reviews on health and public health questions	
	Produces the DARE, NHS EED, and HTA databases and guidelines for undertaking systematic reviews	
The Evidence for Policy and Practice Information and Co-ordinating Centre (EPPI-Centre) at the Institute of Education, University of London	The EPPI-Centre is part of the Social Science Research Unit at the Institute of Education, University of London	http://eppi.ioe .ac.uk/cms
	Provides the main findings, technical summary, or full technical reports of individual EPP-Centre Systematic Reviews	
	Available online: Methods for a Systematic Review	

(continued)

TABLE 5.2 • Online Resources for Evidence-Based Practice (*continued*)

Organization	Description	Web Link
United States National Library of Medicine (NLM)	PubMed (which includes MEDLINE) is the NLM literature search system; it includes more than 20 million citations for biomedical literature from MEDLINE, journals, and online books and includes citations from full-text content	http://www.nlm.nih.gov
	PubMed Central (PMC) is a web-based repository of biomedical journal literature providing free, unrestricted access to more than 1.5 million full-text articles	
	Publishes and provides the following: systematic reviews, meta-analyses, reviews of clinical trials, evidence-based medicine, consensus development conferences, and guidelines	

was written. Reviews are completed using strict inclusion and exclusion criteria, and the aim is to include as much as possible of the research relevant to the research question. The overall objective of an appraisal is to assess the general strength of the evidence in relation to the particular issue studied. The Evidence for Policy and Practice Information and Co ordinating Centre at the Institute of Education, University of London, describes, in detail, the method used for conducting a comprehensive systematic review on its website (Evidence for Policy and Practice Information Coordinating Centre, 2014).

To begin, it is helpful to use a table to group and summarize information according to key areas. Table 5.3 is an example of a tool that can be used to document the critical elements of the evidence such as the design of the study, the study population, and the outcomes. It provides the APRN with a standard method for evaluating the important points gleaned from a literature search and can also act as an audit trail, so that others can judge how well the review was carried out.

An important step in the research review process is the organization and grading of the evidence using a hierarchy. The level-of-evidence approach is a useful method of ranking evidence and helps to remove subjectivity from the assessment of the evidence. In hierarchies, levels of evidence are ranked according to the strengths of the evidence. The strength of the evidence is based on the design of the study used by investigators to minimize bias. Most hierarchies classify the best evidence (studies that provide the most reliable evidence) at the top of the list and the least reliable evidence at the bottom of the list. "Grading systems allow practitioners a tool for determining the best evidence for a given practice or management strategy for a particular disease or condition" (Armola et al., 2009, p. 406).

Many groups have established hierarchies of evidence based on scientific merit. An example of some of the groups that have established hierarchies

TABLE 5.3 • Literature Review and Synthesis for Evidence-Based Practice

Clinical Question:							
Title of Article	Authors With Credentials	Question	Study Design	Level of Evidence	Description of Sample	Measures	Results

TABLE 5.4 • AACN's Evidence-Leveling System

	Description
Level A	Meta-analysis of multiple controlled studies or meta-synthesis of qualitative studies with results that consistently support a specific action, intervention or treatment
Level B	Well-designed controlled studies, both randomized and nonrandomized, with results that consistently support a specific action, intervention, or treatment
Level C	Qualitative studies, descriptive or correlational studies, integrative reviews, systematic reviews, or randomized controlled trials with inconsistent results
Level D	Peer-reviewed professional organizational standards, with clinical studies to support recommendations
Level E	Theory-based evidence from expert opinion or multiple case reports
Level M	Manufacturer's recommendation only

Source: Armola, R., Bourgault, A., Halm, M., Board, R., Bucher, L., Harrington, L., Medina, J. (2009). Upgrading the American Association of Critical-Care Nurses' evidence-leveling system. *American Journal of Critical Care*, *18*(5), 405—409. Used with permission from American Association of Critical-Care Nurses (AACN).

of evidence are as follows: The American Academy of Pediatrics, the Oncology Nursing Association, the Oxford Centre for Evidence-Based Medicine, the Cochrane Institute, and the Joanna Briggs Institute.

The AACN's evidence-leveling system shown in Table 5.4 is an example of this type of system and is a useful tool in the appraisal of research evidence. As with most hierarchal systems, the AACN system classifies the levels of evidence in descending order, with the highest level of evidence placed in Level A and the lowest in Level M.

An evidence-leveling system that includes study designs used in population research (such as case-control and cohort studies) appears in Exhibit 5.1. This system is used by the Centre for Reviews and Dissemination (CRD) at the University of York. Similar to the AACN system, it classifies levels of evidence in descending order, with well-designed RCTs at the top and case studies at the bottom.

The incorporation of many designs into a systematic review can provide valuable insight as it has a direct impact on the complexity of the information. For example, although qualitative studies are not classified as high levels of evidence, they can still provide an APRN with important information for understanding phenomena. The purpose of qualitative studies is to increase the understanding and meaning of a phenomenon when the goal is to describe or understand an experience. A classic example is a qualitative study that was carried out by Beck (1993) using grounded theory to develop an understanding of postpartum depression. Because of the nature of qualitative studies, the results cannot be generalized to the population of all women with postpartum depression; however, the publication of her results does provide the reader with a vivid description of the women in her study and an insight into how the researcher arrived at the theme of "teetering on the edge" to describe the phenomena.

Validity

Once the APRN has completed evidence collection, each individual study needs to be appraised for the internal and external validities of the design. A hallmark of good research is that it is carried out by researchers who are aware of the existence of error and who design studies in such a way that errors are minimized. Table 5.2 is a useful tool to facilitate the appraisal of evidence by providing a method to organize the individual aspects or components of the study design. The APRN needs to use this information to conduct an analysis of the information. Interpreting the findings of a study depends on the design, conduct, and analyses (internal validity), as well the populations, interventions, and outcome measures (external validity) (CRD, 2008).

When appraising the quality of a study, the APRN should attempt to assess how accurate the findings are and whether they are of relevance in the particular setting or population of interest. The appraisal should include the appropriateness of the study design to the research question, the risk of bias, the overall quality of the methods used to carry out the study, the outcome measure, the quality of the intervention, appropriateness of the analysis, the quality of the research report, and the generalizability of the results. Blegen (2009) makes an excellent point that "[p]ersons in training to conduct or apply research must understand the basis for making judgments about the strength of the evidence. It is not about qualitative or quantitative data, but whether the evidence was produced using procedures that promote certainty and to groups whose care we wish to improve" (p. 381). When assessing a qualitative study, the APRN should take into account the theory that was used in the design of the research, analysis, and interpretation of the data. The APRN also needs to decide in advance how qualitative evidence will be used. Qualitative evidence can be used along with the quantitative findings. This is sometimes referred to as "parallel synthesis" (Beck, 2009).

EXHIBIT 5.1 • Hierarchy of Study Designs Used to Assess the Effects of Interventions

Centre for Reviews and Dissemination, University of York, UK
This list is not exhaustive, but covers the main study designs.

Randomized controlled trials
The simplest form of RCT is known as the parallel group trial, which randomizes eligible participants to two or more groups, treats according to assignment, and compares the groups with respect to outcomes of interest. Participants are allocated to groups using both randomization (allocation involves the play of chance) and concealment (ensures that the intervention that will be allocated cannot be known in advance). There are different types of randomized study designs:

> *Randomized crossover trials*
> All participants receive all the interventions; for example, in a two-arm crossover trial, one group receives intervention A before intervention B, and the other group receive intervention B before intervention A. It is the sequence of interventions that is randomized.

> *Cluster randomized trials*
> A cluster randomized trial is a trial in which clusters of people, rather than single individuals, are randomized to different interventions. For example, whole clinics or geographical locations may be randomized to receive particular interventions, rather than individuals.

> *Quasi experimental studies*
> The main distinction between randomized and quasi experimental studies is the way in which participants are allocated to the intervention and control groups; quasi experimental studies do not use random assignment to create the comparison groups.

Nonrandomized controlled studies
Individuals are allocated to a concurrent comparison group, using methods other than randomization. The lack of concealed randomized allocation increases the risk of selection bias.

Before-and-after study
Comparison of outcomes in study participants before and after the introduction of an intervention. The before-and-after comparisons may be in the same sample of participants or in different samples.

Interrupted time series
Interrupted time series designs are multiple observations over time that are "interrupted," usually by an intervention or treatment.

Observational studies
A study in which natural variation in interventions or exposure among participants (i.e., not allocated by an investigator) is investigated to explore the effect of the interventions or exposure on health outcomes.

Cohort study
A defined group of participants is followed over time and comparison is made between those who did and did not receive an intervention.

Case-control study
Groups from the same population with (cases) and without (controls) a specific outcome of interest are compared to evaluate the association between exposure to an intervention and the outcome.

(continued)

EXHIBIT 5.1 • Hierarchy of Study Designs Used to Assess the Effects of Interventions (*continued*)

Case series
Description of a number of cases of an intervention and the outcome (without comparison with a control group). These are not comparative studies.

Source: Centre for Reviews and Dissemination (CRD). (2008). *Systematic reviews: CRD's guidance for undertaking reviews in healthcare [Internet]*. York: University of York. Retrieved from http://www.york.ac.uk/inst/crd/index_guidance.htm. Used with permission from Centre for Reviews and Dissemination, University of York, UK.

Nurses are often intimidated when faced with evaluating the data analysis section in a research article. An important fact to keep in mind is that statistical significance is not synonymous with proof and that sometimes overemphasis is placed on statistically significant findings. It is important to understand the significance of the results and how they apply to clinical practice. According to Hayat (2010), "Statistical significance is not an objective measure and does not provide an escape from the requirement for the researcher to think carefully and judge the clinical and practical importance of a study's results" (p. 219). The APRN should review the results section of a research report carefully to determine whether or not the method of analysis used by the researcher answers the research question(s) or hypothesis and provides enough information to support the interpretation of the results.

Transparency

Transparency is another important concept for consideration during the appraisal of research publications. Transparency in research is a reflection of both the accountability and the integrity of the investigator(s). It also takes into account the clarity and completeness of the research publication. It should be possible, for example, for the study and results to be replicated by others. There should also be a disclosure of relationships that have the potential to cause a conflict of interest. A conflict of interest may occur when a researcher's objectivity is impacted by economic (ownership of stocks or shares), commercial (payouts by companies), or personal interests (when a researcher's status may be impacted by the results of the research) (APA, 2009). For example, an investigator with ties to a company that is closely related to the area of research may stand to profit from steering the results in a particular direction. Even when investigators disclose their conflicts of interest, the APRN should critically review the research for potential bias.

Research Synthesis

The literature review not only provides a historical account of past work in the area of interest but also supports or refutes the necessity for ongoing study. The background for any study is founded on a thorough and comprehensive literature review. It serves as a justification for current research goals and introduces the reader to important past studies that have similar outcomes of comparison. Although not all studies will have an array of historical evidence in the literature, review of similar study designs or interventions can still provide a strong justification if the background is well researched.

The overall purpose of the example described earlier was to determine whether a 6-week CSMP would increase the self-efficacy of mentally ill inmates with diabetes in a state prison setting. All people with diabetes should receive care that meets national standards, and this standard should apply to those who are incarcerated as well as those who are not. The literature review revealed only a few examples of evidence-based models of self-management support delivered to prison populations, but the existing evidence indicated that this model worked well with other diabetic populations. The literature review provided evidence of potential benefit of a disease self-management program for people with diabetes, and also evidence of the relationship between self-efficacy and health behavior. Table 5.5 provides a portion of the research synthesis that was completed using the sample PICO question.

On completion of the systematic review, a proposal was written to pilot study a 6-week self-efficacy course for mentally ill inmates with diabetes. The literature review provided sufficient information to justify the pilot study of the program to corrections officials. As mentioned earlier, outcome measures were self-efficacy and hemoglobin A_{1c} levels. The CSMP proposal was successful, and after receiving a grant from the New Jersey Department of Health and Senior Services (NJDHSS) in October 2009, the CSMP was piloted in January 2010, and has provided workshops to over 1,000 inmates. The prison system currently has three certified master trainers and 50 certified peer leaders who facilitate the program. Currently, there is a waiting list for both staff peer leaders and inmate/patient participants.

There has been an improvement in both outcomes since the implementation of the program. The success of the CSMP can be attributed to the mutual support of the participants, facilitators, and providers; patient referrals from prison healthcare providers; and the collaboration with the New Jersey Department of Corrections site administrators. To assure the success of the program, all staff members were educated about the CSMP and how it would benefit their population. The medical providers were supplied with in-service education about the program. Their belief in and support of the CSMP ensured patient recruitment. Flyers were posted on all the units in the prisons, asking for patient volunteers. From one site, more than 80 requests for one group were obtained from these postings.

During the reaccreditation, the National Commission on Correctional Healthcare (NCCHC) informally commended the organization for raising the healthcare bar in the correctional system and for putting in place practices that are in keeping with the mission of providing medical services that meet or exceed community standards that are accessible, effective, compassionate, accountable, and efficient. The summation of this work from literature review, to research synthesis, to pilot project is an excellent example of how APRNs can use this approach to design interventions to improve population outcomes.

Table 5.5 • Tool Used to Assess Literature Review: Interventions, Purpose, Populations, and Outcomes

Title/Author	Description of Intervention	Purpose and Populations	Outcomes Achieved
1. American Diabetes Association. (2008). Diabetes management in correctional institutions. *Diabetes Care, 31*(Suppl. 1), S87–S93. Retrieved from http://care.diabetesjournals.org/content/31/Supplement_1/S87.full	NA	Not a study A guideline for diabetes management in prisons	NA
2. American Diabetes Association. (2008). Standards of medical care in diabetes 2008. *Diabetes Care, 31*, S12–S54.	NA	Not a study 2008 standards for diabetes care	NA
3. Chiverton, P., Linley P., Tortoretti, D. M., & Plum, K. C. (2007). Well balanced: 8 steps to wellness for adults with mental illness and diabetes [Journal Article, Pictorial, Research, Tables/Charts]. *Journal of Psychosocial Nursing and Mental Health Services, 45*(11), 46–55.	A well-balanced program incorporated health promotion, disease management, and evidence-based practice guideline into a 16-week, 8-steps-to-wellness program for a community-based mental health population.	Seventy-four adults with both serious mental illness and diabetes were evaluated using nursing wellness 8-step model.	Improvements of health risk status, decreased hemoglobin A_{1c} (HbA_{1c}) levels, and an increased satisfaction with the program were noted.

(continued)

Table 5.5 • Tool Used to Assess Literature Review: Interventions, Purpose, Populations, and Outcomes (continued)

Title/Author	Description of Intervention	Purpose and Populations	Outcomes Achieved
4. Chodosh, J., Morton, S. C., Mojica, W., Maglione, M., Suttorp, M. J., Hilton, L., . . . Shekelle, P. (2005). Meta-analysis: Chronic disease self-management programs for older adults. [Meta-Analysis Research Support, U.S. Gov't, Non-P.H.S.]. *Annals of Internal Medicine, 143*(6), 427–438.	To determine the efficacy and important components of CSMP for older adults with diabetes. meta-analysis searched multiple sources dated through Sept 2004; Two reviewers independently identified trials and extracted data.	Meta-analysis searched multiple sources dated through Sept 2004; all RCTs were eligible for inclusion that compared outcomes of self-management interventions with a control or with usual care for diabetes mellitus (DM).	Self-management intervention led to a statistically and clinically significant decrease in HBA$_{1c}$ levels of about 0.81%.
5. Clark, B. (2006). Diabetes care in the San Francisco County Jail [Journal Article, Research, Tables/Charts]. *American Journal of Public Health, 96*(9), 1571–1574.	Retrospective chart review of electronic medical records for 200 inmates identified as diabetic in the San Francisco County Jail system in 2003. The researches systematically sampled 200 inmates from those who met the criteria.	To examine care guideline adherence within the correctional institute. Eligible inmates for inclusion had at least one jail stay of 72 hours or greater and a diagnosis of DM in the medical record, or were prescribed any formulary medications for diabetes.	Of 424 inmates with diabetes, 200 were assessed. Bivariate analysis showed no evidence that adherence rates varied by race, gender, or age; longer stays were associated with greater adherence. A fairly low percentage of diabetic inmates had either HbA$_{1c}$ or lipid profiles checked, although this increased proportionally for those incarcerated longer than 30 days.

(continued)

Title/Author	Description of Intervention	Purpose and Populations	Outcomes Achieved
6. Conklin, T. (2000). Self-reported health and prior health behaviors of newly admitted correctional inmates. *American Journal of Public Health*, 90(12), 1939–1941.	Interviews were conducted with 1,198 inmates on day 3 of incarceration; the 15-minute interviews were conducted in a private room; 130 questions on demographic, household data, health status, health problems, medical facility use, tobacco, alcohol, drug, HIV, other sexually transmitted infections, sexual behavior, prior jail time, and physical abuse were included.	Conducted a baseline health study to better elucidate the extent of inmate preincarceration health problems, health facility use, and health-related risky behaviors. All inmates newly admitted to the facility over a 5-month period were interviewed on their 3rd day of stay.	Data showed that newly incarcerated inmates have a high prevalence of health issues at admission, prior limited access to healthcare, and very high rates of disease and unhealthy behaviors; results of interviews confirmed the significant need for medical, mental, dental, and substance abuse healthcare, with additional prevention and education programs to modify risky health behaviors.
7. Deakin, T. (2005). Group based training for self-management strategies in people with type 2 diabetes mellitus. [Meta-Analysis Review]. *Cochrane Database of Systematic Reviews*, (2), CD003417.	Randomized controlled and controlled clinical trials that evaluated group-based education programs for adults with type 2 diabetes compared with routine treatment. Studies obtained from computerized searches of electronic databases, supplemented by hand searches of reference lists of articles, conference proceedings, and consultation with experts in the field.	To assess the effects of group-based, patient-centered training on clinical, lifestyle, and psychosocial outcomes in people with type 2 diabetes. Studies were only included if the length of the program included follow-up of 6 months or more, and the intervention was at least one session with a minimum of six participants.	Fourteen publications describing 11 studies were included involving over 1,532 participants; the results of the meta-analysis favored the group-based diabetes education programs as reductions in HbA_{1c} were seen. Group-based training for self-management strategies in people with type 2 diabetes were shown to be effective by improving fasting blood glucose levels, HbA_{1c} and diabetes knowledge and reducing systolic blood pressure levels, body weight, and the required diabetes medication.

(continued)

Table 5.5 • Tool Used to Assess Literature Review: Interventions, Purpose, Populations, and Outcomes (*continued*)

Title/Author	Description of Intervention	Purpose and Populations	Outcomes Achieved
8. D'Eramo. (2004). A culturally competent intervention of education and care for black women with type 2 diabetes. [Clinical Trial, Controlled Clinical Trial]. *Applied Nursing Research*, 17(1), 10–20.	A 6-week cognitive behavioral culturally competent DM intervention program was developed and led by an APRN trained in DM care and certified as a DM educator. The Cross Cultural Counseling: A guide for Nutrition and Health Counselors (1987) was used for training and intervention. By using one group, pretest and posttest quasi experimental design, the pilot was tested for feasibility. Twenty-five women were recruited from a local urban community using multiple recruitment strategies such as numerous newspaper and radio announcements, flyers, public-access television announcements, and churches.	This article reports on a pilot feasibility testing of a culturally competent intervention for the education and care of Black women with type 2 DM (CT2DM). Eligible participants were English speaking, between 18 and 60 years old, who had a primary care provider and were diagnosed with type 2 DM and were receiving insulin therapy; excluded persons included anyone who was pregnant or breastfeeding, who had comorbidities or diabetes-related complications such as visual impairment that prevented independence, end-stage renal disease, or lower extremity amputations.	The findings suggested that using a culturally sensitive intervention of nurse practitioners providing diabetes care and education is beneficial for Black women with type 2 DM, resulting in consistent program attendance, fewer missed appointments, improved glycemic control and weight, and decreased diabetes-related emotional distress.

(continued)

Title/Author	Description of Intervention	Purpose and Populations	Outcomes Achieved
9. Duncan, E. (2006). A systematic review of structured group interventions with mentally disordered offenders [Research Support, Non-U.S. Gov't Review]. *Criminal Behaviour & Mental Health, 16*(4), 217–241.	Twenty studies were retrieved that fulfilled the inclusion criteria. All included studies were of participants in hospital settings. Ten of these studies were conducted in British high-security hospitals and six in British medium-security hospital units. The remaining four studies were conducted in Canada or the United States, two of which were unclear regarding the level of security at the location where their study was undertaken.	To evaluate structured group interventions with mentally disordered offenders through systematic review of the evidence for their efficacy and effectiveness Inclusion criteria: 1. Evaluation of the efficacy or effectiveness of structured single-form group interventions applied specifically to offenders with mental disorder. 2. Evaluation of the efficacy or effectiveness of structured complex group interventions applied specifically to offenders with mental disorder. Studies published in English.	Twenty-two studies were retrieved that fitted the inclusion criteria. Four main themes were dominant: problem solving, anger/aggression management, self-harm, and others. Calculated effect sizes gave optimism for the efficacy of structured group interventions with mentally disordered offenders. This review confirmed that there has been some useful research into structured group therapy interventions with mentally disordered offenders.
10. El-Mallakh, P. (2006). Evolving self-care in individuals with schizophrenia and diabetes mellitus [Journal Article, Research, Tables/Charts]. *Archives of Psychiatric Nursing, 20*(2), 55–64.	Clients recruited from five sites of a regional community mental health center The study did not go into detail on how the respondents were chosen. Twenty-six interviews were conducted among 11 respondents with various degrees of ability to care for their coexisting illnesses.	Inclusion criteria: having a comorbid diagnosis of schizophrenia and type 1 or 2 diabetes, self-reported involvement in daily diabetic self-care activities, between the ages of 18 and 72. Exclusion criteria: having any medical problem that prevented the client from participating in the interview and the inability to understand the study's purpose and procedures.	A theoretical self-care model "Evolving self-care for schizophrenia and diabetes" was developed. Findings suggested that the respondents developed realistic and informed self-care health beliefs that accurately reflected knowledge and experiences with self-care of comorbid illnesses.

Source: Conrad, M. (2008). *The effectiveness of a chronic disease self-management program for mentally ill inmates with diabetes.* Unpublished doctoral capstone project, University of Medicine and Dentistry of New Jersey—School of Nursing, Newark, NJ.

INTEGRATION OF EVIDENCE INTO PRACTICE

Time lags commonly occur when applying new research findings to clinical practice. This is the time period between the discovery that an intervention works and the application of new knowledge into actual practice. In 1999, the American Society of Anesthesiology (ASA) revised its practice guidelines for preoperative fasting in healthy patients undergoing elective procedures. "The newer, more liberal recommendations, based on studies showing that pulmonary aspiration occurs only rarely as a complication of modern anesthesia, allow the consumption of clear liquids up to two hours before elective surgery, a light breakfast (tea and toast, for example) six hours before the procedure, and a heavier meal eight hours beforehand" (Crenshaw & Winslow, 2002, p. 36). Crenshaw and Winslow carried out a study to determine whether the guidelines were being followed. They interviewed 155 patients in one hospital about their preoperative fasting, comparing preoperative instructions for fasting, actual preoperative fasting, and ASA-recommended fasting durations for liquids and solids. They found that the majority of patients continued to receive instructions to fast (NPO [nothing per os]) after midnight for both liquids and solids, whether they were scheduled for early or late surgery. They also discovered that, on average, the patients fasted from liquids and solids for 12 hours and 14 hours, respectively, with some patients fasting as long as 20 hours from liquids and 37 hours from solids. These fasts were significantly longer than those recommended by the ASA. Clearly, in this case, the authors discovered a significant lag time between the generation of new knowledge and the implementation of that knowledge into practice.

In 2004, the authors carried out a follow-up study to determine whether the implementation of an evidence-based preoperative fasting policy and the education of healthcare practitioners had improved fasting practices at their facility (Crenshaw & Winslow, 2008). Unfortunately, they determined that unsafe preoperative fasting persisted, although they did find an improvement in the percentage of patients who received instructions on taking medications preoperatively. The authors identified the difficulty of changing entrenched traditions as one reason that preoperative fasting in excess of evidence-based recommendations persisted.

Makic, VonRueden, Rauen, and Chadwick (2011) describe seven practices in nursing that persist in practice despite a lack of evidence that they are effective (and in some cases, evidence that they are harmful). They label these practices "sacred cows." One example that they discuss is the Trendelenburg position for hypotension. They cite studies from as early as 1956 that question its use in hypotension, and point out that a review of the literature indicates that "the evidence does not support the use of the head-down tilt for hypotension" (p. 41). Yet this practice persists in nursing. These are just a couple of examples of the time lag between research and practice and of the difficulty changing traditional practices.

In order to effect change, the APRN needs to understand why these time intervals exist between the development of new knowledge and the incorporation of that knowledge into practice. Investigators have examined the reasons for nurses not keeping up to date in their practice. Jacobson, Ross, and Pravikoff (2005) completed a study to investigate what determines usual nursing practice. They discovered that most nurses practice what they learned in school. Because the average age of nurses at the time the study was completed was more than 40 years, this meant that the majority of nurses in the study had graduated before 1990, making much of what they learned in school out of date. Although nurses in the study acknowledged that an evidence-based practice is important, they expressed discomfort in using health-related data-bases; in fact, the study revealed that 76% of the respondents had apparently never searched CINAHL and 58% had never searched MEDLINE.

A qualitative study of two primary care practices was conducted by Gabbay and le May (2004). The objective of the study was to explore how primary care clinicians derive their healthcare decisions. The results revealed that clinicians rarely accessed or used current evidence but instead relied on what the authors labeled "mindlines." The authors describe mindlines as "internalized guidelines that are formed primarily from interactions with col-leagues and people perceived as opinion leaders." They arise from experience and trusted personal sources. The authors further describe this tendency as "day to day practice based on socially constituted knowledge" (p. 1015).

Makic et al. (2011) quoted Thomas Paine, who in 1776 said, "A long habit of not thinking a thing wrong, gives it a superficial appearance of being right" (p. 58). They point out that tradition is a difficult barrier to overcome, that nurs-ing practice is dynamic, and that science is constantly evolving. Nurses need to question practices based on tradition and instead use evidence whenever pos-sible to guide nursing practice. Depending on the focus of their advanced de-grees, APRNs are educated to fill the roles of highly skilled practitioners and/ or leaders and educators in their fields of expertise. They are in a position to educate other providers, work with direct care nurses to identify and remove barriers to evidence-based practice, and disseminate information. They also receive advanced education in research, and because of this, they are uniquely qualified not only to implement evidence-based care but also to guide direct care nurses in developing PICO questions, searching and synthesizing the lit-erature, and changing practice interventions to reflect current knowledge.

Models of Practice

Several models have been created to facilitate the implementation of evidence-based practice. They provide an organized approach for integrating and sus-taining change. A practice model ensures that professional nursing practice is consistent and minimizes practice variations that can create risk and gaps in care. Some examples of the models in use are the Advancing Research and Clinical Practice through Close Collaboration (ARCC) Model, the Johns Hopkins Nursing Model, the Chronic Care Model (CCM), and the Iowa Model of Evidence-Based Practice to Promote Quality of Care. The overriding characteristic of each is that it provides a structured method for incorporating best evidence into practice.

The focus of the ARCC Model is to bring research experts together with direct care nurses to integrate research with practice. It was developed by Ber-nadette Melnyk and the faculty of the School of Nursing at the University of Rochester, in its School of Medicine and Dentistry, and with community partners. It was originally designed to bring academic communities together with healthcare organizations that provide both acute and community-based care. The APRN as mentor plays a prominent role in this model. An important component is education on evidence-based practice. Fineout-Overholt, Levin, and Melnyk (2004–2005) carried out a study to test the ARCC Model in two pediatric units at acute care facilities. The authors identified the following key strategies for implementing evidence-based practice: administrative support, creation of a clear role for nurses that includes evidence-based practice, adequate infrastructure (such as computer resources and databases), evidence-based practice mentors to work directly with direct care nurses, time and money to carry out studies, and creation of an evidence-based practice culture. Direct care nurses on the study units talked about the importance of working with APRNs to bring about evidence-based practice as opposed to simply being told what to do. The authors point out that APRNs can act as information brokers to create changes based on evidence-based practice while working closely with direct care nurses.

Similar to the ARCC Model, the origin of the Johns Hopkins Nursing Model can be found in a partnership with an academic institution. It was developed in collaboration with the Johns Hopkins Hospital and the Johns Hopkins University School of Nursing. "PET" is an acronym that describes the process used in this model. It stands for practice question, evidence, and translation. The essential cornerstones of the model are practice, education, and research, and the core of the model is evidence. It was developed to ensure that evidence was incorporated into practice (Newhouse, Dearholt, Poe, Pugh, & White, 2007).

The CCM (Group Health Research Institute, 2014) employs a holistic approach to chronic disease management through the use of evidence-based practice. It summarizes the basic elements for improving care in health systems at the community, organization, practice, and patient levels. It has six components: the healthcare delivery system, community, patient self-management support, decision support, delivery system design, and clinical information system. The emphasis of the model is on health promotion. O'Toole et al. (2010) investigated the use of this model in providing primary care to homeless veterans. They used a retrospective cohort design to compare veterans who received their primary care in a clinic that used the CCM to a matched cohort of veterans who received their primary care in "usual care" clinics. Veterans enrolled in the clinic using the CCM for delivery of primary care had fewer emergency department visits and greater improvements in blood pressure and low-density lipoproteins than did the control cohort. The authors cited the importance of the location of the clinic (the clinic was located in an urban Virginia hospital so that it was geographically convenient) and of tailoring interventions to the target population (the clinic addressed issues such as the need for housing and food). They concluded that how primary care is delivered and organized is important in chronic disease management.

The Iowa Model of Evidence-Based Practice to Promote Quality of Care was "developed to serve as a guide for nurses and other healthcare providers to use research findings for improvement of patient care" (Titler et al., 2001, p. 498). Case Study 5.1 presents an example of how one clinic used the Iowa Model to improve practice and population outcomes. Important features of the model are decision points and feedback loops that are characteristic of the ongoing process of improving care through research. Once a problem or new information is identified (step 1), a team is formed to investigate the issue (step 2). A literature review is conducted, and the information is evaluated, critiqued, and synthesized for use in practice (step 3). If the evidence is judged to be sufficient for a change in practice, the change is piloted and monitored. If there is not sufficient evidence to pilot a change, the team may decide to conduct a research study (step 4). Once the evidence is deemed sufficient for a permanent adoption, the organization can move forward to institute the change in practice. The purpose of a pilot is not to test the effectiveness of the intervention but to test whether the intervention is feasible. After a determination is made to change practice, the organization continues to monitor structure, process, and outcome data. Case Study 5.1 illustrates how using a practice model can facilitate change in a clinic setting that ultimately leads to improved patient outcomes.

Ultimately, APRNs need to determine which practice model will best suit their needs. Schaffer, Sandau, and Diedrick (2013) conducted an extensive literature review of practice models. They examined the key factors (characteristics) and usefulness of several. They concluded that in selecting a practice model, nurses should consider "how the model facilitates EBP projects, provides guidelines for evidence critique, guides the process for implementing practice change, and can be used across practice areas" (p. 1206). Their guidelines can be used to help APRNs select a practice model.

CASE STUDY 5.1 • **Use of the Iowa Model to Increase Breastfeeding Initiation Rates of Urban Clinic Mothers**

Trigger
Nurses working in a perinatal clinic determined that the rate of breastfeeding initiation for their patients was 40%. The clinic provides prenatal and maternity services to an ethnically diverse, inner-city population in the northeastern United States.

Form team
A team was created that included a clinical nurse specialist (CNS), the case managers for the perinatal clinic, and a lactation nurse specialist.

Assemble relevant research and related literature
A literature review was carried out by the CNS and the lactation nurse and more than 30 articles were retrieved and appraised.

Critique/synthesize information
The literature search revealed information on the benefits of breastfeeding, breastfeeding rates among inner-city populations, research on effective strategies for increasing rates, and culturally appropriate materials for teaching.
    Among the key findings:
- Breastfeeding can reduce the incidence of many disease states in childhood and throughout adulthood, such as diabetes, sudden infant death syndrome (SIDS), ear infections, allergies, asthma, and obesity (American Academy of Pediatrics, 1999; Chulada, Arbes, Dunson, & Zeldin, 2003).
- The opinions of healthcare providers regarding breastfeeding have enormous impact on urban women, their partners, and families (Philipp, Merewood, Gerendas, & Bauchner, 2004).

(continued)

CASE STUDY 5.1 • Use of the Iowa Model to Increase Breastfeeding Initiation Rates of Urban Clinic Mothers (*continued*)

- Methods to increase the rates of breastfeeding have been unsuccessful for African Americans because these methods are not culturally sensitive (African American Breastfeeding Alliance, 2005).
- The information was summarized, shared, and discussed with team members. The team created a plan to increase the breastfeeding rates of the clinic population.

Pilot change and carryout study

The clinic initiated education programs for clinic staff and community providers and increased lactation services. The clinic environment was changed to include sensitive pictures of ethnically diverse breastfeeding mothers, and improvements were made in bilingual educational brochures. Each clinic counselor was given a protocol book describing specific literature, videos, and discussion to be provided to patients at each trimester. The healthcare providers documented the education that was provided to each patient, and patients completed a postpartum questionnaire that was used to evaluate interventions and factors influencing feeding choice.

Determine whether the change is appropriate for adoption in practice

Five years after the initiation of the evidence-based change, breastfeeding initiation rates had increased to 70%. Analysis of the patient evaluations revealed that counseling and reading material were cited as the most influential factors in making the choice to breastfeed. Other important factors were the opinions of family and healthcare professionals.

The nurses determined that prenatal education interventions that address varied learning styles and delivered in defined segments may be effective in influencing the feeding decisions of new mothers. The educational programs must be culturally sensitive, and staff education is vital to ensure effective and accurate delivery of information.

Continue to monitor structure, process, and outcome data

The team has continued to monitor lactation rates and to review new information on lactation education as it has become available. Educational materials are updated on a regular basis. Eight years after the start of the initiative, their breastfeeding rates placed the hospital among the top 10 in the state. The clinic and its associated hospital achieved Baby-Friendly Designation in 2012, the second in the state. In order to achieve this goal, the clinic needed to demonstrate that they have integrated the "10 Steps to Successful Breast-feeding" into their practice for healthy newborns (Baby Friendly USA, 2010).

Adapted from Procaccini, D., & Mahony, J. (2014). *Survey of educational interventions to increase the breastfeeding initiation rates of urban clinic mothers.* Unpublished manuscript.

SUMMARY

The use of research evidence to guide practice can lead to the implementation of interventions that will improve population outcomes, but this is a complex process. The ability to identify clinical problems and issues, ask clinical questions in a format that allows for study, conduct a search of the literature, appraise and synthesize the available evidence, and successfully integrate new knowledge into practice requires specialized skills and knowledge. This process can be challenging and time-consuming. Researchers have identified many barriers to evidence-based practice, including the lack of belief by practicing nurses that research can make a real difference. APRNs are uniquely situated to influence care through their roles as leaders, educators, and clinical experts. This chapter described some of the basic skills needed to integrate and synthesize information in order to design interventions that are based on evidence to improve population outcomes. APRNs need to use their specialized knowledge and advanced practice roles to identify the barriers to evidence-based practice in order to build the capacity to adopt change. They also require the ability to involve individuals, teams, and organizations in the process. By adopting a culture of evidence-based practice in the work environment, APRNs have the opportunity to facilitate change that can lead to improved quality of care.

EXERCISES AND DISCUSSION QUESTIONS

Exercise 5.1 Write a clinical question using the PICO format.

Exercise 5.2 Carry out a literature review for one of the PICO questions you wrote in Exercise 5.1.
- Establish criteria for inclusion and exclusion of studies.
- Synthesize and appraise the information using Table 5.3.

Exercise 5.3 Determine whether or not you have enough evidence to change current practice using the question from Exercise 5.1.
- Will you need to conduct a study in order to test the effectiveness of the intervention? Provide your rationale.
- If you need to conduct a study, describe the method that you will use to evaluate the effectiveness of the intervention.
- Describe what outcomes of interest you will identify in your study.

Exercise 5.4 Describe how you will incorporate this change into practice.

REFERENCES

African American Breastfeeding Alliance. (2004). *An easy guide to breastfeeding for African American women*. Retrieved November 21, 2005, from http://www.aabaonline.com

American Academy of Pediatrics. (1999). 10 Steps to supporting a parents' choice to breastfeed their baby. In *AAP Task Force on Breastfeeding* (pp. 1–5). Washington, DC: Author.

American Association of Colleges of Nursing. (2006). *The essentials of doctoral education for advanced practice nursing*. Retrieved from http://www.aacn.nche.edu/DNP/pdf/Essentials.pdf

American Psychological Association. (2009). *Publication manual of the American psychological association* (6th ed.). Washington, DC: Author.

Armola, R., Bourgault, A., Halm, M., Board, R., Bucher, L., Harrington, L., . . . Medina, J. (2009). Upgrading the American association of critical-care nurses' evidence-leveling system. *American Journal of Critical Care, 18*(5), 405–409.

Baby Friendly USA. (2010). Ten steps to successful breast feeding. Retrieved from http://babyfriendlyusa.org/

Beck, C. T. (1993). Teetering on the edge: A substantive theory of post partum depression. *Nursing Research, 42*(1), 42–48.

Beck, C. T. (2009). Metasynthesis: A goldmine for evidence-based practice. *Association of Operating Room Nurses Journal, 90*(5), 701–710.

Blegen, M. (2009). Qualitative or quantitative is beside the point. *Nursing Research, 58*(6), 381.

Centre for Reviews and Dissemination. (2008). Systematic reviews: CRD's guidance for undertaking reviews in health care [Internet]. York, UK: University of York. Retrieved from http://www.york.ac.uk/inst/crd/index_guidance.htm

Chulada, P. C., Arbes, S. J., Dunson, D., & Zeldin, D. C. (2003). Breast-feeding and the prevalence of asthma and wheeze in children: Analyses the Third National Health and Nutrition Examination Survey, 1988–1994. *Journal of Allergy and Clinical Immunology, 111*(2), 328–236.

The Cochrane Collaboration. (2014). *About us.* Retrieved from http://www.cochrane.org/about-us

Conrad, M. (2008). *The effectiveness of a chronic disease self-management program for mentally ill inmates with diabetes* (Unpublished doctoral capstone project). Newark, NJ: University of Medicine and Dentistry of New Jersey—School of Nursing.

Crenshaw, J. T., & Winslow, E. H. (2002). Preoperative fasting: Old habits die hard. *American Journal of Nursing, 102*(5), 36–44.

Crenshaw, J. T., & Winslow, E. H. (2008). Preoperative fasting duration and medication instruction: Are we improving? *Association of Operating Room Nurses Journal, 88*(6), 963–976.

DeBourgh, G. (2001). Champions for evidence-based practice: A critical role for advanced practice nurses. *AACN Clinical Issues, 12*(4), 491–508.

EBSCO Publishing. (2014). *CINAHL databases.* Retrieved from http://www.ebscohost.com/nursing/products/cinahl-databases

Editors of the American Heritage Dictionaries. (2000). *The American Heritage Dictionary of the English Language* (4th ed.). Boston, MA: Houghton Mifflin.

Evidence for Policy and Practice Information Coordinating Centre. (2014). *EPPI-Centre methods for conducting systematic reviews.* Retrieved from http://eppi.ioe.ac.uk/cms/LinkClick.aspx?fileticket=hQBu8y4uVwI%3d&tabid=88

Fineout-Overholt, E., Levin, R. F., & Melnyk, B. (2004–2005). Strategies for advancing evidence-based practice in clinical settings. *Journal of the New York Nurses' Association, 35*(2), 8–32.

Gabbay, J., & le May, A. (2004). Evidence based guidelines or collectively constructed "mindlines?" Ethnographic study of knowledge management in primary care. *British Medical Journal, 329*, 1013–1017.

Group Health Research Institute. (2014). *The chronic care model.* Retrieved from http://www.improvingchroniccare.org/index.php?p=Model_Elements&s=18

Hallyburton, A., & St. John, B. (2010). Partnering with your library to strengthen nursing research. *Journal of Nursing Education, 49*(3), 164–167.

Hayat, M. (2010). Understanding statistical significance. *Nursing Research, 59*(3), 219–223.

Houde, S. C. (2009). The systematic review of the literature: A tool for evidence-based policy. *Journal of Gerontological Nursing, 35*(9), 9–12.

Jacobson, A., Ross, J., & Pravikoff, D. (2005). Evidence-based nursing… "Readiness of U.S. nurses for evidence-based practice" (Original research). *American Journal of Nursing, 105*(12), 15, 40–51.

The Joanna Briggs Institute. (2014). *About us.* Retrieved from http://joannabriggs.org/about.html

Lansing Community College Library. (2014). *What is PICOT?* Retrieved from http://libguides.lcc.edu/content.php?pid=280891&sid=2313384

Lippincott Williams & Wilkins (LWW). *Best practices: Evidence-based nursing procedures.* (2007). Philadelphia, PA: Lippincott Williams & Wilkins. Retrieved December 7, 2014, from http://www.r2library.com/Resource/Title/158255532X

Makic, M. F., VonRueden, K. T., Rauen, C. A., & Chadwick, J. (2011). Evidence-based practice habits: Putting more sacred cows out to pasture. *Critical Care Nurse, 31*(2), 38–62. doi:10.4037/ccn2011908

Melnyk, B., & Fineout-Overholt, E. (2005). Evidence-based practice. Rapid critical appraisal of randomized controlled trials (RCTs): An essential skill for evidence-based practice (EBP). *Pediatric Nursing, 31*(1), 50–52.

Melnyk, B. M., & Fineout-Overholt, E. (2010). *Evidence-based practice in nursing and healthcare: A guide to best practice* (2nd ed.). Philadelphia, PA: Wolters Kluwer Health/Lippincott Williams & Wilkins.

Newhouse, R. P., Dearholt, S. L., Poe, S. S., Pugh, L. C., & White, K. M. (2007). *Johns Hopkins nursing evidence-based practice model and guidelines.* Indianapolis, IN: Sigma Theta Tau International.

O'Toole, T., Buckel, L., Bourgault, C., Redihan, S., Jiang, L., & Friedman, P. (2010) Applying the chronic care model to homeless veterans: Effect of a population approach to primary care on utilization and clinical outcomes. *American Journal of Public Health, 100*(12), 2493–2499.

Philipp, B. L., Merewood, A., Gerendas, E. J., & Bauchner, H. (2004). Breastfeeding information in pediatric textbooks needs improvement. *Journal of Human Lactation, 20*(2), 206–210.

Polit, D., & Beck, C. T. (2012). *Nursing research: generating and assessing evidence for nursing practice* (9th ed.). Philadelphia, PA: Wolters Kluwer Health/Lippincott Williams & Wilkins.

Porter-O'Grady, T. (2003). Nurses as knowledge workers. *Creative Nursing, 9*(2), 6–9.

Procaccini, D., & Mahony, J. (2014). *Survey of educational interventions to increase the breastfeeding initiation rates of urban clinic mothers.* Unpublished manuscript.

Schaffer, M. A., Sandau, K. E., & Diedrick, L. (2013). Evidence-based practice models for organizational change: overview and practical applications. *Journal of Advanced Nursing, 69*(5), 1197–1209. doi:10.1111/j.1365-2648.2012.06122.x

Shapiro, S., & Donaldson, N. (2008). Evidence-based practice for advanced practice emergency nurses, Part II: Critically appraising the literature. *Advanced Emergency Nursing Journal, 30*(2), 139–150.

Titler, M., Kleiber, C., Steelman, V., Rakel, B., Budreau, G., Everett, C., . . . Goode C. J. (2001). The Iowa model of evidence-based practice to promote quality care. *Critical Care Nursing Clinics of North America, 13*(4), 497–509.

U.S. National Library of Medicine. (2014). *About the National Library of Medicine.* Retrieved from http://www.nlm.nih.gov/about/index.html

Using Information Systems to Improve Population Outcomes

Ann L. Cupp Curley and David W. Unkle

People access the World Wide Web every day to obtain health information. It is an increasingly popular source of information for both healthcare providers and consumers. According to Internet World Stats (2014), there are over 310,000,000 Internet users in North America, with another 2.7 billion plus users worldwide. In North America, there are over 182,000,000 people on Facebook, whereas outside of North America there are almost 800,000,000 people on Facebook. Among working adults, 50% feel that the Internet is an important part of doing their job.

All of the chapters in this text describe Internet resources and/or online references that are useful for advanced practice registered nurses (APRNs). From online databases that can be used for literature reviews to support evidence-based practice to integrated electronic healthcare records, modern technology provides the APRN with valuable and useful resources. The fourth competency for the doctor of nursing practice (DNP) degree as outlined by the American Association of Colleges of Nursing (AACN, 2006) states, "DNP graduates are distinguished by their abilities to use information systems/ technology to support and improve patient care and healthcare systems, and provide leadership within healthcare systems and/or academic settings" (p. 12). This chapter describes resources that can be found on the Internet and how to evaluate them for quality. It also describes how technology can be used to enhance population-based nursing.

USE OF THE INTERNET TO OBTAIN HEALTH INFORMATION

There are a variety of ways to access information on the Internet. Once available almost exclusively on personal computers, people can now also use smartphones and tablet computers to access health information. According to the Pew Research Center (2013a), 87% of U.S. adults use the Internet and 72% of Internet users report that they have searched online for health information. About 50% of these users report searching for information on behalf of someone else. Information on specific diseases or conditions, treatments or procedures, and searching for physicians or other health professionals are the top topics for research on the Internet. Thirty-five percent of U.S. adults have used the Internet for diagnostic purposes, for themselves or for someone they know. People with chronic conditions are more likely than people without chronic conditions to track symptoms, and people with more than one chronic condition (62%) are more likely to do so than people with one (40%).

There is robust evidence that people around the world use the Internet to obtain health-related information and that this trend is growing. In 2010, 17% of people who owned a cell phone in the United States used it to search for health information online. By 2012, that number had increased to 31%. Among smartphone owners, 52% have reported using their phone to find health or medical information and 19% have downloaded an app to track health or medical information (Pew Research Center, 2013b). An annual survey of breast cancer patients in Germany revealed that the percentage of such patients who searched disease-specific information on the Internet increased significantly from 27% in 2007 to 37% in 2013 (Kowalski, Kahana, Kuhr, Ansmann, & Pfaff, 2014). An international survey commissioned by researchers at the London School of Economics determined that 81% of people with access to the Internet use it to search for advice about health, medicine, and medical conditions, but only about 25% of these users check where the information comes from. The countries that were surveyed for this study included Australia, Brazil, China, France, Germany, India, Italy, Mexico, Russia, Spain, the United Kingdom, and the United States (McDaid & Park, 2010).

There is also ample evidence that certain groups of people are more likely to access the Internet for health information than others. *Digital divide* is the term used to describe disparities in the use of the Internet and other forms of technology. The Pew Internet Project tracks Internet use in many fields, including healthcare. Findings from a U.S. survey completed in 2013 reveal that 29% of people who live in the United States and who prefer to speak or use Spanish are not Internet users, compared with 14% of all U.S. adults. The digital divide can also be defined by age (younger people are more likely to use the Internet than older people), income (wealthier people are more likely to use the Internet than less wealthy people), geography (people living in urban or suburban areas are more likely to use the Internet than people in rural areas), and education (people who use the Internet tend to have attained higher degrees than people who do not) (Pew Research Center, 2013b). APRNs need to know the patterns of Internet use among different aggregates and the types of technology favored by different groups in order to be proactive in educating patients on using the Internet safely and in designing effective and innovative interventions using technology.

The Internet has revolutionized the way that consumers access information and communicate with each other. This is important, because it provides APRNs with fundamental information on who uses the Internet, what types of information they are looking for, and what types of devices and methods they use to search for information. Advances in technology have made it faster and easier than ever before to find information. It is a mistake to believe that people rely solely on healthcare providers for information regarding their health or that they will always confirm the accuracy of what they have found on the Internet with their healthcare provider. Although there is a lot of information on the Internet that is valuable and of high quality, some of the information is dubious at best. It is clear that a digital divide exists and that APRNs need to be aware of this disparity. APRNs also need to acquire the skills to improve access to health technology for populations. It is for these reasons that APRNs need to be proactive in talking to patients about their use of the Internet and other new technologies to better serve and manage their healthcare needs. They need to complete their own assessment of the populations to whom they provide care. When researchers investigated the use of Internet and mobile technology by a population of parents using pediatric care centers that serve primarily urban, low-income, African American patients, they found that a large majority (97.0%) reported owning a cell phone and that of those, 91.1% used their phone to text and 78.5% used it to access the Internet. Although these patients used technology primarily for social networking, the researchers determined that most parents were interested in receiving health information or utilizing social networking to learn more about health topics. They concluded that "[m]obile technology and social networks may be an underutilized method of providing health information to underserved minority populations" (Mitchell, Godoy, Shabazz, & Horn, 2014). This example illustrates how important it is for APRNs to assess the populations that they serve to determine how useful technology might be in providing services.

Accuracy of Internet Sites

APRNs need to be confident that when they direct patients to websites for health information, those sites are current and maintained by a reliable source. They also need to educate patients on how to evaluate Internet resources. An interesting additional finding of the Pew Internet Project is that 42% of all adults report that they or someone they know has been helped by following medical advice or health information found on the Internet, whereas 3% of all adults say they or someone they know has been harmed by following medical advice or health information found on the Internet (Pew Research Center, 2008). In fact, studies show that the Internet provides both accurate and inaccurate information. It is equally important to note that a benefit of obtaining health information on the Internet is that it is more readily accessible, especially for some patients, than access to a physician. Various social networking sites and communication methods, such as Facebook, LinkedIn, Pinterest, Tumblr, Twitter, Instagram, e-mail, chat rooms, and texting, can also be used to exchange information with other people with similar health conditions.

Another report from the Pew Research Center (2011), *Peer to Peer Health-care*, describes the results of a survey intended to determine how people use technology to talk to people with similar problems. One of the revealing findings is that one in four Internet users with chronic conditions, such as high blood pressure and cancer, goes online to find people with similar conditions. Only 15% of Internet users who do not have a chronic health condition have sought similar help online. Other people whom the survey identified as going online to share health concerns are those who have suffered a recent medical crisis or who have had a significant change in health status (Pew Research Center, 2011).

There are many studies that illustrate the importance of being vigilant in knowing the patterns of Internet use by consumers. Modave, Shokar, Penaranda, and Nguyen (2014) completed an analysis of Internet sites that provide information on weight loss. Of the 103 websites that were analyzed, none scored the optimal 16 points on the researchers' scale. Only 5% of the websites scored at least an 8/12 on the section measuring physical activity, behavior, and nutrition content. Although government and university websites scored the highest on the researchers' evaluation scale, these sites tended to appear on pages 2 or 3 of the search. The researchers noted that the information that was most likely to be accessed by searchers is substandard because quality sites posted further down in the search. Moore and Ayers (2011) completed a systematic review to identify websites related to postnatal mental health for both healthcare professionals and patients. Although they were able to identify a number of useful websites based on an evaluation of the accuracy of information, availability of resources, and overall quality, they found that information on many of the sites was incomplete, difficult to read, and of variable quality.

Chan et al. (2012) searched the Internet using three different Internet search engines for websites that provide health-related information for gastrointestinal cancers. They assessed the websites using a scoring system that ranged from −84 (*poor*) to 90 (*very good*). The median score for the websites that they assessed was 53. The highest score was for pancreatic cancer (65) and esophageal cancer (61) sites. Rectal (50), gastric (49), and colon (48) sites scored the lowest. They also found that the best overall sites were charitable websites, which scored a median of 79. The authors noted that gastrointestinal cancers are the most common cancer for which Internet searches are performed.

Ten diabetes-focused social media sites were evaluated for quality of information and privacy protection of users (Weitzman, Cole, Kaci, & Mandl, 2011). The authors noted that only 50% of the sites presented evidence-based information, and inaccurate information about diabetes and ads for unfounded "cures" were found on three sites. In fact, of nine sites with advertising, transparency was missing on five. They also found that privacy protection was poor, "with almost no use of procedures for secure data storage and transmission; only three sites supported member controls over personal information" (p. 5).

Clearly, people use the Internet to seek out information on health-related matters, and just as clearly, the Internet is used as a source of both good and bad information. Websites are also of inconsistent quality and in constant flux. It is critical that APRNs and the patients to whom they provide care understand how to evaluate websites for current and accurate information as is evidenced by studies that show that most Internet consumers do not confirm the validity of the Internet resources that they use. APRNs have an opportunity to better serve their population by helping consumers use the Internet wisely by guiding them to sites that provide evidence-based information and privacy protection.

Evaluating Online Information

The Medical Library Association (MLA), the Health on the Net (HON) Foundation, and the U.S. National Library of Medicine provide guidelines for evaluating online information. Links to these sites can be found in Table 6.1. The NLM has partnered with MedlinePlus to create the tutorial *Evaluating Internet Health Information: A Tutorial from the National Library of Medicine*, which is accessible through the NLM website. The tutorial is useful for both APRNs and consumers.

There are commonalities present in all of the guidelines. The following questions can be used to evaluate Internet sites for healthcare information.

- Who runs the site?
  Check the address (uniform resource locator or URL) of the website. Government sites have *.gov* in the address, educational institutions have *.edu*, and professional sites have *.org* suffixes. Commercial sites have *.com* in

TABLE 6.1 • Links for Evaluating Online Information

Resource	Internet Address	Information Available
Medical Library Association	www.mlanet.org	Use the "For Health Consumers" link to find: MLA user's guide to finding and evaluating health information on the web, MLA's top 10 websites, and Deciphering Medspeak (What Did My Doctor Say?)
U.S. National Library of Medicine	www.nlm.nih.gov/hinfo .html	Use the health information site to find: the guide to healthy web surfing, medical information on the Internet tutorial (from MEDLINE), Health Library Directory, dozens of links for safe health resources for consumers
Health on the Net Foundation	www.hon.ch/HONcode/ Patients/visitor_ safeUse2.html	Includes guidelines for evaluating websites and the criteria for HONcode accreditation

the address. Commercial sites may exist for commercial reasons—to sell products—but many provide useful and balanced information. Go to the "About Us" page. The sponsor and the credentials of the people who run the site should be clearly identified. The site should also include a method for contacting the webmaster or the people responsible for maintaining the site.

- Why have they created the site?
  The site should identify its intended audience. Some sites have separate sections for consumers and for health professionals, whereas other sites are designed exclusively for either health professionals or consumers.
- Who is sponsoring the site? Does the information favor the sponsor?
  The website should disclose all financial relationships such as the source of funding for the site. Advertisements should be clearly labeled as such. Users should examine sites for balanced information that does not favor a sponsor.
- Where did the information come from? Is the information reviewed by experts?
  Websites should provide the credentials of contributors and the process for selecting information that is posted. Look for information on an editorial board; this can usually be found on the "About Us" page. Look for a statement that indicates that it is a peer-reviewed site. The information on the site should be presented clearly and should be factual, not opinion.
- Is it up to date?
  Websites, especially those that provide health-related information, should be current and updated on a regular basis. Dates should be clearly posted.
- What is the privacy policy?
  There should be a privacy policy posted on the site. Check the policy to see whether information is shared. Do not provide personal information unless the privacy policy clearly states what information is and is not shared. You should be comfortable with the policy. (Medical Library Association, 2011; MedlinePlus, 2011)

The HON Foundation is a private organization that has created a code of conduct for medical and health websites (HONcode). It does not rate the quality of information but holds website developers to basic ethical standards in the presentation of information. Both APRNs and patients can look for HONcode certification when searching for reliable websites. Certification is free of charge. All HONcode-certified sites are reviewed annually. In addition to the annual review, the HON Foundation relies on users to report noncompliance with the HONcode and investigates complaints (Health on the Net Foundation, 2010). The HON Foundation code of conduct for medical and health websites can be found at www.hon.ch/HONcode/Webmasters/Conduct.html.

The Internet can be a very helpful tool for APRNs and their patients to use to track and monitor progress or to explore alternative practices for the common goal of improving overall health. But both groups need to be vigilant when using the World Wide Web. APRNs should provide their patients with a list of reliable health websites to visit, and patients should be encouraged to visit more than one site to check information. Patients can be taught to look for the seal of certification from an accrediting organization, such as the HON

Foundation, and they need to be warned "to be careful not to believe claims or promises of miraculous cures, wonder drugs, and other extreme statements unless there is proof to these claims" (HON Foundation, 2010, para. 8). It is critical that APRNs encourage patients to discuss anything they learn on the Internet with their healthcare provider and that they confirm that patients know how to evaluate medical and health websites.

USING TECHNOLOGY TO IMPROVE POPULATION HEALTH

New technologies are creating revolutionary changes in healthcare delivery and how healthcare information is communicated. Although new technologies are not universally available or put into practice, there is evidence that technology offers many possibilities for designing unique interventions to impact population outcomes. Published research provides examples of such technological interventions. One promising use of new technology is telehealth, which is being used by some healthcare providers who serve hard-to-reach populations. Preliminary evidence suggests that telehealth is promising as a way to increase access to populations in rural and underserved areas. Healthcare providers working with various populations have reported excellent results when using technology in their practices to improve patient communication and population outcomes.

Jones, Lekhak, and Kaewluang (2014) described a meta-review of the use of mobile telephony and short message service (SMS) to deliver self-management interventions for chronic health conditions. In their analysis of 11 systematic reviews, SMS texting improved adherence to appointment attendance and adherence with antiretroviral therapy and short-term tobacco smoking quit rates. Texting was considered to be an effective strategy regardless of age or socioeconomic status and allowed for individualization of the delivered message.

Wendel, Brossart, Elliot, McCord, and Diaz (2011) describe a program to increase access to mental health services in a rural Texas community. They cite the many obstacles of rural health, including limited healthcare resources and services and a shortage of healthcare professionals. They also recognized that travel time to medical clinics or hospitals was one barrier to accessing healthcare services for rural residents. Rural settings have significant health disparities compared to urban communities, and one of the contributing factors is limited access to healthcare resources. They designed a program to counteract one such disparity by increasing access to mental health services in a rural community. The researchers used a collaborative effort to improve transportation to services and combined this with a telehealth-based counseling program staffed by doctoral students under the supervision of experienced faculty. Their experience led them to conclude that telehealth is a promising method for providing care to hard-to-reach patients. The authors note that it is imperative that there is a mechanism for secure transmissions and maintaining privacy when technology is used to transmit communications between providers and patients. They also reported that technical difficulties during the study caused some interruption in services. Protecting patient confidentiality and providing reliable services are hallmarks of good care. When planning services using advanced technologies, APRNs need to be aware of both the benefits and the barriers. It is essential that experts in the use of technology are included as team members to help design new interventions that incorporate the use of technology.

In an article by Avdal, Kizilci, and Demirel (2011), the authors acknowledged transportation as a barrier to accessing care in rural communities and in urban areas with poor public transportation. They explain that in Turkey, people with diabetes are monitored and treated in polyclinics, which provide outpatient services for a wide range of health conditions. Polyclinics can be problematic as they can be crowded and diabetic patients often cannot reach healthcare providers in a timely manner. In addition, people in Turkey frequently have to travel long distances to get to polyclinics, also causing problems with access. The result is that people with diabetes are frequently poorly monitored. They designed a study to evaluate the use of telehealth in improving the outcomes of diabetic patients in Turkey. Approximately 25% of people in Turkey have access to the Internet. At the beginning of the study, hemoglobin A_{1c} (HbA1c) levels were similar in both groups (non-telemed group and telemed group). Six months after the study began, HbA1c levels were significantly lower in the experimental group, whereas no changes were detected in the control group. The authors were encouraged by the results and concluded that telehealth is effective as a complementary tool to help patients manage their chronic health conditions.

Access is not always a function of the physical distance between aggregates and healthcare providers. In some cases, patients can become socially isolated because of their physical or financial limitations. The following are examples of how web-based technology has the potential to alleviate problems with access to services and to improve population outcomes.

Oliver, Wittenberg-Lyles, Demiris, and Oliver (2010) carried out a project to engage residents in long-term care in "virtual" sightseeing. Their study was built on the work of earlier researchers who have demonstrated the positive effects of activity programs in long-term care facilities. The authors tested the feasibility of using live videoconferencing to establish communication between residents in a long-term care facility in Iowa and researchers in Athens, Greece. The overall goal of the study was to "open the world of travel for residents confined in long-term care settings and to engage residents in 'virtual' sightseeing of foreign settings" (p. 93). These authors documented that the residents who took part in this feasibility study became clearly engaged in the activity. They noted that through technology, nursing homes can offer residents a way to explore the world outside of their usual environment, and they challenged researchers to build an evidence base to demonstrate the long-term value of this initiative on clinical outcomes for nursing home residents. Other researchers have investigated the use of technology to enrich the environment of people who live in long-term care facilities. Demiris and colleagues (2008) explored the potential of using video phone technology to improve quality of life for long-term care residents and distant family members. The authors propose that technology can redefine the role of distant caregiving for residents and family members in long-term care facilities by increasing opportunities for communication between loved ones. These studies offer tantalizing glimpses into the possibilities of using technology to enrich the lives of people in long-term care.

Many studies have been conducted to determine how the use of technology can improve specific population outcomes. Choi, Lee, Kang, Lee, and Yoon (2014) described the use of a web-based application to assist patients with metabolic syndrome in improving dietary behaviors. The 16-week web-based nutritional program resulted in a decrease in overall body weight, waist circumference, body fat, and body mass index (BMI). Nothwehr (2013) investigated the feasibility of using remote coaching and a handheld electronic device to increase the consumption of fruits and vegetables and decrease television viewing in an adult population, with encouraging results. The author made an important point in writing that "[t]here may be a strong novelty factor to the technology that encourages use" (p. 23). Long-term follow-up and reevaluation are important measures for confirming the results of any intervention in population health. Haze and Lynaugh (2013) described a successful pilot study using smartphone technology to improve nurse–patient communication between nurses and teenagers with asthma who were enrolled in an asthma management program. The teenagers involved in the pilot reported that they felt more comfortable communicating through texting than by telephone calls and that they asked more questions when texting. Nurses were encouraged by the increase in communication with their patients. This is a good illustration of the changes occurring in communication brought about by technology and the need for nurses to use technology to design new methods to carry out interventions that are appropriate for specific populations. Medication adherence is a problem in many patient populations. A group of nurse practitioners completed a study to examine the feasibility of using cell phones to improve medication adherence among a group of homeless individuals. The individuals in the study were given phones, and the results proved promising, as exit interviews indicated that the cell phones were useful in increasing medication adherence and were valued by the participants (Burda, Haack, Duarte, & Alemi, 2012).

Personal health records (PHR) are a set of Internet tools that can be used by consumers to coordinate their personal health information. They are used by individuals to keep track of their complete health histories, including treatments and current medications. The information is maintained online and is accessible to the individual consumer and healthcare providers who have been granted access. PHR facilitate the sharing of up-to-date and accurate health records between consumers and their healthcare providers. Yamin et al. (2011) conducted a cross-sectional study of PHR use in a single health system. They compared consumers who activated a PHR with people who were offered the opportunity but did not activate a PHR. They found that "despite increasing Internet availability, racial/ethnic minority patients adopted a PHR less frequently than white patients, and patients with the lowest annual income adopted a PHR less often than those with higher incomes" (p. 568). They recommended designing interventions to increase the use of PHR by populations that need them. This is yet another example of the digital divide in healthcare and further illustrates the need to be aware of disparities among groups and the need to find ways to increase access to technologically underserved populations.

E-health is a growing field. The Internet can be a very helpful tool for APRNs and their patients to track and monitor progress or to explore alternative practices for the common goal: to improve overall health. Populations are best served when their needs are met using a variety of approaches. There are a number of platforms that can connect APRNs to patients and/or other health providers. Information can be exchanged between health provider and patient via teleconferencing, web casts, podcasting (delivery of audio, text, pictures, and/or video to a computer or mobile device), and Twitter (text-based messages sent through a social networking site), to name just a few. Communication devices range from tabletop home computers and laptops to tablet computers and smartphones. The examples cited in this chapter provide a window into the opportunities open to APRNs to be creative in using technology to improve patient outcomes. Inherent in the fact that this is a relatively new way to provide care, there is a dearth of literature on long-term follow-up and few studies have been replicated. There are also barriers to the use of new technologies such as competency, a poor match between clinical needs and the availability of devices, privacy issues, system downtimes, and disparities among groups related to availability and use patterns. Assessing populations for their patterns of Internet usage and other technologies is an important part of the APRN's role. Equally important is designing interventions that make use of new technologies and measuring the impact on relevant population outcomes. Further research is needed to fully evaluate the advantages and disadvantages of using technology in populations to improve health while maintaining privacy and sustainability.

E-RESOURCES THAT SUPPORT POPULATION-BASED NURSING

There are many resources on the Internet that support population-based nursing. The following list of websites is an example of some of the information and resources that are available. Neither the list nor the descriptions of the sites are meant to be exhaustive. The intent is to provide APRNs with an idea of what is available within different categories of websites and to pique the interest of APRNs so as to encourage them to explore these sites, and more, on their own.

Government Resources

Government sites (which have *.gov* in the URL, as mentioned earlier) are a rich source of information and offer a variety of resources for both consumers and healthcare professionals.

U.S. Department of Health and Human Services: *www.hhs.gov*

The U.S. Department of Health and Human Services (HHS) is the U.S. government's principal agency for protecting the health of all Americans. It provides essential services (such as Medicare) and administers more grant dollars than all other federal agencies combined. The site has a wealth of information on diseases and conditions. An excellent example is *Healthfinder.gov*, which provides easy-to-understand information for consumers to stay healthy. *The Quick Guide to Healthy Living* explains in simple language, recommendations for health screenings and tests. There is even a link for people to help find a physician, health center, or public library. A new addition to the HHS site is StopBullying.gov, which provides information on how children, young adults, parents, and educators can recognize, prevent, or stop bullying. A table provides specific information on how and where to get help for bullying (http://www.stopbullying.gov/). Another recent initiative of the HHS is the National Partnership for Action. This initiative includes a Health Information Disparities Workgroup. The goal of this workgroup is to create projects to combat the digital divide (U.S. Department of Health and Human Services, 2011).

Centers for Disease Control and Prevention: www.cdc.gov

The Centers for Disease Control and Prevention (CDC) is a U.S. government agency. Organizationally, it is under the HHS. Its mission is to "collaborate to create the expertise, information, and tools that people and communities need to protect their health—through health promotion, prevention of disease, injury and disability, and preparedness for new health threats" (Centers for Disease Control and Prevention, 2014, "Mission, Role, and Pledge" section, para 1). The site contains a wealth of information for consumers, health professionals, policy makers, researchers, and educators. The CDC offers a wide variety of helpful resources for these groups, including publications on many health and safety topics, podcasts, and RSS feeds (RSS is the acronym for really simple syndication, which is used to publish recent works, such as blog entries, news headlines, audio, and video, in a standard format and can be sent electronically to subscribers.) The site includes many useful tools, such as photos, a BMI calculator, and slide presentations, that can be used for educational purposes. The CDC also publishes *Emerging Infectious Diseases* (EID), *Morbidity and Mortality Weekly Report* (MMWR), and *Preventing Chronic Disease* (PCD). These publications are free of charge and can be subscribed to on the CDC site. Also available on this site are data on a large range of topics, including FASTSTATS A-Z and trends in U.S. health statistics.

The National Institutes of Health: www.nih.gov

The National Institutes of Health (NIH) is a U.S. government agency. Similar to the CDC, it is under the HSS. Its mission is to "seek fundamental knowledge about the nature and behavior of living systems and the application of that knowledge to enhance health, lengthen life, and reduce illness and disability" (National Institutes of Health, 2014, "Mission, Role, and Pledge" section, para 1). Its primary purpose is to support research for improving the health of the nation. It provides a wealth of material for teachers and students alike on science and health topics. It offers everything from brochures to fact sheets and prepared slide presentations on many health and science topics. *NIH News* provides updated information on U.S. health trends.

FedStats: fedstats.sites.usa.gov

FedStats provides access to a full range of official statistical information produced by the federal government. It links to more than 100 agencies that provide data and trend information on such topics as diseases, demographics, education, healthcare, and crime (FedStats, 2014).

Agency for Healthcare Research and Quality: www.ahrq.gov

The mission of the Agency for Healthcare Research and Quality (AHRQ) "is to produce evidence to make healthcare safer, higher quality, more accessible, equitable, and affordable" (Agency for Healthcare Research and Quality, Mission & Budget section, para 1, 2014). The AHRQ provides information on health so that consumers and healthcare providers can make informed decisions and provide quality healthcare. The information is designed to be useful to consumers, policy makers, healthcare providers, and employers. The site includes extensive information and resources such as information on funding opportunities for research, databases, research findings, and a health information technology (IT) information tool.

The National Guideline Clearinghouse: www.guideline.gov

The National Guideline Clearinghouse (NGC) is a public resource for evidence-based practice guidelines and is housed within the AHRQ. Healthcare providers can search the NGC site to obtain up-to-date guidelines for the provision of evidence-based care.

Let's Move!: www.letsmove.gov

Obesity is a national issue and there are online sites related to obesity springing up all over the Internet. One excellent resource for consumers and APRNs alike is *Let's Move*, the online site related to First Lady Michelle Obama's campaign against obesity. Readers can learn how to prevent childhood obesity, find nutritional facts, get ideas for being active, and learn how you can help schools and communities make healthier foods available to children. *Let's Move* is on Facebook, where individuals can share stories and ideas. There are also connections to Twitter and Meetup (a social networking site that facilitates group meetings among people with common interests and goals).

Educational Sites

Nongovernmental websites are also a source of excellent information for healthcare providers and consumers. Sites with *.edu* in the address are owned by educational institutions. Many universities, particularly those that offer health-related degrees, have extensive resources available for people who are looking for information on health-related topics.

The Nursing Archives, Boston University: hgar-srv3.bu.edu/collections/ nursing

A fascinating glimpse into the history of nursing is provided by the Nursing Archives, which is part of the Howard Gotlieb Archival Research Center at

Boston University. The Nursing Archives includes a collection of personal and professional papers of many nursing leaders, including 250 of Florence Nightingale's letters. There are also records of schools of nursing, public health and professional nursing organizations, histories of various American and foreign schools of nursing, and early textbooks (Boston University, 2014). These materials provide a fascinating look at the early years of nursing and public health.

Institute of Medicine: www.iom.edu

The Institute of Medicine (IOM) is an independent, nonprofit organization that works outside of the government to provide "unbiased and authoritative advice to decision makers and the public" (Institute of Medicine, 2014, "About the IOM" section, para 1). It is an arm of the National Academy of Sciences. It undertakes specific mandates from Congress, federal agencies, and independent organizations. The site makes available a complete list of its reports published after 1998. One such report is "The Future of Nursing: Leading Change, Advancing Health," commissioned by the Robert Wood Johnson Foundation and published in 2010.

Professional Organizations

Professional membership organizations are usually run as not-for-profits and work to further the interests of a profession and to protect the public. They are generally a rich source of information on the healthcare professions. They generally have *.org* in the address. APRNs should search their specialty organizations for resources and information.

American Nurses Association: www.nursingworld.org

The ANA (American Nurses Association; 2014a) is the professional organization for registered nurses in the United States. It has 54 constituent member nurses associations and is affiliated with 35 specialty nursing and workforce advocacy affiliate organizations. It publishes standards of nursing practice for general RN nursing and nursing subspecialty practices. The ANA also lobbies Congress and regulatory agencies on healthcare issues affecting nurses and consumers. The ANA publishes *American Nurse Today* and the *Online Journal of Issues in Nursing* (*OJIN*). The *OJIN* is a peer-reviewed, online publication. Only members have access to current issues, but archived issues are available to anyone. The ANA also distributes the RSS, *ANA SmartBrief.*

The ANA, teamed with seven other organizations, launched an online resource for consumers in 2011. The site HealthCareandYou.org (www .healthcareandyou.org) outlines the provisions in the Affordable Care Act and breaks down the act's benefits by state. Healthcare providers can use the site to obtain information that will be useful for explaining the key points of the Affordable Care Act to patients, and the language and format are kept clear and simple for easy use by consumers (ANA, 2014b).

The American Nurses Credentialing Center (ANCC) is a subsidiary of the ANA. It sets the standards for professional certification, accredits continuing nursing education, and created and oversees the Magnet Recognition

Program. Standards for certification and accreditation are published on the group's website (www.nursecredentialing.org/default.aspx).

American Public Health Association: www.apha.org

Founded in 1872, the American Public Health Association (APHA) is a diverse membership organization of public health professionals. Its mission is to "Improve the health of the public and achieve equity in health status" (American Public Health Association [APHA], 2015, "Our Mission" section, sentence 1). Among its goals are to increase access to healthcare, protect funding for core public health services, and eliminate health disparities. It publishes the *American Journal of Public Health* and *The Nation's Health.* These publications are available free to members and to nonmembers by subscription (APHA, 2014).

Not-for-Profit Organizations

A nonprofit organization uses its earnings to pursue its goals and has controlling members or boards instead of owners. Some examples are the American Heart Association (AHA), the American Cancer Society (ACS), and the Asthma and Allergy Foundation of America (AAFA). Many of these sites have an impressive amount of information and resources that they make available to the public. Most of these groups have *.org* in their URLs.

American Heart Association: www.heart.org/HEARTORG

The AHA has an extensive and eclectic library of information and resources for educators at all levels, consumers, and healthcare professionals. The site includes downloadable lesson plans, risk-assessment tools, and free application software (apps) such as the Walking Path Mobile app. The AHA develops guidelines and course materials for first aid, basic life support, and advanced life support courses.

American Cancer Society: www.cancer.org

Similar to the AHA, the ACS provides extensive information and resources to both consumers and healthcare professionals. Its site includes information on the latest research in cancer prevention and treatment, information and resources for specific cancer topics, information on side effects of different treatments for cancer, and information on funding and paying for treatment.

Asthma and Allergy Foundation of America: www.aafa.org

The mission of the AAFA is to improve the quality of life for people with asthma and allergic diseases through education, advocacy, and research (Asthma and Allergy Foundation of America, 2011). Examples of its extensive online resources are an online "allergy forecast tool," information on its asthma and allergy certification program, an "ask the allergist" online tool, and extensive educational resources on allergies and asthma.

The Pew Research Center: www.pewresearch.org

The Pew Research Center is a subsidiary of the Pew Charitable Trusts. It is a think tank that informs the public about the issues, attitudes, and trends shaping America and the world. It conducts public opinion polling, demographic research, media content analysis, and other empirical social science research (Pew Research Center, 2014).

International Organizations

There are many international organizations described throughout this book. Perhaps one of the most powerful and influential is the World Health Organization (WHO).

World Health Organization: www.who.int

WHO (2014) is an arm of the United Nations. It provides leadership on global health matters and technical support to countries, and monitors and assesses health trends. Its website includes a multilingual page with publications and resources in many languages and on various health topics, and another page with evidence-based guidelines. There is also current information on disease outbreaks and world health trends. WHO publishes the *World Health Report*, *World Health Statistics Report*, and information for international travelers. The multimedia site includes podcasts and videos on various health topics. WHO news can be accessed on Twitter and via RSS.

Commercial Sites

Although only one is listed here, there are many commercial sites that provide balanced and transparent information. Do not dismiss websites because *.com* is in the address. Use the information provided in this chapter to evaluate all websites.

Medscape: www.medscape.com

Medscape (2014) is an online, peer-reviewed resource for health professionals. It features peer-reviewed original articles and provides both continuing medical education (CME) and continuing nursing education contact hours (CH). It also offers a customized version of the NLM's MEDLINE database, a drug interaction checker, and a drug reference, and has free downloadable apps for health professionals. All content in Medscape is available free of charge for professionals and consumers alike, but registration is required. Review the website for information on copyright restrictions and privacy protection.

Analytic Software on the Internet

Epi Info: www.cdc.gov/epiinfo/

Epi Info is a collection of software tools that are available for free download through the CDC website. It can be used to create questionnaires and download data, and allows the user to perform advanced statistical analyses and geographic information system (GIS) mapping. GIS is a technological tool that allows users to map trends in disease or outcomes of interest using such markers as zip codes or city boundaries, and to integrate data into a geographic map that summarizes data to assist users in identifying trends based on geographic location. In healthcare, mapping can be used to show the geographical distribution of specific factors such as obesity or cancer types. By mapping these factors, patterns of occurrence can be identified and specific areas can be targeted for intervention.

The Visual Statistics System: www.uv.es/visualstats/Book

The Visual Statistics System (ViSta) is a free, downloadable statistical system. ViSta can be used for both descriptive and inferential analytic analyses. It performs both univariate and multivariate analyses. Go to the website to learn how to use the program, but be sure to review the copyright restrictions prior to usage.

The Not-So-Hidden Dangers of Social Media in Healthcare

Many professional organizations have written guidelines for the use of social media. It is critical that APRNs remember at all times that patient confidentiality is both a legal and an ethical responsibility. Complaints to state boards of nursing against nurses who use social media usually fall within the following areas (Spector & Kappel, 2012):

- Breach of privacy or confidentiality against patients
- Failure to report others' violations of privacy against patients
- Lateral violence against colleagues
- Communication against employers
- Boundary violation
- Employer/faculty use of social media against employees/students

There are a number of important considerations for APRNs who engage in an online presence. The Internet can be a valuable tool for patient care, communication, and social interaction and for boosting one's career, but nurses have also been fired, lost their licenses, and experienced bullying, all within the context of social media. The National Council of State Boards of Nursing has produced social media guidelines for nurses. A video is available at www.ncsbn .org/347.htm, and *A Nurse's Guide to Professional Boundaries* (*NSBN*) is located at www.ncsbn.org/ProfessionalBoundaries_Complete.pdf. Among the most important facts for people who use social media to remember is that once information is posted on the Internet, it is posted permanently and that privacy settings are not 100% effective.

SUMMARY

Technological innovation has led to a whole new lexicon for healthcare providers and has also provided new methods and opportunities for improving population outcomes. E-mail alerts, RSS, podcasts, videoconferencing, and Twitter are efficient and cost-effective ways to "keep connected" and to deliver healthcare information to both consumers and healthcare professionals. E-health provides a means to bridge distances between patients and healthcare providers and is a creative option for providing patient care. In the fast-moving world of healthcare, technology provides a convenient way to keep up to date. Software applications (apps) that can be downloaded to mobile devices and updated on a regular basis make available immediate and important information (such as drug interactions/calculations) to APRNs and other healthcare providers.

To provide excellent and up-to-date clinical care, APRNs need to be technologically literate and willing to explore new ways to deliver healthcare. APRNs should evaluate their Internet and other technological resources carefully and use them to advance their practices to provide the latest evidence-based care possible. They also need to stay current in their knowledge of the latest technology and guide their patients to resources that are valid and useful. There are both challenges and opportunities to improve patient care through the use of new technology. Of primary concern are the legal and ethical responsibilities related to patient privacy. Regardless of these challenges, technology is here to stay, and it is the responsibility of APRNs to educate themselves and their patients on the many benefits of technology while adhering to patient privacy.

EXERCISES AND DISCUSSION QUESTIONS

Exercise 6.1 Find a website that would be helpful to the population that you serve. Using a search engine, such as Google or Yahoo, type in the name of a disease or condition that is associated with a population to whom you provide care. Eliminate the websites that you find in your search that contain either *.gov* or *.edu* in the address. Evaluate the remaining sites and identify at least two that meet criteria for reliability and transparency using the guidelines in this chapter.

Exercise 6.2 Online databases are a rich source of information for healthcare professionals. Use the following CDC database to research the state that you live or work in: Go to http://wwwn.cdc.gov/sortablestats/

- What is the burden of chronic diseases in your state?
- How do the leading causes of death in your state compare to U.S. figures?
- Identify five important risk factors that need to be targeted in your state.
- Identify vulnerable groups for whom targeted services need to be provided.

Exercise 6.3 Select one vulnerable group identified in Exercise 6.2 and identify an outcome for improvement. Design an interventional study that incorporates the use of technology to improve that outcome.

REFERENCES

Agency for Health care Research and Quality. (2014). *About AHRQ*. Retrieved from http://www.ahrq.gov/cpi/about/index.html

American Association of Colleges of Nursing. (2006). *The essentials of doctoral education for advanced practice nursing*. Retrieved from http://www.aacn.nche.edu/DNP/pdf/Essentials.pdf

American Nurses Association. (2014a). Retrieved from http://www.nursingworld.org/

American Nurses Association. (2014b). *HealthcareandYou.org*. Retrieved from http://www.nursingworld.org/HomepageCategory/Announcements/New-Health-Care-Law-Resource.aspx

American Public Health Association. (2014). *The new APHA*. Retrieved from http://apha.org/about-apha

American Public Health Association. (2015). *Our mission*. Retrieved from https://www.apha.org/about-apha

Asthma and Allergy Foundation of America. (2011). Retrieved from http://www.aafa.org/index.cfm

Avdal, U., Kizilci, S., & Demirel, N. (2011). The effects of web-based diabetes education on diabetes care results: A randomized control study. *Computers, Informatics, Nursing: CIN, 29*(2), 101–106. doi:10.1097/NCN.0b013e3182155318

Boston University, Howard Gotlieb Archival Research Center. (2014). *Nursing archives*. Retrieved from http://hgar-srv3.bu.edu/collections/nursing

Burda, C., Haack, M., Duarte, A. C., & Alemi, F. (2012). Medication adherence among homeless patients: A pilot study of cell phone effectiveness. *Journal of the American Academy of Nurse Practitioners, 24*(11), 675–681. doi:10.1111/j.1745-7599.2012.00756.x

Centers for Disease Control and Prevention. (2014). *Mission, role and pledge*. Retrieved from http://www.cdc.gov/about/organization/mission.htm

Chan, D., Willicombe, A., Reid, T., Beaton, C., Arnold, D., Ward, J., . . . Lewis, W. (2012). Relative quality of Internet-derived gastrointestinal cancer information. *Journal of Cancer Education, 27*(4), 676–679. doi:10.1007/s13187-012-0408-2

Choi, Y., Lee M. J., Kang, H. C., Lee, M. S., & Yoon, S. (2014). Development and application of a web-based nutritional management program to improve dietary behaviors for the prevention of metabolic syndrome. *Computers, Informatics, Nursing: CIN, 32*(5), 232–241.

Demiris, G., Parker Oliver, D. R., Hensel, B., Dickey, G., Rantz, M., & Skubic, M. (2008). Use of videophones for distant caregiving: An enriching experience for families and residents in long-term care. *Journal of Gerontological Nursing, 34*(7), 50–55.

FedStats. (2014). Retrieved from http://fedstats.sites.usa.gov/

Haze, K., & Lynaugh, J. (2013). Building patient relationships: A smartphone application supporting communication between teenagers with asthma and the RN care coordinators. *Computers, Informatics, Nursing: CIN, 31*(6), 266–271.

Health on the Net Foundation. (2010). *The HON code of conduct for medical and health Web sites (HONcode)*. Retrieved from http://www.hon.ch/HONcode/Webmasters/Conduct.html

Institute of Medicine. (2014). *About the IOM*. Retrieved from http://iom.edu/About-IOM.aspx

Internet World Stats. (2010). *Usage and population statistics*. Retrieved from http://www.internetworldstats.com/stats.htm

Jones, K. R., Lekhak, N., & Kaewluang, N. (2014). Using mobile phones and short message service to deliver self-management interventions for chronic conditions: A meta review. *Worldviews on Evidence-Based Nursing, 11*(2), 81–88.

Kowalski, C., Kahana, E., Kuhr, K., Ansmann, L., & Pfaff, H. (2014). Changes over time in the utilization of disease-related Internet information in newly diagnosed breast cancer patients 2007 to 2013. *Journal of Medical Internet Research, 16*(8), e195. doi:10.2196/jmir.3289

McDaid, D., & Park, A. (2010). *Online health: Untangling the web.* Retrieved from http://www.bupa.com/healthpulse

Medical Library Association. (2011). *For health consumers.* Retrieved from https://www.mlanet.org/for-health-consumers

MedlinePlus. (2011). *Evaluating Internet health information: A tutorial from the National Library of Medicine.* Retrieved from http://www.nlm.nih.gov/medlineplus/webeval/webeval.html

Medscape. (2011). Retrieved from www.medscape.com

Medscape. (2014). Retrieved from http://www.medscape.com/multispecialty

Mitchell, S. J., Godoy, L., Shabazz, K., & Horn, I. B. (2014). Internet and mobile technology use among urban African American parents: Survey study of a clinical population [Abstract]. *Journal of Medical Internet Research, 16*(1), e9. doi:10.2196/jmir.2673

Modave, F., Shokar, N., Penaranda, E., & Nguyen, N. (2014). Analysis of the accuracy of weight loss information search engine results on the Internet. *American Journal of Public Health, 104*(10), 1971–1978.

Moore, D., & Ayers, S. (2011). A review of postnatal mental health websites: Help for health care professionals and patients. *Archives of Women's Mental Health, 14*(6), 443–452. doi:10.1007/s00737-011-0245-z

National Guideline Clearinghouse. (2011). Retrieved from http://www.guideline.gov

National Institutes of Health. (2014). Retrieved from http://nih.gov

Nothwehr, F. (2013). People with unhealthy lifestyle behaviors benefit from remote coaching via mobile technology. *Evidence Based Nursing, (16)*1, 22–23.

Oliver, D. P., Wittenberg-Lyles, E., Demiris, G., & Oliver, D. (2010). Giving long-term care residents a passport to the world the Internet. *Journal of Nursing Care Quality, 25*(3), 193–197.

Pew Research Center. (2008). *Pew Internet & American Life Project.* Retrieved from http://www.pewinternet.org/Reports/2009/8-The-Social-Life-of-Health-Information.aspx

Pew Research Center. (2011). *Peer to peer health care.* Retrieved from http://www.pewinternet.org/2011/02/28/peer-to-peer-health-care-2/

Pew Research Center. (2013a). *Pew Internet & American Life Project: Health online 2013.* Retrieved from http://www.pewinternet.org/files/old-media//Files/Reports/PIP_HealthOnline.pdf

Pew Research Center. (2013b). *Who's not online? 5 factors tied to the digital divide.* Retrieved from http://www.pewresearch.org/fact-tank/2013/11/08/whos-not-online-5-factors-tied-to-the-digital-divide/

Pew Research Center. (2014). *About the Pew Research Center.* Retrieved from http://www.pewresearch.org/about/

Spector, N., & Kappel, D. M. (2012). Guidelines for using electronic and social media: The regulatory perspective. *Online Journal of Issues in Nursing, 17*(3), 1. Retrieved from http://nursingworld.org/MainMenuCategories/ANAMarketplace/ANAPeriodicals/OJIN/TableofContents/Vol-17-2012/No3-Sept-2012/Guidelines-for-Electronic-and-Social-Media.html#NCSBN11e

U.S. Department of Health and Human Services (HHS). (2011). Retrieved from http://www.hhs.gov/

Weitzman, E. R., Cole, E., Kaci, L., & Mandl, K. D. (2011). Social but safe? Quality and safety of diabetes-related online networks. *Journal of American Medical Informatics Association, 18*(3), 292–297.

Wendel, M. L., Brossart, D. F., Elliot, T. R., McCord, C., & Diaz, M. A. (2011). Use of technology to increase access to mental health services in a rural Texas community. *Family and Community Health, 34*(2), 134–140.

World Health Organization. (2014). *About WHO.* Retrieved from http://www.who.int/en

Yamin, C. K., Emani, S., Williams, D. H., Lipsitz, S. R., Karson, A. S., Wald, J. S., & Bates, D. W. (2011). The digital divide in adoption and use of a personal health record. *Archives of Internal Medicine, 17*(6), 568–574.

Concepts in Program Design and Development

Ann L. Cupp Curley

Graduates of doctoral education for advanced nursing practice are expected to integrate nursing science with knowledge from other fields in order to provide the highest level of nursing care. They are also expected to develop and provide effective plans for "practice level and/or system-wide practice initiatives that will improve the quality of care delivery" (American Association of Colleges of Nursing, 2006, p. 11). In this chapter, the advanced practice registered nurse (APRN) will learn how to design new programs by addressing factors related to planning and organizational decision making.

Nurse leaders are instrumental in using data to make decisions that lead to program development, implementation, and evaluation. Data used to drive decision making must be accurate, pertinent, and timely in order to be applied appropriately when designing a program. It is critical that a program be constructed in a way that takes into consideration all components that impact that program, both internally and externally. Determining measures of success or desired outcomes when designing a program provides continuous checkpoints for evaluation throughout program implementation. Program development, implementation, and evaluation will vary across geographic and practice settings because of the unique and varied characteristics of an APRN's practice.

CONSUMER AND SOCIETAL TRENDS AND DEMANDS

Consumer and societal trends and demands provide information or data that drive the rationale for designing a specific program. It is not cost-effective to support a program that does not meet an identified consumer need. A simple definition of *trend* is the general direction in which something tends to move. In what direction is healthcare technology moving? In what direction are consumer attitudes and beliefs about disease prevention moving? Consumer and societal trends and demands are constantly changing, making it difficult to know to which trends or demands to pay attention and whether they will continue and for how long. For example, in January 2014, the following trends were identified by Healthcare IT News: (a) security (safe storage of information), (b) healthcare cloud adoption (remote storage of information), (c) telemedicine, (d) integration of genomics and predictive modeling, (e) empowering the increasingly demanding patient (patients want control over health information) (Ratchinsky, 2014). Did these trends continue in 2015? Will they continue through 2020? Is a program designed in 2014, that is based on these trends, still needed and viable in 2015? Will it be needed in 2020? It is critical for APRNs to examine on an ongoing basis the environment in which they practice to confirm the latest trends and demands or identify new ones.

Population demographics can guide APRNs in the development of population-based programs. Communities have their own unique identifying characteristics, including age, socioeconomic status, and ethnic diversity. A program targeting the administration of influenza vaccines during influenza season may look different when implemented in an urban area such as New York City versus a rural community such as farmland in Wisconsin. National information on changing population demographics and implications for healthcare providers can be obtained from national websites such as the U.S. Department of Health and Human Services (HHS; www.hhs.gov/answers/research/find-social-service-research.html) or the Centers for Disease Control and Prevention (CDC; www.cdc.gov/datastatistics).

A starting point for developing a new program might originate in an organization where an APRN is employed. Data that are already collected and easily accessible can be examined and used to design or restructure an existing program. For example, if designing a transitional care program from hospital to home, it would be important to gather information on the number of hospital discharges, number of discharges to home and/or other facilities (e.g., rehabilitation, nursing homes), demographics of clients discharged home, primary discharge diagnoses, rehospitalization rate, and the time from discharge to rehospitalization. Review of the available data might reveal that there is a need for transitional programs for patients with certain diagnoses or certain demographics. If, for example, readmission rates are trending upward for patients with heart failure and are higher than national benchmarks, then an APRN may consider developing a transitional program that minimizes readmission rates in this population. Examination of the patient population (e.g., patient demographics, absence of insurance, access to a medical home, paucity of subspecialists) and processes involved in discharge (e.g., ability to fill discharge medications, clear discharge instructions, medical equipment available for home use) can help guide the APRN in developing a program to reduce the readmission rates while recognizing the characteristics of the patient population that may be contributing to the increase in these rates. A complete assessment of patient/consumer needs and characteristics and comparisons of population outcomes against standard benchmarks provide necessary information for the planning of new programs.

PROGRAM DEVELOPMENT

Justification

Justification for a program helps determine whether it is reasonable or necessary. Information gained from investigating consumer and societal trends and demands contributes to this justification. If a program makes sense, nurse leaders have ammunition to argue their case. Justifying a program requires an understanding of and quantification of the planned scope of the program. Producing a well-defined set of expectations and value propositions will make key stakeholders feel confident about approving and funding a program. The identification of a trend (such as increasing readmission rates for a particular population) is one justification for a program, especially when the trend leads to increasing costs or morbidity/mortality. By conducting a literature search, an APRN might reveal evidence that transitional programs for patients with heart failure are successful in preventing readmissions. Transitional programs that already exist may be adapted to fit an APRN's own patient population rather than designing a new program from scratch. Using evidence from the literature may reinforce the value or justification of such programs, especially those programs that are successful in reducing readmission rates and reducing overall healthcare costs.

Once a program is conceived and a literature review is completed, it is important to consider whether the program is feasible. A feasibility study helps to frame the program structure and identify potential risks associated with the program. Basic questions need to be addressed and answered, such as:

- Are other programs in place that serve a similar purpose?
- Are there other alternatives to the proposed program?
- Is the program economically feasible?
- Does the program make financial sense? A cost–benefit table, such as the one here, can be used to list factors to consider when assessing economic feasibility.

	Potential Costs	Potential Benefits
Quantitative		
Qualitative		

- Is the program technically feasible?
- Is the program operationally feasible to implement?
- Is it possible to maintain and support the program once it is implemented?

Designing a program is different from implementing it; therefore, nurse leaders must determine whether or not the program can be effectively operated and supported. Critical issues such as operational and support issues must be considered. The following is a nonexhaustive list of examples.

Operational Issues	Support Issues
• What tools are needed to support the program? • What skills training does the staff need? • What procedures or processes need to be created and/or updated?	• What support staff will be needed? • What program materials will the staff use? • What training will the staff be provided? • How will changes be managed?

• Is the program politically feasible considering strategic goals and administrative directives? Nurse leaders must be cognizant of the political landscape surrounding the program.
• Will the program be allowed to succeed?

Programs that are seen as having the potential to save money and improve patient outcomes will also often prove to be feasible. The Centers for Medicare & Medicaid Services (CMS) has tied reimbursement to certain key quality indicators. The readmission rate within 30 days for heart failure is one such indicator. Heart failure is the most costly diagnosis in the 65-year-old and older Medicare population (Sherwood et al., 2011). The Affordable Care Act (ACA) established the *Hospital Readmissions Reduction Program*, which requires CMS to reduce payments to inpatient prospective payment system (IPPS) hospitals with excess readmissions. The ACA went into effect on October 1, 2012, and hospitals that were above the national average for 30-day readmission rates saw decreased reimbursement rates (Centers for Medicare & Medicaid Services, 2014). Improving readmission rates makes good financial sense.

The APRN should assess the community to determine whether other, similar programs exist that would compete with the proposed program, or whether the proposed program could be built into an existing program. If a hospital has an existing community outreach department, the APRN could use the existing structure to house a new program.

In summary, justification of a program can be strengthened significantly by providing sound evidence, such as a thorough review of the literature, to establish the background of the problem and by examining currently successful programs that may be applicable to the APRN's population of interest. Additionally, by following trends, APRNs can compare outcome measures to national quality indicators (benchmarks) and follow these measures over time with a goal to improve patient outcomes and reduce costs. And finally, determining whether the program is feasible will further strengthen the justification, as feasibility studies provide a systematic framework in which a program can be assessed and thoughtfully implemented or integrated into current practice.

Identification of Key Stakeholders and Players

Stakeholders

The term *stakeholder* is commonly used in the business arena and refers to a person, group, or organization that has a direct or indirect stake in an organization because it can affect or be affected by the organization's actions, objectives, and policies. The effect can either be positive or negative. Nurse leaders strive to involve stakeholders who will support and facilitate successful program implementation and not thwart efforts. Furthermore, stakeholders can be internal and external, but in either case, there is a synergistic two-way relationship between the organization and its program and the stakeholders. A list of questions can guide identification of key stakeholders:

- Who will be affected by the program?
- Who can influence the program but not be directly involved in its development, implementation, and evaluation?
- What group is interested in the program's success and outcomes?
- Who will be or could be impacted by the program?

There are many stakeholders in healthcare, but there are five important and powerful stakeholders who should not be ignored: patients or clients, medical staff, agency management, professional staff, and the board of directors or trustees. Think broadly when determining key stakeholders and also consider government agencies, professional groups or associations, present and prospective employees, local communities, the national community, the public at large, suppliers, competitors, the media, and future generations.

There may be considerable overlap of stakeholders' expectations, including healthcare quality, support or adequacy of resources, and costs in terms of cost reduction and profitability. Publicly reported indicators may impact consumers' image of a hospital's quality of care. The board of trustees is also invested in the organization's image, which can directly impact a consumer's decision about where to seek care—or a physician's decision about where to admit patients.

The power or influence of stakeholders can vary as a result of the organizational makeup and the stakeholders' philosophy and values. Values drive needs, and when a needs assessment is performed to justify a program, values should be addressed because expectations often arise from values. Understanding expectations of stakeholders and considering expectations when designing a program can result in stakeholder satisfaction and program success. The identification of program outcomes that stakeholders value can help win their support. Healthcare organizations have mission statements that reflect organizational values, and, in many cases, these statements reflect the value placed on the development of community programs.

Key Players

Who are the key players in the program? The lead key player is the program administrator or manager. This role involves common responsibilities, regardless of industry or setting, which include the following:

- Identifies, researches, and solves program issues effectively
- Identifies the resources required for a program's success
- Oversees and directs team members
- Performs team assessment and evaluation
- Recognizes areas for improvement and develops action plans
- Documents and communicates operation of the program
- Ensures that the program complies with standards, regulations, and procedures
- Plans and sets timelines for program goals, milestones, and deliverables

Makeup of the program team will depend on the scope of the program. There are basically two types of staff involved in a program: (a) individuals providing direct program services and (b) staff who support direct providers and program implementation. The type and number of staff members needed to provide direct program services depend on the nature of services provided and number of program locations. The same is true for the type and number of support staff needed for program implementation and evaluation.

Regardless of the number and type of team members, the program manager or administrator plays a critical role in building a successful team. A team that is effective and focused contributes to the success of the program. A useful framework for building successful teams is described best by the acronym "together (T) everyone (E) achieves (A) more (M)." The origins of the model are difficult to trace, but its concepts are sound and used by many. Successful teambuilding requires attention to the following:

- Clear communication of expectations
- Team members' understanding of why they are participating on the team
- Commitment
- Competence
- Understanding of the program charter
- Control or sense of ownership
- Collaboration
- Communication
- Creative thinking
- Awareness of positive and negative consequences
- Coordination
- A cultural shift that is team based, empowering, and enabling

Stakeholders, team leaders, and team players all play a critical role in the success and/or failure of a program. Each member has a role and an expectation based on the anticipated outcome of a new program. Values sometimes play a role, and it is important to share these values and address them early on to ensure success. Ultimately, commitment, communication, and collaboration are some of the most important characteristics a team requires for a successful program.

Structure

Program structure can be as simple or complex as desired as long as specific outcome measures and sustainability are considered in the planning phase. APRNs must be careful when employing complex approaches to program structure, as complex designs can lead to failure if discrete outcomes are not easily measured or if too many measures or variables are being studied. For example, a simple approach might structure the program around the following six areas:

1. WHAT
   - What is the title of the program?
   - What is the focus of the program?

- What are the goals of the program?
- What are the objectives of the program?
- What outcomes will be measured?
- What is the budget for the program?
- What is the timeline for program development, implementation, and evaluation?

2. WHERE
- Where will the program take place?
- Where is the program's base location?
- Where will staff be housed?
- Where will supplies or resources for the program be stored?

3. WHO
- Who are the stakeholders?
- Who is in charge of the program?
- Who are the staff members involved in program development, implementation, and/or evaluation?
- Who is the program attempting to reach?
- Who will fund this program?

4. WHEN
- When will the program be implemented?
- When will the program end?

5. WHY
- Why is the program needed (justification)?
- Why might the program succeed or fail?

6. HOW
- How will data be collected?
- How often will data be collected?
- How often will outcomes be examined?
- How will the program be developed? Implemented? Evaluated?
- How will the program sustain its funding or obtain future funding?
- How will the program's success be determined?

This structure is the "skeleton" on which a program can be designed and can serve as a reference when planning resources, budgets, staffing, and operational procedures. A program's structure consists of the program's goals and objectives, which follow directly from strategic planning. The plan should include a description of the resources needed to achieve the goals and objectives, including necessary funding. A major component of these resources may include human resources described in terms of required skills and scope of practice. Technical resources for data, including their analysis and storage, will need to be considered when designing a program budget. Initial budget proposals for new programs usually estimate costs in broad categories. Final program budgets require careful attention to all aspects of program planning, implementation, and evaluation, and should estimate yearly costs as closely as possible. Funding is determined after a program budget is created. The source may be a state or federal grant, or it may be self-financed through health insurance held by consumers or a combination of funding sources. Whatever the source (or sources) for financing costs, a method of funding must be identified before the program can move forward.

Outcomes

Outcomes are often defined by regulatory, governmental, or certifying agencies such as The Joint Commission, the AHRQ, and the American Nurses Credentialing Center (ANCC). The AHRQ, for example, has identified a number of quality indicators that can be used as outcome measures of quality of care (for a complete list, go to www.qualityindicators.ahrq.gov/Default.aspx). The Joint Commission defines an outcome measure as the end result of a function or process in a patient population over a set period of time, often expressed as a rate or percentage.

The ANCC manages the Magnet designation program and describes outcomes as results, impacts, or consequences of actions. Agencies that have received the Magnet designation or are seeking it must compare data collected for a specific outcome against cohort groups at national levels and demonstrate that the majority of nursing units or practice arenas outperform the national benchmarks the majority of the time (American Nurses Credentialing Center, 2014).

Before establishing outcomes, one must revisit the mission and objectives of the program. What does the program do? Why does the program exist? Outcomes are the measurable results of the program objectives. They provide a method of evaluating the success of a program. State and national statistics can be used as benchmarks when examining outcomes. Comparisons to quality indicators (discussed in Chapter 2) can also serve as benchmarks to evaluate success or progress in a program. Outcomes should be established for short-term, intermediate, and long-term objectives. The mnemonic SMART provides a template for writing such objectives (Centers for Disease Control and Prevention, 2013).

- *Specific*: The outcome is well defined and unambiguous.
- *Measurable*: Concrete methods and criteria for assessing progress are used.
- *Achievable*: The goal stretches you, but is reasonable given the program's resources and sphere of influence. Reasonable goals and objectives must be motivational; they should provide incentives for success of program staff and stakeholders.
- *Relevant*: The outcome must be relevant to the program's vision, mission, and goals. Outcomes must also be relevant to all people affiliated with or impacted by the program.
- *Time*: The time period for accomplishing goals and evaluating outcomes is reasonable.

Outcomes can be incremental and subtle. Trying to turn personal or subjective experiences into concrete, specific, observable measures can be a daunting task. Hence, both quantitative and qualitative outcomes may be helpful and necessary.

Impact is another tool used to measure program success in recent years. It uses qualitative and quantitative measures to establish its success by looking at broad-based outcomes. It is viewed in broader terms and is less specific than outcomes. Impact is defined as the difference in the changes in outcomes between those involved with the program and those not involved (Baker, 2000). It is the evaluation of the effects, both positive and negative, caused by a program. Impact evaluation is an effort to determine, in broad terms, whether a program has the desired effects on individuals, households, and institutions, and whether those effects are attributed to the interventions associated with the program. The following are examples of how the impact of a transitional program intended to reduce readmission rates for heart failure patients might be articulated in quantitative and qualitative terms:

- Within 1 year of the inception of the program, the hospital's heart failure readmission rate was reduced and outperformed the national benchmark.
- In a recent 10-month tracking period, more than 20 patients successfully completed the program.
- A patient's wife describes its value this way: "Thank you so much for your excellent program! I sincerely believe you and your team deserve an award for excellence in patient care. I don't know what we would have done without your support and guidance."
- The personal impact of the program and its professional staff is acknowledged by one participant: "[T]he staff helped me realize I was not eating as well as I should and got me moving in the right direction. Also, I noticed that when I eat so many fruits and vegetables, I don't have room for so much junk food. Before this program I didn't realize how much salt was in the food I was eating."

Program outcomes illustrate what you want your program to do. Outcomes should provide information that can be used for quality improvement. After defining program outcomes, consider applying the following questions as a critique:

- Is it clear what the program is assessing?
- Is the outcome measurable?
- Is the intended outcome measuring something useful and meaningful?
- How will the outcome be measured?
- Are the outcomes realistic for the time frame of the program?

Outcome data can be collected continuously throughout the program implementation or at specific points in time, such as quarterly, or at the completion of a particular time-limited program.

When designing programs, outcome measures must be clear, concise, measurable, and easily compared to quality indicators when possible. They should be realistic and time delimited. Evaluation of the impact of a program can also be helpful when dealing with qualitative and quantitative measures. In summary, the outcomes selected should show the progress (or ineffectiveness) of a program and allow for objective evaluation.

Policies and Procedures

Well-designed policies and procedures (P&P) should document structure, processes, and outcomes and are essential for a successful program. They ensure compliance, manage risks, and drive improvement. P&P help describe the program—the way business is done, how situations are handled—provide legal protection, mandate compliance, and guide consistent performance. A program does not need a policy for every contingency, thus providing more latitude in operations. When developing P&P, the APRN should consider the following:

- Writing of the P&P
- Providing administrative support and possible legal review
- Reviewing and discussing the P&P with the program staff
- Ensuring P&P are supported by evidence
- Interpreting and integrating the P&P into program practices
- Ensuring compliance with the P&P

Using the earlier example, if a program was designed for transitioning patients with heart failure from hospital to home, it would require a review of the literature to determine evidence-based strategies that have been used by other organizations to prevent or delay readmissions. Program planners would also need to review state and federal regulations related to important factors such as reimbursement for services and zoning requirements for program facilities. The synthesis of evidence would provide a framework for the development of P&P for clinical services and program implementation.

A carefully constructed P&P manual is critical for program success. It can be modeled after evidence-based protocols and can provide the framework for consistent training of staff and community outreach workers. P&P also serve as a guideline for staff to follow to ensure delivery of quality care and consistent practices in the program.

Marketing

The American Marketing Association (2013) defines *marketing* as "the activity, set of institutions, and processes for creating, communicating, delivering, and exchanging offerings that have value for customers, clients, partners, and society at large" ("Marketing" section, para 1). Marketing requires activity and is not passive. It is a group effort involving a variety of individuals and groups, internal and external to the program or organization. Marketing is also process driven. Without processes, nurse leaders cannot plan effectively and can have difficulty determining what is working and what is not. A well-mapped-out process is critical for success. Marketing is not advertising. Advertising is only one part of marketing. Market research is accomplished by identifying consumer and societal trends and demands. Marketing is delivering on the promise made to key stakeholders. At the very least, the promise needs to be delivered. A nurse leader acting as a marketer can impress program customers by achieving desired outcomes.

The concept of "positioning" can be applied to a nurse-led program. Positioning is how you differentiate your program from the competition and present your brand in the marketplace. Positioning happens in one place, in the mind of the consumer, and occurs in a moment. You have to get the attention of the consumer who becomes interested in your program. The consumer will spend energy evaluating your program in relation to others and will make a choice to participate in your program or not. Ask yourself the following questions related to the concept of positioning (McNamara, 2010):

- Who is the target market?
- Who are the competitors for the program?

- What should be considered when determining the logistics of the program, including costs?
- What should be considered when naming the program?

Marketing is an important component to consider in program design and development. It is important to be aware of not only your competitors but also what will appeal to your audience (e.g., potential participants). A strong marketing campaign can lead to long-term successes not only for your program but for future programs as well. Stakeholders will see the value in a well-constructed marketing plan, which ultimately is important for program sustainability.

Communication

If a tree falls in the forest, but no one is around to hear it fall, does it make a sound? This question highlights a realistic problem faced when communicating about a program. You may have the best program in the world, but if you do not communicate the benefits and features of the program to the right audience, how are consumers going to find out about it? How are stakeholders and program team members going to buy into the program?

Communication consists of a sender, a receiver, and a medium. Communication is important to marketing a program and can come in many forms. Consider the following basic questions when engaging in strategies to communicate about a program:

- Who will be responsible for communicating information about the program?
- What is the message being communicated?
- Who is the intended recipient of the communication?

The medium for the message can include verbal and nonverbal communications. Verbal communication may include word of mouth, telephone voice messages, and presentations at meetings. Communication through nonverbal means includes ads in newspapers, information on an organization's website and Twitter account, newsletters, posters, text messages, and e-mails.

Programs are successful only if they have the participation of the target population. There must be buy-in by its members, and without effective communication by a variety of modalities, this message may never reach the intended population. As noted earlier, there are verbal and nonverbal forms of communication; verbal communication is probably the most effective for some populations, as the value of face-to-face interaction and relationship building cannot be replaced using nonverbal methods. With that said, many of these forms of communication require an investment of time and money, and these costs need to be included in the program budget.

Models for Program Design

The Logic Model

The *Logic Model*, developed by the W. K. Kellogg Foundation (2004), is commonly cited in the literature as a model for program planning. The model is used in program evaluation but is also useful and appropriate for program planning and management. It is a tool used to help shape a program. Additionally, logic models help leaders identify factors that may impact a program and enable them to forecast needed data and resources to achieve success. A logic model is a graphic display or "map" depicting the relationship among resources, activities, and intended results that identify underlying theory and assumptions.

The Logic Model is aligned with the scientific method. Just as a hypothesis is tested in research, program objectives are tested through program development, implementation, monitoring, and evaluation. The following steps outline the Logic Model program planning—clarifying program theory:

- Describe the problem(s) your program is attempting to solve or the issue(s) your program will address.
- Specify the needs and/or assets of your community that led your program to address the problem(s) or issue(s).
- Identify desired results by describing what you expect to achieve, short and long term.
- List factors you believe will influence change in the population or community.
- List successful strategies or "best practices" your research identified that helped address the targeted population and achieved results your program hopes to achieve.
- State assumptions underlying how and why the identified program will work.

The Logic Model provides a focus for leaders and helps to clarify program progress. Goals are easily identified, task responsibilities are assigned, and outcomes are clearly communicated. Because of the Logic Model's graphic display, key stakeholders and players visually see their roles and accountability can be measured. As a result, collaboration and communication are enhanced.

Lane and Martin (2005) have described the successful use of the Logic Model by three APRNs who designed and evaluated a breast health program for rural, underserved women. According to the authors, "The Logic Model was most useful in outlining the program, guiding the first year, and identifying needed direction for the future of the program. It was at the heart of the program development and served as the visual schemata" (p. 110). A diagram of the completed Logic Model for this program can be found in Figure 7.1.

Developing a Framework or Model of Change

Another approach, built on the Logic Model and incorporating best processes from the literature that guides the development of programs to promote community change and improvement, is referred to as *Developing a Framework or Model of Change* (Community Toolbox, 2014). This model is an innovation created by Community Toolbox, a public service sponsored by the University of Kansas. Community Toolbox is an online resource that provides information to people who are interested in promoting community health and development. Developing a Framework or Model of Change provides a road map for creating a new program by outlining the relationships among inputs, such as resources, outputs or the proposed interventions, impact (e.g., immediate results), and outcomes, including community or behavioral change. It is a 12-step process that organizes thinking and orients program development through intended outcomes. The steps include the following:

- Analyzing information about the problem or goal
- Establishing a vision or mission
- Defining organizational structure and operating mechanisms
- Developing a framework or model of change

FIGURE 7.1 • Logic Model

Define the problem.	Some rural women in the region lack knowledge about and access to malignancy screening techniques.

↓

Identify the intervention.	Create a model-based program to meet the malignancy screening needs of women in a rural community.

↓

State the goal.	Increase the knowledge and practice of malignancy screening techniques and increase linkages for rural women in this region by creating a cancer health network with initial focus on breast health.

↓

Outline key objectives.	1. Develop the infrastructure for a cancer health network and establish linkages. 2.. Provide annual screening opportunites, including education and referral information. 3. Identify and secure ongoing funding for the cancer health network to sustain annual screening.

↓

Determine desired outcomes.	1. Increase awarness of early detection screening techniques by rural women. 2. Increase the screening resource (i.e., access to and finances for) in the geographic area. 3. Increase community support for screening activities. 4. Stabilize a recognized program for providing the screening activities. 5. Track demographic data and screening results of the women participating in the program. 6. Disseminate the knowledge gained.

Source: Lane, A., & Martin, M. (2005). Logic model use for breast health in rural communities. *Oncology Nursing Forum, 32*(1), 106. ONS disclaims any responsibilities for inaccuracies in words or meaning that may occur as a result of translation from English.

- Developing and using action plans
- Arranging for community mobilizers
- Developing leadership
- Implementing effective interventions
- Ensuring technical assistance
- Documenting progress and using feedback
- Making outcomes matter
- Sustaining the work

Activities outlined in the Developing a Framework or Model of Change process assist nurse leaders in bringing together diverse people to summarize collective thinking in an organized manner. As a result, a common understanding is created and commitment is enhanced. Additionally, these steps, together, set the stage for strategic action with the likelihood of comprehensive interventions reflective of experience and research. Organized thinking through the Developing a Framework or Model of Change approach results in a clear rationale for programs, which can facilitate funding opportunities, guide support staff, and direct the identification of outcomes and data collection. Using and developing best practices ensures that interventions will have the desired impact on outcomes and, more important, advance the science of healthcare. Several examples of how the model has been used to plan, develop, implement, and evaluate successful community programs are available on their website (www.ctb.ku.edu).

The PRECEDE–PROCEED Model

The *PRECEDE–PROCEED Model* of health program planning and evaluation is another design model evolved at Johns Hopkins University based on the work by Green and Kreuter (1992). It is founded on epidemiological principles; social, behavioral, and educational sciences; and health administration. There are two fundamental propositions underlying this model: (a) health and health risks are caused by multiple factors, and (b) because of this, efforts to impact change must be multidimensional. The goals of the model are twofold: (a) to explain health-related behaviors and environments and (b) to design and evaluate interventions that influence both behaviors and the environment. The model follows a continuous cycle. Information gathered in the PRECEDE steps drives actions in the PROCEED process, which in turn provide additional information for the PRECEDE process.

PRECEDE (*Predisposing, Reinforcing, and Enabling Constructs in Educational Diagnosis and Evaluation*) outlines the planning process that aids in the development of targeted and focused programs. PRECEDE consists of five steps:

1. Determine population needs.
2. Identify health determinants of these needs.
3. Analyze behaviors and environmental determinants of health needs.
4. Outline factors that predispose, reinforce, or enable behaviors.
5. Ascertain interventions best suited to change behaviors.

PROCEED (*Policy, Regulatory, and Organizational Constructs in Educational and Environmental Development*) guides program implementation and evaluation. PROCEED is a four-step process.

1. Implement interventions.
2. Evaluate interventions.
3. Evaluate the impact of the interventions on factors that support the behavior as well as the behavior itself.
4. Evaluate outcomes.

Ahmed, Fort, Elzey, and Bailey (2004) used the PRECEDE–PROCEED Model to study the barriers that underserved women had to overcome in order to be screened for breast cancer. Once these barriers were identified, recommendations were made to improve healthcare system procedures. Table 7.1 summarizes how the model was used by these researchers. Another example of how the PRECEDE–PROCEED Model can be used was illustrated by Allegrante, Kovar, MacKenzie, Peterson, and Gutin (1993), who implemented and evaluated a walking program for patients with osteoarthritis of the knee. They found success with their program and suggest that the intervention strategies designed around this model are readily adaptable for a wide range of settings.

An Evaluation Framework for Community Health

Produced by the Center for Advancement of Community Based Public Health and based on work by the CDC, Framework for Program Evaluation in Public Health (2000) is another model that can be used for program development, implementation, and evaluation. This systematic approach involves procedures that are useful, feasible, ethical, applicable, and accurate. Evaluation is the driving force for planning effective programs, improving existing programs, and demonstrating results to justify investment in resources. The framework comprises six interdependent steps that build on one another and facilitate understanding of the program context, including its history, setting, and organization. The steps are as follows:

- Engage stakeholders
  - Those involved in the program, those served or affected by the program
- Describe the program
  - Program needs, expected effects, activities, resources, stages of program development, operational chart
- Focus the evaluation design
  - Program purpose, users, uses, questions, methods, agreements
- Gather credible evidence
  - Program indicators, sources, quality, quantity, logistics of data collection
- Justify conclusions
  - Program standards, analysis and synthesis, interpretation, judgments, recommendations
- Ensure use and share lessons learned
  - Program design, preparation, feedback, follow-up, dissemination, additional uses

Models serve as organizing frameworks for developing a program from beginning to end, including planning, implementation, and evaluation. Nurse leaders may tailor these models to guide them in the design and development

TABLE 7.1 • Application of the PRECEDE–PROCEED Model

Case Study: Use of the PRECEDE Model to Explore How Underserved Women Overcame Barriers to Mammography Screening. What Must Precede the Outcome?

PRECEDE

Step 1: Determine population needs.

The authors note that mammography can reduce breast cancer mortality and that rates of regular screening are very low in the general population. Efforts to improve rates have had varying results.

Step 2: Identify health determinants of these needs.

The authors conducted focus group discussions with women from underserved populations who themselves obtain regular screenings. The goal of the focus groups was to identify facilitators and barriers to mammography screenings.

Step 3: Analyze behaviors and environmental determinants of health needs.

Two themes emerged from the discussions. The first is related to the environment and the second to behavior: (a) the role of the healthcare system in preventive health behaviors and practices and (b) personal factors (the woman's responsibility).

Step 4: Outline factors that predispose, reinforce, or enable behaviors.

The authors note that lack of insurance used to be viewed as one of the major barriers to obtaining mammography—but even with the removal of this barrier, rates remain low. The focus of this study was on the behavioral factors influencing mammography screening. The authors report that the women in the focus groups described characteristics that influence them to obtain regular screenings: (a) awareness, knowledge, and trust—they understood cancer risks (some had personal experiences with family members who had cancer; some had healthcare providers who were receptive and encouraging); (b) personal responsibility—they demonstrated attitudes that support proactive behaviors, and this behavior developed within their families or through interaction with others; and (c) pride in self and satisfaction—these women found satisfaction with being role models for others.

Step 5: Ascertain interventions best suited to change behaviors.

To increase screening rates in underserved populations, the authors recommend providing information on risks and the importance of mammography in early detection (education) and inviting adherent women to act as role models. They further emphasized the importance of involving the media in providing information, as many of the women in the focus groups reported getting their information about mammography from television.

Adapted from Ahmed, N., Fort, J., Elzey, J., & Bailey, S. (2004). Empowering factors in repeat mammography: Insights from the storied of underserved women. *Journal of Ambulatory Care Management, 27*(4), 348–355.

of their own programs. APRNs can use these models to best serve their populations by either following the steps of a specific model or using various components from a number of models. All of the approaches are strongly focused on outcomes or program results. Outcomes drive evidence-based practice and best practices and therefore are a critical part of program design and success.

Care Delivery Models

As societal and healthcare demographics change, the APRN must consider new approaches to healthcare delivery. Implementing programs designed by nurse leaders requires innovation to promote health, decrease costs, and improve outcomes while maintaining quality, safety, and satisfaction. Care delivery models or systems operationalize the philosophy, values, and mission of an organization and its programs. These must be value driven. Values might focus on clinical practice, financial costs and viability, functional outcomes, and/or patient/client and provider satisfaction. They must provide rules and structures that define accountability and operational processes. Specifically they should identify who is accountable for expected outcomes and work to maintain strong relationships among key stakeholders and players.

A white paper commissioned by the Robert Wood Johnson Foundation outlined innovative care delivery models (2008). Twenty-four models were identified and categorized into acute care, bridging the continuum, or comprehensive care. Eight common elements or themes were noted throughout the models (Joynt & Kimball, 2008):

1. Elevated roles for nurses: nurses as care integrators
2. Migration to interdisciplinary care: team approach
3. Bridging the continuum of care
4. Pushing the boundaries: home as setting of care
5. Targeting high users of healthcare: elderly plus
6. Sharpened focus on the patient
7. Leveraging technology in care delivery
8. Driven by results: improving satisfaction, quality, and costs

How patient/client care, outlined in a specific program, is delivered will depend on the type of care being provided. Regardless of the type of care or method of its delivery, nurse leaders need to incorporate the following concepts reflective of the common elements identified in the innovative care delivery model white paper:

- A specific population focus
- A team approach
- Consideration of the continuum of care, including the home environment
- Strategies to engage the patient/client
- Teaching or education
- A focus on results or outcomes

The delivery of healthcare is an ever-changing process. Changes in the healthcare needs of a population should be addressed and reassessed on a regular basis to ensure patients' needs are still being met. Programmatic changes may need to be made, but the end result can lead to improved patient health, decreased costs, and overall improved patient satisfaction.

OVERCOMING BARRIERS AND CHALLENGES

The first step in overcoming barriers is assessing and identifying obstacles to program development, implementation, and evaluation. Insight into obstacles can pave the way toward developing action plans to overcome barriers and challenges. Is the challenge in the design of the program? Is the challenge the competition? Is the challenge related to resources, including time? Is the challenge due to the data being collected or the process of data collection?

The plan–do–check–act (PDCA) model used in quality improvement can be used to identify obstacles and plan subsequent actions. In 1980, NBC TV aired a program called "If Japan Can…Why Can't We?" It highlighted Japan's rise as an economic power from not just virtual, but actual, ashes. The program featured W. E. Deming, a statistician who taught quality control to Japanese manufacturers. That program and Deming are often credited with bringing quality-improvement initiatives to the attention of corporate America (Walton, 1991). Deming believed that American thinking was too "linear" and that it should be more circular fashion. The PDCA model is a Deming creation based on work by Andrew Shewhart.

- *Plan*: Plan the change.
- *Do*: Do it.
- *Check*: Check the results, then tailor your action based on the results.
- *Act*: Act to stabilize the change or begin to improve on the change with new information.

An example of the successful use of the PDCA model to improve the quality of care in an acute care hospital is provided by Saxena, Ramer, and Shulman (2004). A collaborative team was formed in an acute care hospital and charged with improving blood-administering practices using the FOCUS-PDCA method. FOCUS is the acronym for Finding a process to improve, Organizing a team familiar with the process, Clarifying the current situation, Understanding causes of variation, and Starting the PDCA cycle. The hospital identified a need to improve blood-administering processes (F) and formed a collaborative team that included nursing representatives, quality improvement, and laboratory and pathology personnel (O). They reviewed all of the P&P related to blood transfusions (C), had independent auditors assess current practices (U), then trained nurses to observe and assess the dispensing and administering of blood products to determine adherence to policy and procedure (S). They found that continuous, direct observational audits using the PDCA method improved compliance with P&P, thus reducing risk related to transfusion error.

The PDCA model is a process. The point is to strive toward continuous improvement or quality through ongoing assessment and improvement. Quality-improvement models such as this can provide a framework to assist APRNs in addressing some of the barriers that may be encountered in program development.

SUMMARY

In this chapter, APRNs and nurse leaders were given the tools to design and develop comprehensive programs that address multiple components of program development ranging from the identification of key stakeholders to marketing and communication strategies. Successful programs must incorporate knowledge from many fields in order to address issues related to the structure, process, and outcomes involved in program planning, development, implementation, and evaluation. Program models provide a standard and tested method for helping nurse leaders throughout the process of program implementation. Program designs that address consumer and societal trends are more likely to be successful and can lead to improved quality of care and ultimately improved patient outcomes.

EXERCISES AND DISCUSSION QUESTIONS

Exercise 7.1 Using data that can be found on the HHS or the CDC websites, identify trends in population demographics and health in an area that you serve.
- What are the implications for healthcare providers?
- What type of healthcare services and programs are needed right now?
- What type of services do you believe will be needed in 10 years?
- From a demographic point of view, in 10 years, what will be the important characteristics of the population that you serve if you stay where you are right now?

Exercise 7.2 You work in a family center that is part of a large hospital system with a catchment area that covers three counties. In the course of your usual work, you note that there has been an increased rate of childhood communicable diseases in your community and a decrease in immunization rates. You want to convince your employer to start a program to increase vaccination rates in the community that you serve.
- How would you justify such a program?
- How would you determine the feasibility of the program?
- Who are the stakeholders?
- How would you create the structure of the program?
- Identify the program outcomes.
- Using the "SMART" method, write short-term, intermediate, and long-term objectives for the program.
- How might you use the PRECEDE–PROCEED Model to plan, implement, and evaluate the program?
- How will you market the program?

REFERENCES

Ahmed, N. U., Fort, J., Elzey, J., & Bailey, S. (2004). Empowering factors in repeat mammography: Insights from the storied of underserved women. *Journal of Ambulatory Care Management, 27*(4), 348–355.

Allegrante, J. P., Kovar, P. A., MacKenzie, C. R., Peterson, M. G., & Gutin, B. (1993). A walking education program for patients with osteoarthritis of the knee: Theory and intervention strategies. *Health Education Quarterly, 20*(1), 64–81.

American Association of Colleges of Nursing. (2006). *The essentials of doctoral education for advanced practice nursing.* Retrieved from http://www.aacn.nche.edu/DNP/pdf/Essentials.pdf

American Marketing Association. (2013). *About AMA.* Retrieved from https://www.ama.org/AboutAMA/Pages/Definition-of-Marketing.aspx

American Nurses Credentialing Center. (2014). *Magnet recognition program® FAQS: Data requirements.* Retrieved from http://www.nursecredentialing.org/Magnet2014FAQ

Baker, J. L. (2000). *Evaluating the impact of development projects on poverty: A Handbook for prac-titioners*. Washington, DC: The World Bank.

Center for Advancement of Community Based Public Health. (2000). *An evaluation framework for community health*. The Center for Advancement of Community Based Public Health, University of North Carolina. Retrieved from http://prevention.sph.sc.edu/Documents/CENTERED%20Eval_Framework.pdf

Centers for Disease Control and Prevention. (2013). *Writing SMART objectives*. Retrieved from http://www.cdc.gov/healthyyouth/evaluation/pdf/brief3b.pdf

Centers for Medicare & Medicaid Services. (2014). *Readmissions reduction program*. Retrieved from http://www.cms.gov/Medicare/Medicare-Fee-for-Service-Payment/Acute InpatientPPS/Readmissions-Reduction-Program.html

Community Toolbox. (2014). *Tools to change our world*. Retrieved from http://ctb.ku.edu/en

Green, L. W., & Kreuter, M. W. (1992). CDC's planned approach to community health as an application of PRECEED and an inspiration for PROCEED. *Journal of Health Education, 23*(3), 140–144.

Joynt, J., & Kimball, B. (2008). *Innovative care delivery models: Identifying new models that effectively leverage nurses* [white paper]. Princeton, NJ: Robert Wood Johnson Foundation. (No longer available.)

Lane, A., & Martin, M. (2005). Logic model use for breast health in rural communities. *Oncology Nursing Forum, 32*(1), 105–110.

McNamara, C. (2010). *Designing and marketing your programs*. Retrieved from http://managementhelp.org/np_progs/mkt_mod/market.htm

Ratchinsky, K. (2014). *Top HIT trends for 2014: Accelerated change is coming*. Health care IT News. Retrieved from http://www.health careitnews.com/blog/top-hit-trends-2014-accelerated-change-coming

Saxena, S., Ramer, L., & Shulman, I. (2004). A comprehensive assessment program to improve blood-administering practices using the FOCUS-PDCA model. *Transfusion, 44*, 1350–1356.

Sherwood, A., Blumenthal, J. A., Hinderliter, A. L., Koch, G. G., Adams, K. F., Jr., Dupree, C. S., Bensimhon, D. R., . . . O'Connor, C. M. (2011). Worsening depressive symptoms are associated with adverse clinical outcomes in patients with heart failure. *Journal of the American College of Cardiology, 57*(4), 418–423.

Walton, M. (1991). *Deming management at work*. New York, NY: Perigee Books.

W. K. Kellogg Foundation. (2004). *Using logic models to bring together planning, evaluation, and action: Logic model development guide*. Retrieved from http://www.uwsa.edu/edi/grants/Kellogg_Logic_Model.pdf

E • I • G • H • T

Evaluation of Practice at the Population Level

Barbara A. Niedz

Early in their careers, nurses often have an enthusiasm and energy for caring for one patient at a time. Over the years that focus broadens as the more experienced nurse embraces a role that is more expansive and addresses issues at a population level. As administrators, leaders, educators, and managers, the advanced practice registered nurse's (APRN's) scope of practice widens even further. Quality nurse professionals expand their view to the entire organization and across departments. Nurses have, over the years, moved in many diverse directions. We not only care for patients at the bedside, but in their homes, businesses, schools, prisons, rehabilitation settings, as well as in outpatient and mental health facilities. Nurses also serve in settings that may be considered more "nontraditional": for example, working for managed care organizations (MCOs) by providing utilization management, and designing and implementing case and disease management programs. Another critical responsibility of APRNs is the oversight of clinical outcomes at the population level.

The advancement of many educational opportunities for nurses has moved our profession into new and exciting places. The advent of the advanced practice licensure designation has opened doors for nurses that did not exist 20 years ago. Nursing has become proactive and more responsive to the needs of the healthcare environment and to the needs of our patients. APRN status and licensure expand the nursing role to include status as primary care providers, and APRNs are recognized in many preferred provider networks across the country, receiving appropriate reimbursement. Our potential to influence the health of patient populations has expanded accordingly.

This chapter describes ways to evaluate population outcomes, systems' changes, as well as effectiveness, efficiency, and trends in care delivery across the continuum. Strategies to monitor healthcare quality are addressed, as well as factors that lead to success. Most important, these concepts are explored within the role and competencies of the APRN.

MONITORING HEATHCARE QUALITY

Nurses have been concerned about the quality of patient care for many years. Although our definitions of quality have varied, at the heart of this discussion is our collective desire to continuously improve patients' health and management of various disease states, regardless of where a given patient fits on the continuum.

Definitions of Quality and Theoretical Models

Just as nurses have cared for one patient at a time, initial models for quality dealt with individual patient reviews. Donabedian (1980) defines quality in broad terms: "Quality is a property that medical care can have in varying degrees" (p. 3). His definition holds that "attributes of good care ... are so many and so varied that it is impossible to derive from them either a unifying concept or a single empirical measure of quality" (p. 74). This notwithstanding, Donabedian's (1980) model of structure, process, and outcome addressed how quality can be maximized in organizations, and continues to be used today to structure research on quality methods throughout the globe (Chen, Hong & Hsu, 2007; Gardner, Gardner, & O'Connell, 2013; Handler, Issel, & Turnock, 2001; Schiller, Weech-Maldonado, & Hall, 2010; Wubker, 2007).

In recent years, Donabedian's influence continues in the way organizations are required to demonstrate their quality endeavors. For example, most accrediting bodies, such as The Joint Commission (TJC), the National Committee for Quality Assurance (NCQA), and URAC, all require evidence of a quality structure. Trilogy documents (a program description for quality, the annual work plan, and an annual program evaluation) are developed and reported through a committee structure that provides insight into the quality program from frontline staff through governance. In addition, process indicators of quality, such as whether or not the patient with an elevated ST segment and positive troponin is provided with aspirin on admission to the emergency department (ED), are a mandate within the core measure set for acute myocardial infarction (AMI). Finally, the emphasis of outcomes in recent years also emerges from the Donabedian model. The model provides for a robust relationship between structures and processes, which, taken together, enhance the potential for maximizing outcomes, such as reducing the incidence of significant cardiac damage in AMI.

Nash, Reifsnyder, Fabius, and Pracilio (2011) explain that the concept of population health includes an integrated system of care across the continuum. The population health model "seeks to eliminate healthcare disparities, increase safety, and promote effective, equitable, ethical and accessible care" (p. 4). They explain that quality is defined in terms of clinical data and outcomes, both economic and patient centered. In their view, "quality is founded on evidence based medicine" (p. 5) and describes the relationship between quality of care and the cost of care; if the quality of care improves, the cost of care is reduced (Nash et al., 2011). Nash et al. (2011) describe the importance of prevention, screening, and patient self-care management. They describe the importance of identifying risk factors to the development of chronic illness and the influence of the community, the availability of and access to various programmatic elements that can help manage and reduce the cost of care. The incidence of diabetes mellitus could potentially be reduced by getting control of the rampant obesity problem across the United States. As an example of a prevention indicator of quality for health plans, monitoring the patient's body mass index (BMI) is an important Healthcare Effectiveness Data and Information Set (HEDIS) measure and is also included in the Centers for Medicare & Medicaid Services Five-Star Quality Rating System (CMS STARs) measures. Preventing the incidence of diabetes mellitus can potentially result in reducing its short- and long-term complications, which could subsequently save thousands, perhaps hundreds of thousands, of healthcare dollars. As an example, consider the impact of preventing the incidence of type 2 diabetes mellitus on end-stage renal disease (ESRD), and the cost of dialysis alone. In 2012, Medicare expenditures for outpatient dialysis were $10.7 billion (Medicare Payment Advisory Committee, 2014).

The Institute for Healthcare Improvement (IHI) puts the ideas of Nash et al. (2011) into action in the Triple Aim initiative. The goals of the Triple Aim are (a) better health, (b) better experience of care, and (c) lower cost. The Triple Aim framework serves as the model for many organizations and communities (Bisognano & Kenny, 2012). The Triple Aim site can be accessed at www.ihi .org/Topics/TripleAim/Pages/default.aspx.

Juran (DeFeo, 2014; DeFeo & Juran, 2010) offers a definition of quality that is both parsimonious and applicable across disciplines. He defines quality in terms of the customer and explains that a product or service has quality if it is "fit for use" in the eyes of the customer. Goonan (1995) and Dienemann (1992) have applied Juran's definition to healthcare scenarios. Patients, as consumers of healthcare products and services, fit the definition of customers, regardless of the payment source. Juran (DeFeo, 2014; DeFeo & Juran, 2010) explains that for a product or service to meet the needs of the customer, it must have the right features and must be free from deficiencies.

In Juran's view (DeFeo & Juran, 2010), new features (such as new cardiac surgical equipment or the capacity to provide outpatient dialysis) may require capital and operating expenses. Deficiencies or defects in our healthcare products or services always contribute to the cost of poor quality. The cost of one hospital-acquired infection has been estimated at $15,000 by McCaughey (2006) and may range from as low as $500 to as much as $50,000 (Hassan, Tuckman, Patrick, Kountz, & Kohn, 2010). Hospitals are no longer reimbursed for the cost associated with the development of a third- or fourth-degree pressure ulcer in a patient if that ulcer was hospital acquired and not present on admission. The Centers for Medicare & Medicaid Services (CMS), which functions under the aegis of the U.S. Department of Health and Human Services (HHS), promulgated rules to this effect in 2008 (see www.cms. gov/HospitalAcqCond). The development of a hospital-acquired third- or fourth-degree pressure ulcer is also included in the National Quality Forum's list of "never events" ("The Power of Safety," 2010). In recent years, CMS has dictated by law and regulation that hospitals will not be reimbursed for care related to 14 of these never-event conditions that occur during an inpatient admission (CMS, 2014a). Other preventable outcomes that contribute to the cost of poor quality have consequences that go beyond dollars and cents.

Deficiencies that result in complications and even death arise from poor systems and human failures. These have gotten significant and appropriate attention through the patient safety movement (Institute of Medicine [IOM], 1999, 2001). Through TJC and the National Patient Safety Goals, attention to hospital and other healthcare organizations has resulted in significant strides toward reducing deficiencies. The importance of improving quality by avoiding the "never events" and reducing deficiencies has reinforced the necessity of accurate and thorough documentation and medical decision making by all healthcare providers.

Although Juran's definition of quality does have merit and application in healthcare (Kaplan, Bisgaard, Truesdell & Zetterholm, 2009; Muerer, McGartland-Rubio, Counte, & Burroughs, 2002), capturing ways and means to measure both outcome and process indicators of quality have emerged from an evidence-based approach. For example, research literature has shown that in order to decrease the incidence of congestive heart failure (CHF) hospital readmission rates, inpatient discharge instructions should capture key components, including (a) discharge medications, (b) the importance of weight tracking and documenting daily, (c) diet control, (d) what to do if symptoms worsen, (e) activity level restrictions, and (f) follow-up care instructions (Agency for Healthcare Research and Quality [AHRQ], 2014). Lack of any of these components is clearly seen as a "deficiency" and should be captured across aggregate data sets in hospitals (see http://www.jointcommission.org/). Thus, measurement mechanisms emerge from Juran's definition of quality (2010), which also fit with Donabedian's (1980) framework of structure, process, and outcome and Nash et al.'s (2011) view of population health.

Organizational Models for Excellence

Nurses provide the backbone of healthcare organizations, whether inpatient, outpatient, rehabilitation, home care, community health, or in an MCO. Services can be provided in person or sometimes via the telephone. In certain circumstances, nurses provide support by developing and monitoring telehealth programs. As such, understanding the organizational framework that can maximize positive outcomes and minimize deficiencies through the role of the nurse has value. The APRN, in particular, adds value, particularly through oversight and development of these newly emerging models of care.

Both Defeo and Juran (2010) and Donabedian (1980) put the concept of quality into the framework of an organization. Care of a patient across the wellness–illness continuum requires consistent and cogent processes and systems. Accordingly, Donabedian's view is that healthcare organizations require appropriate structure and key processes. Taken together, the structure and processes assist the organization in producing desired outcomes for their patients (Donabedian, 1980). Juran characterizes organizations as high functioning and marked by positive outcomes if features are maximized and deficiencies are minimized. In order to accomplish this, organizations plan for, control, and continuously improve quality. Both clinical and service quality characteristics are defined in terms of customers' needs and expectations. Others have made similar observations in applying Juran's organizational model in healthcare organizations (Best & Neuhauser, 2006; Goonan & Scarrow, 2010; Maddox, 1992). In 1987, the federal government instituted the Malcolm Baldridge Award, which recognizes those organizations that demonstrate principles characteristic of high performance and achieve significant business results through quality-improvement techniques. This award is based on seven key guiding principles and embodies the theoretical model of quality that Juran honed throughout his career (DeFeo & Juran, 2010; National Institute of Standards and Technology [NIST], 2015). In the late 1990s, this award was opened to healthcare organizations. Between 2002 and 2014, there were 17 winners of the Baldridge Award in the healthcare division (NIST, 2015).

In order for organizations to maximize positive outcomes and minimize deficiencies, planning must take on a strategic focus. Leadership and governance have responsibility and oversight for quality, and are essentially responsible for organizational planning. Quality planning, according to Juran (DeFeo, 2014; DeFeo & Juran, 2010), provides depth, breadth, and scope of how the product or service is designed, developed, and implemented. Key quality characteristics in the form of measurable goals and objectives for the organization and for patient outcomes are designed in the system or process before that product or service begins. Once that product or service is in operation, customers' needs and expectations (whether in the form of clinical quality, customer satisfaction, core business processes, or utilization of healthcare resources) can be understood, defined, and measured. External benchmark comparison data can be helpful in goal setting and in evaluating the extent to which a product or service meets customers' expectations. Juran's model (DeFeo, 2014; DeFeo & Juran, 2010) holds that all products and services are delivered to the customer employing various processes and systems. High-performing organizations design processes and systems to meet customer needs consistently, reducing variation in outcomes and minimizing defects. Juran calls this piece of the puzzle "quality control." For example, hospitals have put tremendous effort into improving patient flow in recent years: meeting patient (as customer) expectations for reducing delays in the ED and physician (as customer) expectations for radiology results reporting in a timely manner. The advent of the electronic health record (EHR) in hospitals and other healthcare organizations is another example of an efficient way to capture documentation and evidence of the patient's history across the continuum of care as well as contribution to overall patient safety and reduction of medical error. These complex operational processes in hospitals exemplify organizational processes and systems that can address key customer groups' needs: patients and providers.

W. Edwards Deming (Moen & Norman, 2010) developed similar theories of quality and consistently modeled the theme of reducing variation, and building quality into a product or system so that there is less need to depend on inspection (after the fact). Deming's model was also influenced by the work of other quality giants, like Shewhart and Feigenbaum ("Guru Guide," 2010). Ishikawa ("Guru Guide," 2010) paved the way for Japan's economic turnaround after World War II, largely based on the work of both Juran and Deming, who were sent by the U.S. government to support Japan after the war. These models rely heavily on the theory that all of quality is measurable and that reducing variation in processes holds a vital role in reducing the incidence of defects and, ultimately, assuring better outcomes.

Berwick, Godfrey, and Roessner (1990) were pre-eminent in applying these theoretical models to healthcare. Six leading healthcare organizations were armed with a national demonstration grant from the Robert Wood Johnson Foundation; within this seminal work, the authors cataloged the experiences of these organizations in applying this theoretical approach to quality. Their experiences clearly indicate that the models and tools had merit and value in reducing defects, improving processes, and maximizing outcomes (Berwick et al., 1986). This landmark work demonstrated that what had been shown repeatedly in manufacturing and in service industries throughout the country (and, in fact, worldwide) could be repeated in healthcare, and laid the groundwork for potential application throughout the healthcare industry. Deming's model has been applied in nursing, and the literature is replete with references depicting its application (Gavrilof, 2012; Institute for Healthcare Improvement, 2015a).

The IHI has put Deming's model into action. The IHI rapid cycle improvement model is based on iterative cycles of "plan, do, study, act" (PDSA). This model encourages small tests of change; implementation of bundles is built on this concept. The bundle concept is the development of a small number of evidence-based key components, which, implemented organizationally using iterative PDSA cycles, result in a desired outcome. There are five key components in the central line bundle: (a) hand hygiene, (b) maximal barrier precautions, (c) chlorhexidine skin antisepsis, (d) optimal catheter site selection, and (e) daily review of line necessity. The "how to guide" includes detail as to how an organization can successfully implement the bundle, using iterative PDSA cycles. For example, the CLABSI (central line-associated bloodstream infection) bundle encourages the use of a checklist. So, one of the PDSA cycles included to guide the implementation of the bundle relates to the use of this checklist. Other implementation strategies include developing measurement mechanisms and assuring adequate supplies to guarantee sterile technique on insertion and availability of chlorhexidine and other important adjuncts to reducing the CLABSI rate in hospitals (Centers for Disease Control and Prevention, Healthcare Infection Control Practices Advisory Committee, 2011).

Deming (Moen & Norman, 2010), Juran (2010), Crosby ("Guru Guide," 2010), and others explain that reducing variation is a continuous task, even when a given product or service is exceeding the needs of customers and especially when a given product or service is not competitive in the marketplace. The Six Sigma movement (DeFeo & Barnard, 2004; Pyzdek & Keller, 2009) emerged from a quality-improvement initiative at General Electric in the 1980s and set out to reduce defects or deficiencies to fewer than 3.4 defects per 1,000,000 opportunities. In essence, this model for quality improvement and planning is built on the work of Juran, Deming, Crosby, Ishikawa, Feigenbaum, and others ("Guru Guide," 2010). Although it is clear that Donabedian's work is theoretically sound, it also resonates with this thinking. In designing an influenza vaccination process for employees using the Six Sigma approach, Kaplan, Bisgaard, Truesdaell, and Zetterholm (2009) applied the model to a population health issue. Many others have applied the Six Sigma theoretical model to various healthcare processes. This model has significant application for process improvement across the spectrum of healthcare processes (Corn, 2009). To illustrate the application of process improvement theory and the use of Six Sigma models, consider the studies presented in Table 8.1.

Developing a Six Sigma approach works best when it is done broadly, across the entire organization. When a Six Sigma approach is well defined for a given organization, the impetus and funding source for the program comes directly from governance and cascades from the senior leadership team throughout, to the frontline employees, who use the systems and processes within them on a day-to-day basis. Deciding which projects are convened and which are not is also a governance process, and would likely emerge out of the quality infrastructure. Governance provides for an educational process to learn and apply the use of the many tools in the Six Sigma tool chest, many of which have a heavy statistical process control overlay. Six Sigma leadership uses an educational process in the form of various "belts" for certification. For example, a master black belt possesses the skills to oversee multiple Six Sigma projects simultaneously. The black belt is typically the project facilitator; green belts are often process business owners and may serve as the team lead in a Six Sigma team. The yellow belt is the team member who will also be schooled in the use of many of the tools (Pyzdek & Keller, 2009).

The patient safety movement in healthcare has given rise to a wider application of the Six Sigma model. In addition, the language of defects and deficiencies, though developed out of manufacturing and other type of product development, has resulted in consistent thinking that complications heretofore considered risks of procedure or hospitalization are now considered preventable (Courtney, Ruppman, & Cooper, 2006). The patient safety movement in the United States emerged largely due to the TJC and their attention to sentinel events (Joint Commission Resources, 2003). In addition, the consensus report of the Institute of Medicine "To Err Is Human," published

TABLE 8.1 • **Examples of Process Improvement Theory and the Use of the Six Sigma Model**

1. Anderson-Dean (2012) described the application of lean (which is a variation of Six Sigma model, focusing on eliminating waste and "nonvalue added" steps in a given process) principles in nursing informatics.

2. Drenckpohl, Bowers, and Cooper (2007) used the method to reduce errors related to breast milk identification processes in the neonatal intensive care unit (NICU).

3. Breslin, Hamilton, and Paynter (2014) applied the Lean Six Sigma model to care coordination processes.

4. Corn (2009) described the history of the model and its application in healthcare.

5. Fairbanks (2007) applied Six Sigma and Lean methodologies to improve operating room delays in throughput

6. Stankovic and DeLauro (2010) used the model to improve timeliness and reduce errors in the laboratory, in processing specimens.

7. Yun and Chun (2008) applied the design aspect of Six Sigma to telemedicine service processes.

by the IOM in December 1999, provides a focus on the potential for preventable error. One of the most telling comments early in the book explains that there are between 44,000 and 98,000 preventable medical errors annually in the United States that lead to patient deaths (IOM, 1999). The variability in the range is significant. Measurement mechanisms that would provide accurate descriptions of these sentinel events did not exist at that time. In the language of the process improvement gurus, these are defects and deficiencies. Applying these theoretical models to healthcare has tremendous potential in accurately describing quality of care by improving outcomes through attention to process.

Kaplan and Norton (1996, 2001) take measurement in organizations a step further and link progress against the strategic planning cycle to organizational goals and objectives. Their "balanced scorecard" model lends itself to healthcare well, and has been applied internationally (Chu, Wang, & Dai, 2009; Moulin et al., 2007; Potthoff & Ryan, 2004; Yap, Siu, Baker, Brown, & Lowi-Young, 2005). In fact, the Malcolm Baldridge Award has several specific criteria (see www.nist.gov/baldrige/publications/hc_criteria.cfm), and one of the most important is the recognition of "results." The results criteria require evidence of measurement and improvement of quality across organizations and systems. A well-defined scorecard at the enterprise level, which is balanced across several categories relating to the customer's experience, is a useful and important tool for senior leadership and governance. As we move into a discussion about planning, controlling for and improving quality across the entire patient population, understanding theoretical models for process improvement and their application becomes not only useful and accepted, but necessary and, most important, leads to improved outcomes of care.

Process Improvement Models and Tools

The literature provides applied evidence of various process improvement models that have many commonalities. Deliberate and thoughtful use of applied evidence and the use of process improvement models can result in reduction of defects and deficiencies to levels that meet and exceed customers' expectations, whether those expectations surround clinical quality, customer satisfaction, core business process, or utilization of healthcare resource expectations. The "plan, do, check, act" (PDCA) process improvement model (Moen & Norman, 2010); the Juran Six-Step Quality Improvement Process model (DeFeo & Juran, 2010); or Six Sigma's define, measure, analyze, improve, and control (DMAIC) model all have common features and they are all problem-solving models that drive measurable improvement when used properly. They can facilitate a thought process and require a team initiative. They will work whether the problem is related to clinical quality, customer satisfaction, core business processes, or utilization of healthcare resources. They work inside and outside of healthcare, whether the problem is simple or complex and whether one is concerned about the care of patients or developing tangible products for retail sale. Table 8.2 describes characteristics that are commonly found in process improvement models.

TABLE 8.2 • Characteristics and Commonalities of Process Improvement Models

1. The problem is defined in measurable terms.

2. The problem is stated in terms of the customer's needs and expectations.

3. External comparative benchmark data are sometimes drawn on to help set the goal for the project.

4. Members of the team have well-defined responsibilities.

5. Most teams should have 6–10 members. Larger teams may not be able to control the problem process and might need to break into smaller groups to be effective. Smaller teams may have inadequate representation to fully address all facets of the problem.

6. The team includes an executive sponsor to usher the project as a priority in the organization.

7. Other team roles include business process owner as team leader, internal or external consultant as facilitator, and clearly described roles for remaining team members.

8. There is an analysis phase. This phase employs both qualitative and quantitative methods to arrive at barriers, obstacles, and root causes of the problem.

9. The analysis phase should be well supported with qualitative data (like a cause–effect diagram) and quantitative "theory testing" data (like a diagnostic study of the root causes of the process problem).

10. Remedies that address both the qualitative and quantitative barriers are designed.

11. A plan for piloting or testing the remedies is well defined, engages the full team, considers the cost of implementation and decision making therein, and defines whether or not they are sufficient to achieve the desired improvement.

12. A measurement mechanism is designed to evaluate the effectiveness of the change strategy and the degree to which an additional remedial plan is needed.

13. A mechanism for evaluating ongoing data collection, day to day and month to month, is put in place, to assure that the gains are held constant.

14. In order to provide an effective use of a process improvement model, the focus must be clear and well defined. Teams must sometimes winnow down a larger project to its smaller component parts. At the end of a successful process improvement project, consider going back to revisit other improvement opportunities, which may have been set aside from the focal interest.

All process improvement models have these common characteristics. In addition, a variety of tools support the quality professional along the process improvement path. Tools such as process flow charting, barriers and aids charts, cost–benefit analyses, data-collection tools and statistical methods, SIPOC (suppliers–inputs–process–outputs–customers) analyses, project planning tools, lean thinking, and many others provide useful insight and drill closer to improvement goals (Balanced Scorecard Institute, 2014; DeFeo & Barnard, 2004; Pyzdek & Keller, 2009; Womack & Jones, 2003).

Population-Based Models

On a continuum from health and wellness (H&W) products to complex care management, a variety of population-based models have emerged over recent years (Table 8.3). Patients move across a continuum from good health to the end of life and enter a variety of settings in doing so. Programs are designed

TABLE 8.3 • Population Health Models

1. *Health and Wellness (H&W):* These programs are primarily telephonic, and may have a biometric screening component; program awareness and patient education materials are often part of a direct-mail campaign. These programs aim at identifying patients with significant health risk and encourage patient participation in screening. Completion of a health risk assessment is often a key component of lifestyle management programs. Smoking cessation, weight reduction, and attendance at preventive care visits are examples of desired outcomes for this patient population. Although significant health risks may emerge here, this patient population is essentially healthy without the presence of diagnosed disease states; the focus of H&W programs is aimed at identifying risks, with prevention of chronic illness as the ultimate target.

2. *Disease Management (DM):* These programs are likely to be telephonic, field based, or a combination of both. Patients qualify for DM programs on the basis of identified disease states, singly or in combination. Most DM programs target at least five or six disease conditions: persistent asthma, COPD (chronic obstructive pulmonary disease), CAD (coronary artery disease), diabetes mellitus, CHF (congestive heart failure), and depression. Other programs are broader and capture superutilizers, high-risk patients with varied chronic disease states. DM programs often have a care coordination component, which can provide such things as assistance in placing patients in a medical home and medical transportation (to help reduce the overuse of emergency medical services and ED [emergency department] care), or help in finding funding sources for medication management (to avoid disease exacerbations due to medications not being filled), etc. Examples of outcomes for this patient population include, but are not limited to, (a) assuring that a diabetic patient gets HbA1c testing done at least annually, (b) assuring that a patient with persistent asthma has a prescription for controller medications, and (c) confirming that a CHF patient knows the importance of measuring his or her daily weight and what to do if symptoms worsen. For example, when discharging from the inpatient setting a patient who has CHF and an ejection fraction of less than 40%, with proper discharge plans and instructions we assure that the patient is appropriately prescribed an angiotensin-converting enzyme (ACE) inhibitor and knows the importance of weighing himself or herself daily. In summary, care coordination assures that the patient has the ability to fill the prescription (has transportation to obtain and financial resources to buy), has a scale at home or the means to purchase one, and has transportation to the doctor's office for follow-up or preventative care.

3. *Case Management (CM):* These programs capture patients who have complex needs and multiple health conditions. These patients are often high risk and high cost, and come to the surface in stratification and predictive models because of overutilization of EDs and multiple admissions due to poor outpatient management or lack of a medical home. These patients account for a very small percentage of the total population, but account for more than 60% of the total healthcare dollar. Models that integrate care across various specialties for a given patient set (e.g., patients with severe mental illness who also have multiple medical disease conditions) are emerging.

to offer both telephone care and field-based approaches to prevention, disease management (DM), care coordination, case management (CM), and care integration. Patients are identified through predictive models and other stratification methods. The extent of outreach is determined by various levels of acuity, and the frequency of patient contact may depend on clinical assessment and care planning. Motivational interviewing and health education are primary strategies to engage patients into modifying their behaviors, but a hallmark of all of these programs is ultimately a change in health behaviors, which leads to desired outcomes. Preventive strategies such as smoking-cessation programs, as well as care coordination strategies such as identifying a medical home and assuring medical transportation to an outpatient facility, combined with condition-specific strategies in the presence of various chronic disease states, to reduce the incidence of ED usage for primary care and reduce inpatient admissions are all examples of ways to improve access to care in the hopes of ensuring overall quality of care (Fetterolf, Holt, Tucker, & Khan, 2010; Moreo & Urbano, 2014; O'Toole et al., 2010; Rice et al., 2010). Research has shown that disease and CM programs are effective in reducing the trajectory of chronic disease by providing less utilization of healthcare resources and providing enhanced patient satisfaction by improving the patient's ability to perform activities of daily living and improving her or his ability to manage chronic diseases (self-efficacy) Baicker, Cutler, & Song, 2010; Bedell & Kaszkin-Bettag, 2010; Govil, Weidner, Merritt-Worden, & Ornish, 2009; Lamb, Toye, & Barker, 2008; Rantz et al., 2014).

One of the most interesting recent trends in population-based care management is care integration. Care integration is a concept that is well known to nurses, but may not be as familiar to other health professionals. Here's an example: A patient is admitted to an inpatient acute care hospital with a significant drug overdose, subsequent to an attempted suicide. This long-standing behavioral health (BH) patient has been managed "on and off" by a variety of BH professionals, and has been receiving various psychotropic medications. In addition, the patient has a medical history that includes long-standing diabetes and CAD; other healthcare professionals have managed these aspects of the patient's healthcare. In fact, the medical professionals have not been in touch with the BH professionals, at the patient's request. In the ED, the BH professionals' role is pre-empted as the patient's overwhelming medical needs are the priority. When the patient is admitted to the intensive care unit (ICU), a host of consultants are brought to the case, and after being "cleared medically," the patient is transferred to the inpatient BH unit. Care is sometimes fragmented and the BH needs are addressed separately and apart from the medical needs of the patient. The primary care physician may not be involved until after discharge and may not have a clear sense of the many issues that play a role in the complete care of this patient. Although there is no question about the prioritization of care, there is also no integration of care. The patient's experience is divided into two distinctly different phases, in some ways compromising effective use of healthcare resources. This is where the importance of the medical home comes into play. Length of stay is clearly segmented into two sequential phases rather than managed in parallel. Although this inpatient example is a familiar one, lack of care integration is a common problem also on the outpatient side of the care continuum.

Processes of care that appropriately integrate care have been somewhat problematic in the U.S. healthcare system in the past. In recent years, it has become apparent that care integration needs to improve, which would improve the quality of care, resolve access issues, and reduce overutilization of healthcare resources (Gill, Swarbrick, Murphy, Spagnolo, & Zechner, 2009; Godchaux, 1999; Santos, Henggeler, Burns, Arana, & Meisler, 1995; Weinstein, LaNoue, Collins, Henwood, & Drake, 2013).

Two recent initiatives bring these ideas into sharp perspective. The first is the concept of the patient-centered medical home (PCMH). Within this model, care integration services are well defined and the process of bringing care to the patients where, when, and how they need them becomes not only possible but practical. The NCQA promulgates standards that describe this initiative (see www.ncqa.org/tabid/1302/Default.aspx). Accountable care organizations (ACOs) provide another model that incorporates these ideas into organized systems of care with healthcare providers, PCMHs, and hospitals partnering together. This is a program furthered by the CMS (see www.cms .gov/PhysicianFeeSched/downloads/10-5-10ACO-WorkshopAMSession Transcript.pdf and www.cms.gov/Medicare/Medicare-Fee-for-Service-Payment/ACO/index.html?redirect=/ACO).

Nurse-Sensitive Process and Outcome Indicators at the Population Level

Many authors have promulgated ways to organize measures, as taken together they represent a picture of quality. Kaplan and Norton (1996, 2001) suggest four generic categories that could work for any organization, including organizations that focus on healthcare. These perspectives include (a) internal business processes, (b) customer focus, (c) learning and growth, and (d) financing. The NCQA places the HEDIS measures into categories as well. The HEDIS categories include (a) effectiveness of care, (b) access/availability of care, (c) satisfaction with the experience of care, (d) use of services, and (e) cost of care (HEDIS, 2014).

Although the list of possible indicators used to measure population health and population health nursing may seem endless, four categories of measures, metrics, and indicators emerge. These broad categories are clinical quality, customer satisfaction, core business processes, and utilization of healthcare resources. Loosely based on Kaplan and Norton (1996, 2001) and the NCQA HEDIS frameworks, an organizing framework for evaluating population health nursing emerges. As these categories are of use in organizing our thinking regarding quality in the inpatient setting, they also have merit in outpatient settings, and as we consider care of the entire population with a given disease condition, these categories continue to add value to this discussion as an organizing framework. For the purpose of this discussion, the words "measures," "metrics," and "indicators" are used interchangeably. As we have put forward a definition of quality that is "measurable," our measures are quantifiable, a set of metrics that indicate the presence or absence of quality, and degrees on that continuum.

Whenever possible, standardized data definitions are essential. This sets up a level playing field for comparisons. Since the late 1990s, data sets, external comparisons, and guidance for standardized numerator and denominator have emerged across the patient continuum of care. As our industry has become more accountable to the public for outcomes, this kind of standardization has been essential, facilitating external comparisons on the basis of data sets. In addition, these numerators and denominators are described in detail, right down to the technical specifications. These technical specifications describe what types of codes are included in the numerator and which are included and excluded in the denominator. These codes have become widely accepted, the application of which results in fair and appropriate comparisons and rankings. Various groups (both governmental and private) have defined measures, specified the technical mechanics of counting and determining rates, and applied these measures across the industry. These include, but are not limited to, (a) CMS (www.cms.gov/center/quality.asp), (b) TJC (www.jointcommission. org), (c) the Agency for Healthcare Research and Quality, (d) NCQA (www. ncqa.org), (e) the National Quality Forum (NQF; www.qualityforum.org), and (f) the National Database of Nursing Quality Indicators (NDNQI; http:// www.pressganey.com/ourSolutions/performance-and-advanced-analytics/ clinical-business-performance/nursing-quality-ndnqi).

Measures have also emerged over time. As our foray into this area of accountability for outcomes has been heightened by legislators, policy makers, and the public at large, the connection between the cost of poor quality in healthcare and healthcare reform has become more explicit. Although it might require capital and operational outlay of funding to develop a specific product or service with the right features within the healthcare industry, the cost of poor quality adds a substantial burden to the cost of healthcare. For example, when a patient in a hospital setting experiences a delay in obtaining a diagnostic procedure that is essential to the appropriate management of his or her disease state, this core business process can delay decision making, causing a longer length of stay for the patient in the hospital. This delay may also lead to disease progression and result in complications that otherwise might have been prevented. Another question that should be addressed is whether these types of delays are due to the type of insurance, underinsurance, or lack of insurance. As discussed in Chapter 2, an important component of APRN practice is the need to recognize and address issues related to healthcare disparities.

When patient safety is compromised in hospitals, the result can be substantial. The example of delayed diagnostic testing may not only hinder the determination of a patient's diagnosis but may lead to patients receiving inaccurate medications or treatments or errors, such as a patient identification mix-up, that can result in loss of life. Over time, we are better able to identify the impact of the cost of poor quality by capturing and quantifying these indicators of quality in the aggregate. Sorting out "what counts and what doesn't" helps to provide clarity and a clearer view of quality across the board.

Clinical Quality

Nurse-sensitive indicators of population health that relate to clinical quality can be seen in a number of the metrics recognized by external organizations with available external benchmarks. In the HEDIS (NCQA, 2014a) data set created and maintained by the NCQA, there are several benchmarks that relate to chronic disease conditions. Nurses, who are in the field or on the phone in telephone call centers, reach out to patients with the intention of helping them wade through the various resources made available to them through private and public means to manage their overall health, given the presence of various disease states. The most common disease states managed by DM programs include (a) diabetes mellitus, (b) persistent asthma, (c) COPD, (d) CAD, and (e) CHF. Other chronic disease conditions also may be of interest. In CM programs, the complexity of care is heightened by the number and acuity of the chronic conditions coexisting in a patient's profile. Social problems, housing, transportation, and pharmacy costs often emerge in CM programs. Similarly, the emphasis from a clinical quality perspective in H&W programs is on preventive care, early recognition of emerging disease, and use of appropriately placed screening tools.

With the agreement of the NCQA, CMS has adopted the use of HEDIS in its Star rating program for various types of MCOs. For example, each Medicare Advantage Health Plan licensed by CMS is rated on a five-point star system. Clinical quality measures include process indicators collected through administrative means that contribute to a given health plan's Star rating. For example, whether or not the patient with a diagnosis of diabetes mellitus has a hemoglobin A1c (HbA1c) test done at least annually tells us something about the care that a patient with diabetes receives. CMS weights each one of the Star measures as to its importance. This process indicator of clinical quality that is determined by the presence or absence of an administrative claim or encounter for an outpatient laboratory test (in this case HbA1c) is weighted with 1 point toward the health plan's overall Star rating. However, the actual value of the HbA1c is a component of "comprehensive diabetes care," a HEDIS measure, which is included in HEDIS, and another Star measure for Medicare Advantage health plans in Part C. We know from scientific research that patients who maintain lower HbA1c levels (less than 8.0%) have fewer complications, a better quality of life, and longer life expectancy than do patients who are poorly controlled (AHRQ, 2014b). This makes HbA1c levels a significant clinical outcome indicator. Health plans collect actual HbA1c levels through a rigorous process and through a variety of means, including EHR data, providers' outpatient medical records, or actual laboratory data feeds. Most importantly, these data are weighted at three times the value of a process indicator in the overall Star rating. In order to score at the highest, 5-star rating, Medicare Advantage health plans strive to have a significant percentage of their patients score less than 8% on the HbA1c test.

Table 8.4 lists several examples of clinical quality measures that are sensitive to the APRN role at the population health level in DM, CM, and lifestyle management or H&W programs, whether their intervention is on the telephone, in person in any setting, or via a telehealth program. APRNs who have responsibilities regardless of the setting can strengthen a program design by assuring that outcomes measures are used in evaluating program effectiveness and incorporating a blend of process and outcome measures in quality program development.

TABLE 8.4

Sample Nurse-Sensitive Clinical Quality Measures in DM, CM, and H&W Programs

1. HEDIS Comprehensive Diabetes Mellitus Care: Did the patient have at least one HbA1c level drawn in a 12-month period?
2. CMS STARs HEDIS: Comprehensive Diabetes Care: Did the patient, aged 65 or older, show good control, through HbA1c levels of 8% or less?
3. HEDIS Asthma Care: Did the patient diagnosed with chronic persistent asthma have prescriptions for the appropriate medications to manage chronic persistent asthma?
4. AHRQ Prevention Quality Indicator of Congestive Heart Failure: What is the annual inpatient admission rate per 100,000 (at the population level) for CHF?
5. AHRQ Prevention Quality Indicator of Chronic Obstructive Pulmonary Disease: What is the annual inpatient admission rate per 100,000 (at the population level) for COPD?
6. HEDIS: Did the patient diagnosed with CAD (coronary artery disease) and an LDL (low-density lipoprotein) level of >100 mg/dL have a prescription for a statin or HMG-CoA (3-hydroxy-3-methylglutaryl-coenzyme A) reductase inhibitor?
7. HEDIS: Did the infant have appropriate well-child visits during their first year of life?

Adapted from HEDIS (2014).

Utilization of Healthcare Resources

One of the many important goals for nurses who work in DM, CM, and H&W programs is to direct patients to use healthcare resources in the most cost-effective way. In the context of population health, the most expensive healthcare resources include the use of the ED and inpatient stays. By ensuring that the patient's discharge plan coming out of the inpatient setting is fully executed, one can reduce the risk of rehospitalization. By assuring that patients have transportation and other care coordination needs met, it is to be hoped that we can reduce or eliminate emergency medical service (EMS) utilization for a ride to the local ED for primary care issues. The two metrics that are the most useful and sensitive to the nursing role in DM and CM programs are inpatient admissions per 1,000 members and ED visits per 1,000 members. In some ways, this work is an extension of the work that nurses have participated in for years, in utilization management (UM) programs based in hospitals, for health plans and for other providers of healthcare benefits. However, DM, CM, and H&W nurses take UM to the next step and assure that patients have the means, insight, and knowledge to carry out their healthcare needs with some degree of independence and autonomy. By reviewing care needs and targeting the right level of care, and matching it to the appropriate venue, we reduce the inappropriate use of these very costly services.

An evaluation of the utilization of healthcare resources is often included in a given DM or CM contract as a "return on investment" (ROI) analysis as evidence of financial performance. The bulk of the healthcare dollar primarily resides in the use of two resources: ED visits and inpatient stays. Both may be misused in the absence of an effective medical home or with poor access to primary care. At the population level, measuring the impact of population health models on the utilization of these two key healthcare resources is a very important component of any population health evaluation method. Three possibilities present themselves in an ROI evaluation; rigorous methodology is a component of well-designed DM and CM models. First, an estimation of cost avoidance involves using historical data to predict the number and percentage of ED utilizers and inpatient admissions in a given patient population that are likely to occur after a year of DM intervention. For example, after 1 year of investment in a telephonic nursing DM program, it is reasonable to predict that patients will be linked into a medical home and lessen their risk of admissions for preventable primary care conditions such as uncontrolled diabetes, asthma, or even CHF. These strategies also have the potential to prevent the use of EDs for primary care. Another method to evaluate ROI is to predict a trend and trajectory based on the baseline history of a given set or population of patients. A typical data set for comparison is a 12-month period of time, used as the starting point or baseline for comparisons moving forward. A third option to calculate the ROI of a DM, population health nursing program, posits that as a result of DM intervention, certain specific events will not occur. These are examples of rate changes that could (potentially) be the subject of an ROI calculation: a reduction in the readmission rate, reduction of the rate of patients per 1,000 with multiple admissions in a given year, or reduction of patients with admissions for ambulatory-sensitive conditions (ASCs). ASCs are also described by AHRQ as preventive quality indicators. (Visit www.ahrq.gov for more information on these important indicators.)

In recent years, two additional areas were identified for cost savings indicators: reducing the incidence of readmissions to the inpatient setting within 30 days of discharge and reducing the cost of pharmaceuticals by developing an appropriate formulary and applying rigorous criteria for medical necessity of pharmaceuticals. APRNs can take a key role in reducing inappropriate use of healthcare resources by assuring that care coordination tasks are addressed across the continuum, particularly at the point of transition from one setting to another, and by building and tapping into community resources (Brock et al., 2013; McCarthy, Bihrle Johnson, & Audet, 2013). All-cause readmissions within 30 days are emerging as a significant measure of healthcare resource usage, and is another example of a CMS STARs outcome measure that is weighted more heavily in a given health plan's overall STAR rating. Finally, although readmission after discharge from an acute care facility has long been an area of focus, in recent years, unplanned acute care readmissions within 30 days of discharge from a rehabilitation setting and from long-term care hospitals (LTCHs) have also received attention (CMS, 2013). Additionally, significant efforts have been made to reduce the utilization of expensive medications in pharmacy benefit programs and specialty pharmacy programs alike. Innovative programs, driven by pharmacists, that target long-term control of chronic conditions and the role of the clinical pharmacist are emerging. Medication therapy management (MTM) programs for patients with chronic illness and complex medication profiles are becoming more of a mandate and less of a luxury (CMS, 2014b).

Measures that relate to medication usage such as medication reconciliation, particularly in the chronically ill and the elderly, are included in CMS

STARs, as Plan D measures (part of the pharmacy benefit) and selected measures in Plan C, the medical benefit. There are also pharmacy measures that relate to special needs patient population plans, for those patients who are dually eligible for both Medicare and Medicaid (CMS, 2015a).

It could be argued that many of these measures fall into both the clinical quality and the utilization of healthcare resource categories. They not only improve the clinical quality of care received, and serve to prevent short- and long-term complications, but also reduce inpatient hospitalizations for patients with chronic illness and an acute need, as well as reduce the cost of care. It is also interesting that many of these clinical and utilization of healthcare resource measures also emerge for Medicare patients who are members of ACOs. ACOs are formed to address the needs of direct, fee-for-service Part A and Part B Medicare patients. These ACOs mandate at least 5,000 Medicare patients for a 3-year term. In order to achieve the incentives, these ACOs must demonstrate the same type of improvement in similar measures as Medicare Advantage health plans (CMS, 2015b).

Customer Satisfaction

For many years, patients have been identified as important consumers of healthcare products and services and, accordingly, have been defined as "customers" and important stakeholders in DM and CM organizations (NCQA, 2014b; The Utilization Review Accreditation Committee, 2014). Accordingly, key metrics that are sensitive to the nursing role can tell us something about the degree to which our patients, as customers, have had a positive experience with our nurses, whether those nurses practice in hospitals, in DM organizations, or at MCOs. How frustrating is it when a customer makes a telephone call to any company and ends up in a hold queue for long periods of time? Two call center metrics are often cited as important: (a) average speed of answer (ASA) and (b) call abandonment rate (ABN) (Cross, 2000; Del Franco, 2003; Formichelli, 2007; Gustafson, 1999). This literature is replete with guidance on how long it should take to answer inbound telephone calls in order to meet or exceed customers' expectations. The industry standard for ASA is fewer than 30 seconds and that for ABN is less than 5%. That is, less than 5% of calls should be lost when a customer abandons the call due to a prolonged waiting time (Cross, 2000; Del Franco, 2003; Formichelli, 2007; Gustafson, 1999). Akin to waiting for a response to a call light in an inpatient setting, prolonged wait times on the phone are a primary source of customer dissatisfaction. In recent years, the advent of multiple phone trees, predictive dialing, and interactive voice response (IVR) use in call centers has added technology and options aimed at improving the customer's experience. Call wait times and abandonment rates continue to be important drivers of customer satisfaction (Khudyakov, Feigin, & Mandelbaum, 2010; Mandelbaum & Zeltyn, 2013; Whiting & Donthu, 2009). Assuring that staffing levels (for both licensed and nonlicensed staff members) are appropriate and that technology provides adequate tools for observing the call queue, and using data down to the level of the staff member are important oversight supervisory functions for ensuring telephonic DM or CM care in a way that meets or exceeds customer satisfaction.

Monitoring, managing, and measuring complaints are additional ways to tap into the customer's experience. Customer complaints, whether from patient as customer or provider as customer, can be an insightful means to understanding patterns and trends of care delivery, and can be the key to improvement. Customer complaints can be very serious and can lead to a written complaint or, if a patient is not satisfied with the resolution offered, the launching of a formal grievance process. Customer complaints that are resolved by the nurse on the call are important to document and are worth tracking. Sometimes, complaints come into a DM call center that might be serious, but the target of the complaint is not the DM organization. In this case, these complaints are also valuable indicators of quality and should be referred to an appropriate authority or organization. Again, tracking and trending the nature of the complaint and the agency or organization to which the complaint was referred (rather than resolution) may be all that is required.

Various techniques are available for tracking patient, provider, and client satisfaction for DM programs. Annual surveys are the most frequent vehicle used, and the Care Population Health Alliance provides patient and provider surveys to organizational members (www.populationhealthalliance.org). These surveys have established reliability and validity. The surveys include items that measure the overall satisfaction of the patient with the services provided by the DM organization, but also tap into the "likelihood to recommend." Satisfaction with the skills and techniques employed in the service of DM programs by the individual nurse can also be assessed. Accordingly, these items are "nurse sensitive." Examples include items that evaluate the nurse's willingness to "listen" as well as provide information that can influence the patient's behavior in the interest of better management of specific chronic disease states.

Measuring customer satisfaction through a survey process has long been established as an important function, whether that measurement occurs in a hospital or in a population health setting, like a DM program. Many hospitals use a variety of prominent vendors for patient satisfaction monitoring such as Press Ganey™ Associates (www.pressganey.com/index.aspx), Healthstream® Research (www.healthstream.com/index.aspx), and many other research groups that specialize in healthcare survey processes. In recent years, the CMS has mandated the use of an agreed-upon set of questions administered in a consistent way regardless of the vendor. In the inpatient venue, the CMS survey titled the Hospital Consumer Assessment of Healthcare Providers and Systems (HCAHPS) is widely used (Hospital Consumer Assessment of Healthcare Providers and Systems, 2015). Although individual vendors, such as Press Ganey, offer comparisons based on various methods, the HCAHPS survey offers broad comparisons across the country on an agreed set of questions, worded the same and applied using the same, mandated research methods.

Surveys targeted at physicians and other providers of healthcare services that evaluate the extent to which the DM organization provides services to them, in the interests of their patients, are another important tool to gauge overall effectiveness. Annual surveys of providers as customers can also be insightful to a DM organization. The IHI also provides some insight into the usefulness of provider satisfaction assessment (Institute for Healthcare Improvement, 2015b). Other proprietary organizations provide additional insight (see also www.rand.org/content/dam/rand/pubs/research_reports/RR400/RR439/RAND_RR439.pdf).

Phone automated surveys and IVR surveys are also available, and a variety of telephone services provide this capability. This type of data collection and these methods have been used extensively because they provide timely feedback that is relevant on an ongoing basis. They do present advantages over annual surveys, in that a data stream is available with data summaries on six to eight items at weekly, monthly, even daily frequency, with assignment right to the level of the nurse. Survey research is fraught with both opportunity and challenge. Careful attention must be paid to sample size, response rate, generalizability of the findings, frequency of assessment, reading level of written surveys, and so on. In short, survey research requires the same rigor as a well-designed research study if the results are expected to reflect services rendered accurately and point to quality-improvement initiatives.

In recent years, the CMS has launched a customer satisfaction survey that taps into a given patient's level of satisfaction with the benefits and administration of the health plan. This tool, titled the Consumer Assessment of Healthcare Providers and Systems (CAHPS), has been developed in conjunction with the NCQA (2014). Technical specifications on the use of this survey tool can be found at HEDIS (2014). Some of these measures do evaluate patients' health behaviors (e.g., if the patient has obtained a flu shot) and their overall experience with the healthcare industry in general. Although the CAHPS tool does not specifically measure DM or CM, some of the items on the instrument may be nurse sensitive and may be of value because of available comparative data and because some health plans bundle DM into their services. For example, some of the questions on the adult CAHPS tool refer to specific aspects of care rendered by your doctor or other healthcare provider (nurses are not included as a separate type of healthcare provider). Other questions refer to the extent to which advice has been offered by healthcare providers on such things as smoking cessation and hypertension and cholesterol management, all of which may relate to the nursing role in disease prevention/management or H&W programs that encourage self-care management.

Patient self-reported outcomes are captured in survey form by the CMS in the form of the Health Outcomes Survey (HOS), which is administered to a defined cohort of CMS members every 2 years. These self-reported outcomes include measures on the extent to which patients perceive their overall physical and emotional health status over the 2-year period of time. HOS measures also contribute to CMS STAR measures for managed Medicare health plans and for special needs plans for the dually eligible (CMS, 2012).

Core Business Processes

Nurses are supported in many ways by the systems and processes through which they provide care. Although this is true in any direct care setting, it also has merit in telephone care and field-based DM and CM programs. While in hospitals, there might be some value to considering how acuity influences staffing levels; in the DM industry, acuity levels and ratios of staff to patients in DM programs are useful data. At the same time, because nurses are supported by job descriptions that are accurate and competency based, they are evaluated on their performance on a regular and ongoing basis. This is sound human resource practice, regardless of the setting or care type. Similarly, productivity levels are very important in all settings in which nurses practice. Can a given nurse manage a patient care assignment that is appropriate to the setting and meet all of the patient care requirements in a given time frame? This important question in the DM and CM industry might be answered by examining not only how many patients can be cared for per nurse per day but how many active minutes of the day the nurse is talking with patients on the telephone. Although in hospitals, outpatient settings, and rehabilitation facilities there is a "hands on" nature to the care, in telephonic DM programs both "calls per nurse per day" and "talk time in minutes" are direct measures of nursing productivity. Clinical quality and utilization of healthcare resource outcomes may be the best overall indicators of the quality of care, but these indirect measures also have merit. In other words, for a nurse to be effective in managing the care of an entire population of patients, across the continuum of care, volume and focus matter. In order to measure overall effectiveness of a group of nurses in DM programs, these measures of core business processes, when taken with clinical quality, customer satisfaction, and utilization of healthcare resources, can add to the panel of metrics that bring depth and understanding to managing the care of hundreds of thousands of patients across an entire population.

Other measures that are reflective of core business processes have value in evaluating the role of the nurse. In population health, DM, and CM processes, APRNs are interested in finding those patients for whom they can have an impact on their healthcare behaviors and make a difference in the way in which they manage their day-to-day care. A patient with diabetes and advanced comorbidities, who has not been in an ED or admitted (even for short- or long-term complications) to an inpatient facility, may not have obvious gaps in treatment (i.e., this patient is well managed without any help from the DM nurse). Suppose that a given diabetic patient is well managed (on his or her own), has an annual checkup with the physician, and his or her last HbA_{1c} was less than 7%. This patient may have very little actionable need for a conversation with a nurse in a DM program other than an introduction, consent, a condition-specific assessment, written materials, and encouragement to stay the course. Contrast this to a newly diagnosed 55-year-old patient with an HbA_{1c} of over 11%, with poor nutritional habits, who has just started on insulin and was just discharged from the hospital for "uncontrolled diabetes." Patients such as these have more actionable needs and are at risk for readmission if no DM assessments and interventions are put into place. Finding these patients, teeing them up for the nurse, and assuring that we have accurate call information are all strategies that are collectively called "patient identification" and "acuity stratification" processes. Oftentimes, DM and CM companies and MCOs use sophisticated information technology processes to identify patients for the nurse to call. A resulting engagement rate that measures the percentage of patients who are identified with one or more of the disease conditions under study and the percentage of patients who complete an enrollment and condition-specific assessment process with a nurse is a useful indicator of the degree to which the DM and/or CM programs are reaching the intended population.

This is a type of volume indicator that, when taken together with productivity metrics, can provide some evaluation of the impact of the role of the nurse on population health in DM and CM programs.

In summary, about 20 to 25 metrics in the four categories of (a) clinical quality, (b) customer satisfaction, (c) utilization of healthcare resources, and (d) core business processes taken together would provide an organization with a keen and parsimonious panel of metrics. This panel of metrics described in the earlier pages provides the reader with possibilities for evaluating the totality of any given population health nursing program, whether DM, CM, or all three program types. Kaplan and Norton (1996, 2001) describe this idea of a panel of metrics to guide the strategy of the organization as "the balanced scorecard." The examples provided earlier and from these four categories fit the evaluation need in DM, CM, and H&W programs, but neither the categories nor the example metrics are the only possibilities. In general, metrics and measures should be easily found using existing measurement mechanisms and standardized data definitions, which can be compared against national standards and are representative of the nurse's role in improving the health of the population. A parsimonious set is useful; it is often the case that in healthcare we measure too many things. In tracking countless indicators without intention or purpose, we lose the ability to make the measures meaningful and may miss the overall strategic goals of the organization.

Data Sources

Administrative data sets have been criticized in the past for not providing useful information and for not serving as accurate measures of quality ("Case-Mix Measurement," 1987). However, a broader understanding of the usefulness of administrative data has emerged in more recent times, particularly when evaluating quality at the level of the population (Jha, Wright, & Perlin, 2007; Schatz et al., 2005). Claims data have also been called "administrative data." Encounter data are another type of administrative data that are captured for patients in "at risk" health plans, that is, plans that are capitated or partially capitated. Administrative data are rich in various coding types, including, but not limited to, the *International Classification of Diseases*, 9th Edition (ICD-9; World Health Organization, 20xx), codes, Current Procedural Terminology or CPT codes, or CMS's Healthcare Common Procedure Coding System (HCPCS) codes. Used as the basis for electronic billing, these codes are rich in information about the patient and have been refined through the years to provide even more information (American Academy of Professional Coders, 2015). In DM, the ICD-9 codes, demographics, and patient experiences as captured through the administrative process provides an outline of care that affords the opportunity not only to identify patients with the most actionable need but also to find patients with those gaps in treatment. In the past, the evaluation of quality required detailed and sometimes tedious chart reviews, with random samples of charts pulled from various patient types. The effective use of administrative data is providing a rich source of information on the effectiveness of DM programs in shaping patients' health behaviors and habits over time (HEDIS, 2014).

In most DM programs, some type of documentation is required to track the patient's progress with an educational approach and the degree to which a behavior is shaped. So, although it is most important for the nurse to document an educational session on, for example, the importance of asthma controller medications, it may be just as important to hold a three-way call with the patient's primary physician to identify the need to move from frequent use of a short-acting beta agonist to an inhaled corticosteroid and to document this action. The measure of the true outcomes (such as the claim for the prescription or no documented ED visits for the remaining year) may come through that administrative data set later on, but the role of the nurse is and should be accurately captured in written or electronic documentation. The review of the nurse's documentation from a clinical perspective is no less important in call center and field-based DM programs than it is in the hospital, in an outpatient setting, or in a direct-care home setting. This documentation needs to be audited on a regular and ongoing basis; this supervisory function can also provide rich evidence of the productivity and role of the nurse. It is an important precursor to those outcomes, which may be measured through claims or other sources.

Patient self-reported data may also be useful, but this source of information may be risky as it introduces bias (recall bias, information bias, etc. [see Chapter 4]). Patients' recollection of a given result may be colored by their own resistance to a change in health behavior, by their lack of knowledge, or by very strong denial defense mechanisms that develop along what may be a very difficult diagnosis to accept. Consequently, there are times when self-report data may not be useful. For the NCQA to award the status of Accredited With Performance Reporting, certain measures must be met that include actual laboratory results, and patient self-report is not permitted. Data-collection methods using the HEDIS "hybrid" method require actual provider-held chart reviews (for a random sample) or data on laboratory results that come directly through a link to the laboratory that performed the test. Two examples that exemplify the use of laboratory data include the collection of HbA_{1c} annual results in the patient with diabetes and the annual LDL levels in the CAD patient. The HEDIS technical specifications provide a depth of rigor on these data-collection methods that is intense and appropriate. On the other hand, HEDIS recognizes that claims data on flu shots are very unreliable. Appropriately, patients are offered flu shots on a seasonal basis at health fairs, county-run clinics, during an inpatient stay, or at a local pharmacy (Pollert, Dobberstein, & Wiisanen, 2008). It may be the case that in these venues, there may be no claim submitted for the flu shot, considerably reducing the accuracy of the claims data on the incidence of obtaining flu shots in various patient populations. For most adults, the accuracy of the data on whether or not a patient has received a seasonal flu shot may be maximized by asking them. Self-report may be the best source of data available but is still not ideal. Data sources abound for key metrics in a panel of indicators that are both nurse sensitive and descriptive of population-based nursing. CMS recognizes the value of self-reported data and has incorporated a variety of measures in the Health Outcomes Survey (Health Services Advisory Group, 2014).

Quantitative Strategies for the Evaluation of Outcomes

One significant advantage of the study of health at the population level is the ample access to large populations of electronic data, allowing for a large sample size for analysis. Certainly, nursing's role in population health is enhanced by our ability to measure and track key characteristics of the patient population that are indicative of clinical quality and utilization of healthcare resources. Administrative data sets and access to an electronic medical record (EMR) in a given venue, or an EHR that has the potential to "follow" the patient across various inpatient and outpatient settings, have enhanced our collective ability as a profession to evaluate nursing's role in providing care and service by allowing us to use large data sets to analyze patterns of care and disease in the populations we serve.

Data Availability

The advent of the universal electronic billing process became a reality many years ago in the United States with the advancement of Medicare legislation. CMS, known at the time as the Healthcare Financing Authority (HCFA), launched an electronic billing process for hospitals in the early 1990s. The electronic format emerged from a device called the "universal bill." This universal bill, issued in 1992 (UB92), was the first vehicle to provide a rich source of demographic, diagnostic, and procedural data. In more recent years, ways and means to measure quality through this data set and other claims from individual providers, from outpatient venues of all types, as well as from rehabilitation settings and other posthospital venues, have been continually refined. Administrative data do provide some practical application. Although the usefulness of these data have been qualified and challenged over time, there is a fair amount of consensus that the information included in claims and encounters can be useful in determining the overall health of a given population of patients with certain chronic conditions (e.g., CHF, CAD, asthma, COPD, and diabetes). These data also illustrate nursing's role regardless of venue in influencing outcomes for these patients (Brock et al., 2013; "Case-Mix Measurement," 1987; Jha, Wright, & Perlin, 2007; McCarthy, Johnson, & Audet, 2013; Schatz et al., 2005).

Because of the very nature of lifestyle management (H&W), DM, and CM programs, data collection on large data sets becomes possible. Although there are methodological considerations for appropriate hypothesis testing of these data, developing processes for determining the impact of the nursing role on outcomes becomes possible without extensive and tedious chart review and manual data collection.

Electronic systems for facilitating both EMR and EHR also raise the bar on the potential for outcomes research related to nursing's role in population health. In H&W, DM, and CM programs, the nursing role in providing guidance for patients' self-management of their disease conditions is documented in such a way that these "self-reported" data on milestones for patient care management are adequately captured for electronic reporting, theory testing, and hypothesis evaluation. For example, nurses who are involved in lifestyle management, H&W programs that include such things as smoking-cessation programs, are able to interact with patients telephonically to ascertain their progress with smoking cessation, and these interactions are captured in electronic reporting for later analysis. Our ability to evaluate whether or not the patient has filled a smoking-cessation prescription or is using a smoking-cessation treatment may be facilitated if pharmacy claims are available, but in general, we have no idea whether the patient filled the prescription and is taking it without a self-report. The patient's report on 7-day prevalence ("Have you smoked a tobacco product in the past 7 days?") is the type of data available only through self-report or direct observation. These data can also be easily captured in EMR databases, and although it is still patient self-reported data, it is extremely useful and can be used in measurement submission, for example, in selected HEDIS measures (NCQA, 2015).

In 2010, and through the Affordable Care Act (ACA), incentive monies became available to organizations to implement electronic means and to advance the use of the EMR and EHR systems. The program was called "Meaningful Use," and organizations were required to use these information systems and, once implemented, submit data to CMS on quality process and outcomes measures (CMS, 2014c).

Hybrid data collection is a method proffered in the HEDIS data-collection model. For some of the metrics, securing the data may require samples of outpatient charts with designated data collectors to provide specific data that are not available through electronic means. Here is an example. Some programs may have the ability to secure electronic results of laboratory data. So, the HEDIS measure called "comprehensive diabetes care" includes several components. One measure includes the extent to which patients who have been diagnosed with diabetes were able to secure an HbA1c test within a 12-month period. This HEDIS metric can easily be compiled through quantitative methods if claims data are available. However, unless laboratory data are also available, the actual value of the HbA1c is not forthcoming. An alternative to this is found in the hybrid method of data collection. HEDIS provides for a method of random sample selection and sample size. Data collectors are deployed, who collect the needed information by hand. For this measure and for several others in the HEDIS data set, patient self-reported data are not acceptable. In order to sort out the impact of a nursing DM strategy on patients' ongoing diabetes management, it is essential to be able to determine not only whether the patients have an annual HbA1c test performed but also the results of that test. More important, once you have those data, one has the ability to analyze which patients have good control (HbA1c less than 7% or 8% depending on defined metrics for your population) and which patients have poor control (HbA1c > 9%), and this can lead to identification of the strengths or weaknesses in a DM program. Without actual laboratory results in an electronic feed or hybrid data collection, claims data are limited in providing this insight. With good reason, and because of the significant dollars at risk, as incentives are provided for those organizations demonstrating improved outcomes in population health, audit validation procedures are rigorous.

CMS has, over time, refined billing practices and requirements for appropriate documentation in the electronic invoicing processes for inpatient facilities and independent providers of care. Accordingly, these changes have helped to capture useful information not only in claims and encounters but also in provider practices, and to make connections for patients across the continuum of care. Incentives have been developed in recent years to reward positive practices and to better align payment with outcomes. For example, years ago UM practices for Medicare required payment only when the appropriate patient placement and level of care in an acute care setting occurs, whereas individual provider reimbursement for an inpatient stay occurs regardless of denied payment to the facility. The TJC and CMS have now aligned their processes around the core measures project, holding hospitals accountable for process of care measures (e.g., getting the AMI patient with ST elevation to the catheter laboratory within 90 minutes of arrival to the hospital). In the past, no incentives were given to physicians who achieved the less-than-90-minute goal. Similarly, keeping a patient in the hospital longer for a hospital-acquired complication (e.g., removal of a retained instrument) had no consequences. In 2009, CMS began to limit reimbursement to hospitals that demonstrate these "never events" (CMS, 2015c). As a result, 14 conditions were identified in this category. Similarly, in 2006 a drive by CMS to "pay for performance" was launched, encouraging individual providers to capture data in their billing practices that demonstrate patient outcomes and preventive measures in their outpatient practices, with a resultant financial reward (CMS, 2015d). For example, providers who can demonstrate (through their CMS billing) that a certain percentage of their diabetic patients have had an HbA1c test done annually, and a significant proportion of that patient population has results below 7% or 8% depending on the nature of their patient population, receive additional reimbursement.

The ease of access to administrative data sets and claims data has appropriately led to legislation that is intended to protect the integrity of these electronic data. The Health Insurance Portability and Accountability Act (HIPAA) was passed in 1996, and has resulted in a number of requirements across the country and in any venue or service related to the patient's right to confidentiality and privacy protections. Highlights of these regulatory requirements include the following concepts: (a) annual training for all staff members (whether involved in patient care or not) regarding protected health information; (b) signed business associate agreements assuring that these protections transverse various vendors and clients; (c) adequate auditing, policies, and procedures are in place to assure that the extent and spirit of the regulations are met (Brown, 2009).

National Trends and Healthcare Reform

Data availability, whether from electronic, self-report, or hybrid data, has changed the nature of the healthcare landscape, and the accessibility and reliability of these data have been influenced by powerful market pressures. Certainly, CMS has had a significant impact on healthcare in the United States since Medicare legislation in the 1960s first guaranteed healthcare as a right to all Social Security recipients over the age of 65 (Social Security, n.d.). In recent years, evolving legislation linked the issue of availability of healthcare to the quality of healthcare and recognized the inherent relationship between cost and quality. As quality improves, the cost of care is reduced. As measurement mechanisms and the availability of data have developed over the past 20 years, so has the collective wisdom. At the end of 2009, it was almost impossible to pick up a newspaper or read about the latest political debate without time and attention brought to "healthcare reform." Although pundits deconstruct the key elements of the current need for healthcare reform, all agree that the cost of providing healthcare in the United States has escalated. One can only hope that accessibility has improved for increasing segments of our society, but there are still significant disparities throughout regions of the country with a shortage of both primary care and subspecialty providers. There continues to be broad disagreement over the way in which healthcare reform was enacted despite legislation passed in 2010. Regardless of the ongoing debate about this legislation, data availability as a result of claims, in patient self-reporting, in hybrid data collection, and as a result of provider P4P (pay for performance) initiatives makes the measurement of quality considerably more elegant, more reliable, and clearer than it has ever been in the United States in estimating the impact of nursing's role in improving population health.

Since its enactment in 2010, the debate regarding healthcare reform has continued to mark the political landscape. By the end of 2014, a number of states have chosen to refrain from opting into the program. The consequences of these state decisions remain controversial 4 years after the ACA was signed into law. Regardless of the political debate, data on clinical outcomes are equally available for Medicare and Medicaid programs across the United States.

Standardized Data Definitions and Comparative Databases

A theme that is consistent in this chapter on evaluation methods is that measurement methods have evolved for the better over the course of the past 20 to 30 years. Clearly, the information technology age and the availability of administrative data sets are related to the present state. In addition, clinicians have provided adequate guidance through professional organizations on both process and outcome indicators of quality and have evolved data definitions that have methodological rigor and standardization (AHRQ, 2014a, 2014c). This agreement and standardization give rise to the potential for comparisons on a level playing field.

Standardized data definitions are made available by the NCQA (HEDIS volumes are available for purchase at www.NCQA.org) and include detailed technical specifications. NCQA is a leader in the field and provides not only technical specifications and guidance on hybrid data collection and sample size but certifications for HEDIS auditing capabilities. In addition to this functionality, the NCQA provides annual data comparisons with actual percentile rankings on the HEDIS measures for Medicare, Medicaid, and commercial lines of business. These are published on their website annually. Purchase of the Quality Compass makes regionalized comparisons possible and provides the percentile ranking comparisons a little sooner than they become public.

The AHRQ (www.AHRQ.gov) provides technical specifications as a free service for many of their measures and provides the technical specifications and free software for either IBM SPSS or SAS,[1] which facilitates access to actual comparative database information. An interesting website provided by AHRQ is called the "National Clearinghouse for Indicators." This website provides search capabilities on various topics, including specific disease states and conditions, and provides a collection of hundreds of metrics submitted by various specialty groups, some of which are international. The indicators are provided in a standardized format, but the technical specifications are not nearly as detailed as those provided by NCQA through its HEDIS initiative and through AHRQ. The format includes information about the name of the indicator, the owner or author, the broad inclusions in the numerator and the denominator, with typically extensive bibliographic support from the evidence-based literature on why this indicator accurately describes some aspects of clinical quality for a given condition or disease state (AHRQ, 2014a). This national clearinghouse includes metrics from private and public groups, including, but not limited to, the NQF (www.qualityforum.org/Home.aspx), CMS (www.cms.gov/center/quality.asp), TJC (www.jointcommission.org/), and specialty groups such as the American College of Cardiology, the Society of Thoracic Surgeons, and many others.

Qualitative Strategies for the Evaluation of Program Outcomes

Significant strides in nursing have been made (that did not exist 40 years ago) to improve measurement methods and use quantitative means to evaluate population health. This notwithstanding, qualitative methods are also a source of rich and useful information in this evaluation process.

Accreditation and Certification

Accreditation and certification programs offer a systematic review of a given organization's ability to provide evidence of compliance with standards. Standards define the required elements to accreditation success, and these organizations provide both rigor and agreed-upon methodologies in pursuit of organizational distinction. Although many would argue that the process itself is more quantitative than qualitative, most would agree that the result is a credential that is desirable, often sought after, and sometimes a mandate. Most accreditation and certification programs provide various levels of review and accept both depth and breadth in terms of evidence permitted. Regardless of the type of program reviewed, these accrediting bodies have a number of common elements.

A set of standards is the primary hallmark of an accrediting program. Whether evaluation of a given program is housed in a facility (like an acute

---

[1] IBM SPSS and SAS are both powerful statistical software programs that permit data mining and statistical analysis with a full range of descriptive, inferential (both parametric and nonparametric), and trending capabilities. They are available for purchase and used extensively in large organizations, government programs, and academic institutions. Individuals can also purchase various modules and needed statistical analytic capabilities. See www-01.ibm.com/software/analytics/spss/and http://www.sas.com/en_us/home.html

care hospital accredited through TJC) or a DM program that is made up of telephonic call centers, accreditation or certification is considered to be a measure of quality. For example, TJC's certification program for CHF is offered in conjunction with the American Heart Association and offers this certification based on standards and outcomes (The Joint Commission, 2015). As nurses practice and provide nursing care within and throughout these facilities and programs, accreditation is an indirect measure of the quality of nursing practice. The processes used within an accrediting program are also variable, but are often characterized by common features: (a) written documentation is submitted for review; (b) site visits comprise overview of the program, its capabilities and outcomes, and staff interviews; and (c) chart or file reviews of some kind are included in the accreditation process validating that as nurses we provide evidence-based care.

As part of the accreditation process, there is hardly a time when an organization must not produce metrics that are sensitive to the nursing role, demonstrate patient characteristics, and quantify patient outcomes. The accrediting process becomes qualitative as the evaluation of the quality program may or may not show actual improvement in defined patient care indicators. Many accrediting bodies are not prescriptive in the application of their standards; this is in no way a detracting characteristic. In fact, the latitude in the application of the standards (the "how") is often desirable as there are many ways to achieve the same outcome. Examples of accrediting bodies and the type of programs that they accredit or certify are provided in Table 8.5. This list is not intended to be exhaustive but simply illustrative. Each includes standards that evaluate the outcome of nursing care in some way.

Community Advisory Boards

As DM, CM, and UM programs have within their essential construct the total health of the population at large as a key benefit, oftentimes, representative members of that patient population are sought after to provide insight into the effectiveness and usefulness of these programs as benefits. These committees or boards meet on a regular basis (as frequently as quarterly to as seldom as annually or "ad hoc," depending on the need) and provide qualitative insight as to the impact of the program on patients' lives, as well as insight into enhancements. Telephonic services, written materials, field-based options, communication devices, and program changes are often reviewed with these boards to anticipate patient response. Certainly, members of the benefit program (patients and families) and local community groups representing the various segments of the community affected by the benefit might be included in the membership roster.

Provider Advisory Committees

Providers across specialties and venues, from nurses to physicians to hospitals, are key components to the overall success in improving the health of the patient population in its entirety. Telephonic nursing provides options for care that did not exist in the past. However, face-to-face communications from

TABLE 8.5 • Examples of Accrediting Bodies and the Types of Programs They Accredit

1. The Joint Commission accredits acute care hospitals and provides certification to a number of specialty hospitals and programs, many of which have a patient focus that goes well beyond the patient's inpatient experience. Accordingly, these accreditation programs have an influence on the health of the total patient population as well as nursing's role in the experience. TJC is often designated by state licensure for hospital review. TJC holds deemed status for CMS; hospitals seeking to achieve or maintain provider status must be both accredited and licensed. Find more information about TJC at www.jointcommission.org.

2. The National Committee for Quality Assurance offers numerous recognition, accreditation, and certification programs, including, but not limited to, health plans, UM programs, DM programs, HEDIS auditing, and many other types. Information regarding the programs offered by this organization can be found at www .ncqa.org.

3. The Utilization Review Accreditation Committee formally adopted the acronym URAC in 1996. It is an organization with a long track record in offering accreditation for total population health. UM, DM, and CM programs and other types of accreditations that are related to the nursing role in total population health are among the many types offered. More information on this organization can be found at www.urac.org.

4. The Commission on Accreditation of Rehabilitation Facilities (CARF) is yet another organization with a focus on evaluating the quality of various programs, including behavioral health services across the rehabilitation continuum, durable medical equipment providers, aging programs, and other program types. The CARF website provides a wealth of useful information (www.carf.org/Accreditation).

5. DNV NIAHO: This organization provides an accreditation based on the International Organization for Standardization (ISO) 9000 (www.asq.org/learn-about-quality/iso-9000/overview/overview.html) and achieved deemed status from CMS in September 2008 (www.dnv.com/industry/healthcare). Although this organization specializes in managing risk for many types of industries, a recent focus on healthcare and CMS deemed status has opened a new option for accreditation. This organization has focused on accrediting hospitals, primary stroke centers, and critical access hospitals. More information can be sought at www.dnvaccreditation .com/pr/dnv/default.aspx.

nurse to physician provider become more complex in this environment. In addition, quantitative methods have the potential to supply providers with data on their care practices that may or may not demonstrate the achievement of improvements in patient outcomes. Providing feedback to physicians in a systematic and patient-centered way is a strategy that can be of tremendous benefit. Consequently, devising a vehicle to enhance communications with healthcare providers in a formal setting, such as through committees, can be of significant value.

Provider advisory committees come in all shapes and sizes and meet with varying frequency. Shalala (2010) advises that APRNs who are in private practice represent an important enhancement to our ability to extend primary care capacity across the country (Naylor & Kurtzman, 2010). Representative providers, including APRNs, can "weigh in" on data presentation; they can provide advice on ways and means to make sound use of these data in a global way, as well as help to anticipate reaction. These forums serve as educational opportunities for the DM program and can enhance practice management as well as demonstrate how the EHR across the continuum of care can enhance communication processes among all members of the healthcare team as well as maximize patient outcomes. Provider advisory committees provide depth to a DM program, which is not easily found through quantitative methods.

SUMMARY

APRNs play an increasingly important role in evaluating the quality and effectiveness of healthcare delivery systems. As APRN roles have expanded into this area, it is paramount that APRNs understand the ways and means used to evaluate population health outcomes, as well as the systems of care that provide population health services. Various definitions of quality have been presented, and several theoretical frameworks are available for evaluating quality. Nurse-sensitive indicators of quality can be described using the following categories: (a) clinical quality, (b) utilization of healthcare resources, (c) core business processes, and (d) customer satisfaction. APRNs hold various roles, both clinical and administrative, in a variety of settings. Regardless of role or setting, measurement and improvement of quality with its broad definitions remain paramount. In the past, measurement systems were limited, and manual data collection was the primary method of gaining insight and information as to the outcomes of clinical care, management of chronic illness, and the patient's experience. As nurses strive to make an impact on the overall health of the population, reduce the cost of care, and improve the patient's experience of their healthcare, APRNs' roles expand.

EXERCISES AND DISCUSSION QUESTIONS

Exercise 8.1 Measuring quality often depends on one's definitions, and it is quite appropriate to provide a glossary of terms to ensure a common understanding. Imagine that you are a clinical director at an organization with a contract for Medicaid Disease Management in a rural Midwestern state. You have oversight responsibility for eight registered nurses who serve in the capacity as health coaches in a telephone call center located in an office setting in the state's capital. Your patients live in rural areas of the state, there are no urban settings, and there are few primary care providers who accept Medicaid. However, there are five primary hospitals spread throughout your state, a number of 25-bed "critical access" hospitals, and a few federally qualified health centers (FQHCs). Your DM program focuses on five disease conditions: CHF, COPD, asthma, diabetes, and CAD. Your program is guided by a very competent medical director, who is a physician, and you report to an executive director, who is also an APRN. You have sound information technology support, and the state sends claims data weekly with eligible patients who have already been identified with one or more of the various disease states for entry into your DM program. Consider your customer (the state in the Midwest) and the role of the telephone nurse and answer the following questions for discussion.

- What are some examples of customers' expectations that might emerge from this contract?
- How might the state in the Midwest define quality in measurable terms? At the end of the 3-year term? On an ongoing basis?
- What would represent the features of your program?
- What patient outcomes might be considered of value to your customer?
- What would constitute a deficiency?

Exercise 8.2 As an APRN, you are serving in the capacity as the executive director of an office that proudly holds commercial contracts with health plans all over the country to provide DM and CM services to their members. In approximately 40 different contracts, some large and some small, your site houses a telephone call center that employs over 40 RNs, "on call" with patients in health plans across the country. Your leadership team is made up of a full-time medical director, six supervisors in both clinical and nonclinical roles, and another 40 people who serve various administrative and nonclinical functions. You have access to claims data for every contract and a fully functioning EMR for your DM and CM documentation. Most of your contracts are 3-year contracts.

- Brainstorm at least three metrics for each of the four categories that we've discussed in this chapter.
- Consider goal setting. What will you set for annual goals for clinical quality outcome measures selected in the previous question?
- How will you track your nurses' progress on the core business process measures?
- What resources will you consider using to capture data on customer satisfaction?
- Your contracts are, for the most part, 3 years in length. At the end of the first year, describe where you'd like to go with HEDIS measures when compared to the rest of the commercial PPO (preferred provider organization) and HMO (health maintenance organization) patients? The second year? The third year?

Exercise 8.3 Imagine that you are the vice president for quality improvement in a national DM company with contracts and interests in 26 states across the country. Your health coaches are RNs who work in telephone call centers across the country and focus on patients with gaps in their treatment program. These nurses work under the supervision of clinical managers, who are also RNs with advanced degrees. Quality managers in these local sites are seeking your input and guidance on a matter of measurement. In addition, your company is preparing a balanced scorecard and is interested in monitoring quality in four categories: clinical quality, utilization of healthcare resources, core business processes, and customer satisfaction. Your contracts consistently include patients with diabetes mellitus, COPD, CHF, asthma, and CAD; you serve primarily commercial clients with HMOs and a PPO. You will need access to the Internet for this exercise.

- Name at least two clinical quality or utilization of healthcare resource (condition-specific) metrics for each of the five aforementioned conditions. Choose at least two HEDIS metrics.
- Consult the NCQA website and the data that are available which provide percentile rankings. If you were to set a quality goal for the coming year at the 75th percentile using HEDIS guidance for commercial PPO plans, what

average score for your two selected HEDIS clinical metrics would your contracts each need to achieve?

- Think about how these measures "connect" to the RN/health coach role. What functions does the nurse perform day to day on a call with a patient that drives toward the outcomes you've chosen to measure?

Exercise 8.4 As an APRN you have an expanding role as an actively practicing primary care clinician. You are in private practice with two other similar APRNs and a primary care physician. Your practice has a large number of Medicaid recipients who have, as a benefit, eligibility and enrollment in a DM program. Your practice has achieved recognition by the NCQA for diabetes care (www.ncqa.org/tabid/139/Default.aspx). You don't know much about the DM program (at all), but you know that (a) you've been contacted by a nurse on the phone representing the needs of your patients, (b) you've seen some data on your patient outcomes (and they are not as high as you'd expected them to be), and (c) your practice has been invited to serve on a provider advisory committee. You are really pressed for time in your busy practice, but you are intrigued. You are deciding whether or not to participate. Consider the following questions in making a contribution.

- What questions would you bring to the table?
- How would you like to see the agenda take shape?
- Your practice is already recognized by the diabetes association with "provider status." Would you be expecting contact hours for your participation? Why or why not?
- How can this data possibly be correct?

REFERENCES

American Academy of Professional Coders. (2015). *What is medical coding?* Retrieved from https://www.aapc.com/medical-coding/medical-coding.aspx

Agency for Healthcare Research and Quality. (2014a). *National Quality Measures Clearinghouse.* Retrieved from http://www.qualitymeasures.ahrq.gov/content.aspx?id=46440

Agency for Healthcare Research and Quality. (2014b). *National Quality Measure Clearinghouse, measure summary.* Retrieved from http://www.qualitymeasures.ahrq.gov/content.aspx?id=46980&search=hemoglobin+a1c

Agency for Healthcare Research and Quality. (2014c). *Clinical guidelines and recommendations.* Retrieved from http://www.ahrq.gov/professionals/clinicians-providers/guidelines-recommendations/index.html

Anderson-Dean, C. (2012). The benefits of lean six sigma for nursing informatics. *American Nursing Informatics Association, 27*(4), 1, 6–7.

Baicker, K., Cutler, D., & Song, Z. (2010). Workplace wellness programs can generate savings. *Health Affairs, 29*, 304–311.

Balanced Scorecard Institute. (2014). *Handbook for basic process improvement.* Retrieved from https://balancedscorecard.org/Resources/Articles-White-Papers/Process-Improvement-Tools

Bedell, W., & Kaszkin-Bettag, M. (2010). Coherence and health care cost—RCA actuarial study: A cost-effectiveness cohort study. *Alternative Therapies, 16*(4), 26–31.

Berwick, D. M., Godfrey, A. B., & Roessner, J. (1990). *Curing health care: New strategies for quality improvement.* San Francisco, CA: Jossey-Bass.

Best, M., & Neuhauser, D. (2006). Joseph Juran: Overcoming resistance to organizational change. *Quality and Safety in Health Care, 15*(5), 380–382.

Bisognano, M., & Kenney, C. (2012). *Pursuing the triple aim.* San Francisco, CA: Jossey-Bass, Wiley.

Breslin, S. E., Hamilton, K. M., & Paynter, J. (2014). Development of lean six sigma in care co-ordination: An improved discharge process. *Professional Case Management, 77*(2), 77–83.

Brock, J., Mitchell, J., Irby, K., Stevens, B., Archibald, T., Goroski, A., & Lynn, J. (2013). Association between quality improvement for care transitions in communities and rehospitalizations among Medicare beneficiaries. *Journal of the American Medical Association, 309*, 381–391.

Brown, J. (2009). *The healthcare quality handbook* (24th ed.). Pasadena, CA: JB Quality Solutions.

Case-mix measurement and assessing quality of hospital care [Annual supplement]. (1987). Health Care Financing Review, 39–48.

Centers for Disease Control and Prevention, Healthcare Infection Control Practices Advisory Committee. (2011). *Guidelines for the prevention of intravascular catheter-related infections.* Retrieved from http://www.cdc.gov/hicpac/pdf/guidelines/bsi-guidelines-2011.pdf

Chen, C. M., Hong, M. C., & Hsu, Y. H. (2007). Administrator self-ratings of organizational capacity and performance of healthy community development projects in Taiwan. *Public Health Nursing, 24*, 343–354.

Chu, H. L., Wang, C. C., & Dai, Y. T. (2009). A study of a nursing department performance measurement system: Using the balanced scorecard and the analytic hierarchy process. *Nursing Economic$, 27*, 401–407.

Centers for Medicare & Medicaid Services. (2012). *Health Outcomes Survey (HOS).* Retrieved from http://www.cms.gov/Research-Statistics-Data-and-Systems/Research/HOS/index.html?redirect=/hos/

Centers for Medicare & Medicaid Services. (2013). *Specifications for the All-Cause Unplanned readmission measure.* Retrieved from http://www.cms.gov/site-search/search-results.html?q=All%20cause%20readmissions%20within%2030%20days

Centers for Medicare & Medicaid Services. (2014a). *Hospital acquired conditions (present on admission indicator).* Retrieved from http://www.cms.gov/HospitalAcqCond/

Centers for Medicare & Medicaid Services. (2014b). *Part C reporting requirements.* Retrieved from http://www.cms.gov/Medicare/Health-Plans/HealthPlansGenInfo/ReportingRequirements.html

Centers for Medicare & Medicaid Services. (2014c). *2014 definition stage I of meaningful use.* Retrieved from http://www.cms.gov/Regulations-and-Guidance/Legislation/EHRIncentivePrograms/Meaningful_Use.html

Centers for Medicare & Medicaid Services. (2015a). *Part C and D performance data.* Retrieved from http://www.cms.gov/Medicare/Prescription-Drug-Coverage/PrescriptionDrugCovGenIn/PerformanceData.html

Centers for Medicare & Medicaid Services. (2015b). *Quality measures and performance standards.* Retrieved from http://www.cms.gov/Medicare/Medicare-Fee-for-Service-Payment/sharedsavingsprogram/Quality_Measures_Standards.html

Centers for Medicare & Medicaid Services. (2015c). *Quality of care center.* Retrieved from http://www.cms.gov/center/quality.asp

Centers for Medicare & Medicaid Services. (2015d). *Physician quality reporting system.* Retrieved from http://www.cms.gov/pqri/

Corn, J. B. (2009). Six sigma in health care. *Radiologic Technology, 81*(1), 92–95.

Courtney, B. A., Ruppman, J. B., & Cooper, H. M. (2006). Save our skin: Initiative cuts pressure ulcer incidence in half. *Nursing Management, 37*(4), 36, 38, 40.

Cross, K. F. (2000). Call resolution: The wrong focus for service quality? *Quality Progress, 33*(2), 64–67.

DeFeo, J. A. (2014). *Juran's quality essentials for leaders.* New York, NY: McGraw-Hill.

De Feo, J. A., & Barnard, W.W. (2004). *Juran Institute's Six Sigma's breakthrough and beyond: Quality performance breakthrough methods.* New York, NY: McGraw–Hill.

DeFeo, J. A., & Juran, J. M. (2010). *Juran's quality handbook: The complete guide to performance excellence* (6th ed.). New York, NY: McGraw-Hill.

Del Franco, M. (2003). Cutting back on call abandonment. *Catalog Age, 20*(7), 59–60.

Dienemann, J. (Ed.). (1992). *Continuous quality improvement in nursing.* Washington, DC: American Nurses Publishing.

Donabedian, A. (1980). *The definition of quality and approaches to assessment.* Ann Arbor, MI: Health Administration Press.

Drenckpohl, D., Bowers, L., & Cooper, H. (2007). Use of the Six Sigma methodology to reduce incidence of breast milk administration errors in the NICU. *Neonatal Network, 26,* 161–166.

Fairbanks, C. B. (2007). Using six sigma and lean methodologies to improve OR throughput. *AORN Journal, 86*(1), 73–82.

Fetterolf, D., Holt, A. E., Tucker, T., & Khan, N. (2010). Estimating clinical and economic impact in case management programs. *Population Health Management, 13,* 73–82.

Formichelli, L. (2007). By the numbers. *Multichannel Merchant, 24*(4), 44–45.

Gardner, G., Gardner, A., & O'Connell, J. (2013). Using the Donabedian framework to examine the quality and safety of nursing service innovation. *Journal of Clinical Nursing, 23*(1-2), 145–155.

Gavriloff, C. (2012) A performance improvement plan to increase nurse adherence to use of medication safety software. *Journal of Pediatric Nursing. 27,* 375–382.

Gill, K. J., Swarbick, M., Murphy, A. A., Spagnolo, A. B., & Zechner, M. R. (2009). Co-morbid psychiatric and medical disorders: Challenges and strategies. *Journal of Rehabilitation, 75*(3), 32–40.

Godchaux, C. W. (1999). Case managers drive care integration. *Nursing Management, 30*(11), 32B, 32F.

Goonan, K. J. (1995). *The Juran prescription.* San Francisco, CA: Jossey-Bass.

Goonan, K. J., & Scarrow, P. (2010). Interview with a quality leader: Kate Goonan and performance excellence. *Journal for Healthcare Quality, 32*(3), 32–35.

Govil, S. R., Weidner, G., Merritt-Worden, T., & Ornish, D. (2009). Socioeconomic status and improvements in lifestyle, coronary risk factors and quality of life: The multisite cardiac lifestyle intervention program. *American Journal of Public Health, 99,* 1263–1270.

Guru guide: Six thought leaders who changed the quality world forever. (2010). *Quality Progress, 43*(11), 14–21.

Gustafson, B. M. (1999). A well-staffed PFS call center can improve patient satisfaction. *Healthcare Financial Management, 53*(7), 64–66.

Handler, A., Issel, M., & Turnock, B. (2001). A conceptual framework to measure performance of the public health system. *American Journal of Public Health, 91,* 1235–1239.

Hassan, M., Tuckman, H. P., Patrick, R. H., Kountz, D. S., & Kohn, J. L. (2010). Cost of hospital-acquired infection. *Hospital Topics, 88*(3), 82–89.

Hospital Consumer Assessment of Healthcare Providers and Systems. (2015). *CAHPS hospital survey.* Retrieved from http://www.hcahpsonline.org/home.aspx

Health Services Advisory Group. (2014). *Medicare Health Outcomes Survey.* Retrieved from http://www.hosonline.org/Content/Default.aspx

Healthcare Effectiveness Data and Information Set. (2014). *Narrative, technical specifications, and survey measurement* (Vols. 1–3). Washington, DC: National Committee for Quality Assurance. Retrieved from http://ncqa.org/tabid/59/Default.aspx

Institute for Healthcare Improvement. (2015a). Retrieved from http://www.ihi.org/Pages/default.aspx

Institute for Healthcare Improvement. (2015b). *Provider and Staff Satisfaction Survey.* Retrieved from http://www.ihi.org/resources/Pages/Tools/ProviderandStaffSatisfactionSurvey.aspx

Institute of Medicine. (1999). *To err is human; building a safer health system. A consensus report.* Retrieved from http://iom.edu/Reports/1999/To-Err-is-Human-Building-A-Safer-Health-System.aspx

Institute of Medicine. (2001). *Crossing the quality chasm: A new health system for the 21st century.* Retrieved from http://iom.edu/~/media/Files/Report%20Files/2001/Crossing-the-Quality-Chasm/Quality%20Chasm%202001%20%20report%20brief.pdf

Jha, A. K., Wright, S. M., & Perlin, J. B. (2007). Performance measures, vaccinations, and pneumonia rates among high-risk patients in Veterans Administration health care. *American Journal of Public Health, 97,* 2167–2172.

Joint Commission Resources. (2003). *Root cause analysis in health care; tools and techniques* (2nd ed.). Oakbrook, IL: Author.

The Joint Commission. (2010). Retrieved from http://www.jointcommission.org/

The Joint Commission. (2015). *Advanced certification in heart failure.* Retrieved from http://www.jointcommission.org/certification/heart_failure.aspx

The Joint Commission & Centers for Medicare & Medicaid Services. (2010). *Specifications manual for national hospital inpatient quality measures.* Retrieved from http://www.jointcommission.org/specifications_manual_for_national_hospital_inpatient_quality_measures/

Juran, J. (1993). Made in U.S.A.: A renaissance in quality. *Harvard Business Review, 71*(4), 42–50.

Kaplan, S., Bisgaard, S., Truesdell, D., & Zetterholm, S. (2009). Design for six sigma in healthcare: Developing an employee influenza vaccination process. *Journal for Healthcare Quality, 31*(3), 36–43.

Kaplan, R. S., & Norton, D. P. (1996). *The balanced scorecard.* Boston, MA: Harvard Business School Press.

Kaplan, R. S., & Norton, D. P. (2001). *The strategy-focused organization.* Boston, MA: Harvard Business School Press.

Khudyakov, P., Feigin, P. D., & Mandelbaum, A. (2010). Designing a call center with an IVR (Interactive Voice Response). *Queueing Systems, 66,* 215–237.

Lamb, S. E., Toye, F., & Barker, K. L. (2008). Chronic disease management programme in people with severe knee osteoarthritis: Efficacy and moderators of response. *Clinical Rehabilitation, 22,* 169–178.

Maddox, P. J. (1992). Successful implementation of a CQI process. In J. Dienneman (Ed.), *Continuous quality improvement in nursing* (pp. 115–124). Washington, DC: American Nurses Publishing.

Mandelbaum, A., & Zeltyn, S. (2013). Data-stories about (im)patient customers in tele-queues. *Queueing Systems, 75,* 115–146.

McCarthy, D., Bihrle Johnson, M., & Audet, A. M. (2013). Recasting readmissions by placing the hospital role in community context. *Journal of the American Medical Association, 309,* 351–352.

McCaughey, B. (2006). Saving lives and the bottom line. *Modern Healthcare, 36*(5), 23.

Medicare Payment Advisory Commission. (2014). *Report to the Congress: Medicare payment policy.* Retrieved from http://www.medpac.gov/documents/reports/mar14_ch06.pdf?sfvrsn=0

Meurer, S. J., McGartland-Rubio, D., Counte, M. A., & Burroughs, T. (2002). Development of a healthcare quality improvement measurement tool: Results of a content validity study. *Hospital Topics, 80*(2), 7–13.

Moen, R. D., & Norman, C. L. (2010). Circling back: Clearing up myths about the Deming cycle and seeing how it keeps evolving. *Quality Progress, 43*(11), 22–28.

Moreo, K., & Urbano, F. L. (2014). Are we prepared for affordable care act provisions of care coordination? *Professional Case Management, 19*(1), 18–26.

Moulin, M., Soady, J., Skinner, J., Price, C., Cullen, J., & Gilligan, C. (2007). Using the public sector scorecard in public health. *International Journal of Health Care Quality Assurance, 20,* 281–289.

Nash, D. B., Reifsnyder, J., Fabius R. J., & Pracilio, V. P. (2011). *Population health; Creating a culture of wellness.* Sudbury, MA: Jones and Bartlett Learning.

National Committee for Quality Assurance. (2014a). *Standards and guidelines for the accreditation and certification of disease management.* Washington, DC: Author.

National Committee for Quality Assurance. (2014b). *Tell us your opinion!* Retrieved from http://ncqa.org/

National Quality Forum. (2010). Retrieved form http://ncqa.org/

Naylor, M. D., & Kurtzman, E. T. (2010). The role of nurse practitioners in reinventing primary care. *Health Affairs, 29,* 893–899.

National Institute of Standards and Technology. (2015). *Baldridge performance excellence program.* Retrieved from http://www.nist.gov/baldrige/publications/hc_criteria.cfm

NCQA (2014). *Technical specifications for health plans* (Vol. 2). Washington, DC: NCQA.

O'Toole, T. P., Buckel, L., Bourgault, C., Blumen, J., Redihan, S. G., Jiang, L. M., & Friedmann, P. (2010). Applying the chronic care model to homeless veterans: Effect of a population approach to primary care on utilization and clinical outcomes. *American Journal of Public Health, 100*, 2493–2499.

Pollert, P., Dobberstein, D., & Wiisanen, R. (2008). Jumping into the healthcare retail market: Our experience. *Frontiers of Health Services Management, 24*(3), 13–22.

Population Health Alliance. (2015). Retrieved from http://www.populationhealthalliance.org/

Potthoff, S., & Ryan, M. J. (2004). Leadership, management, and change in improving quality in healthcare. *Frontiers of Health Services Management, 20*(3), 37–41.

The power of safety: State reporting provides lessons in reducing harm, improving care. (2010, June). *National Quality Forum Quality Connections.* Retrieved from http://www.qualityforum.org/Publications/2010/06/Quality_Connections__The_Power_of_Safety__State_Reporting_Provides_Lessons_in_Reducing_Harm,_Improving_Care.aspx

Pyzdek, T., & Keller, P. (2009). *The six sigma handbook* (3rd ed.). New York, NY: McGraw-Hill.

Rantz, M., Popejoy, L. L., Galambos, C., Phillips, L. J., Lane, K. R., Dorman-Marek, K., . . . Ge, B. (2014). The continued success of registered nurse care coordination in a state evaluation of aging in place in senior housing. *Nursing Outlook, 62*, 237–246.

Rice, K. L., Dewan, N., Bloomfield, H. E., Grill, J., Schult, T. M., Nelson, D. B., . . . Niewoehner, D. E. (2010). Disease management program for chronic obstructive pulmonary disease: A controlled random trial. *American Journal of Respiratory Critical Care Medicine, 182*, 890–896.

Santos, A. B., Henggeler, S. W., Burns, B. J., Arana, G. W., & Meisler, N. (1995). Research on field-based services: Models for reform in the delivery of mental health care to populations with complex clinical problems. *American Journal of Psychiatry, 152*, 1111–1123.

SAS. (2011). Retrieved from http://www.sas.com

Schatz, M., Nakahiro, R., Crawford, W., Mendoza, G., Mosen, D., & Stibolt, T. B. (2005). Asthma quality-of-care markers using administrative data. *Chest, 128*, 1968–1974.

Schiller, K. C., Weech-Maldonado, R., & Hall, A. G. (2010). Patient assessments of care and utilization in Medicaid managed care: PCCMs vs. PSOs. *Journal of Healthcare Finance, 36*(3), 13–23.

Shalala, D. (2010). *Group recommends expanding nurses' role in primary care.* Retrieved from http://thefutureofnursing.org/recommendations

Social Security. (n.d.). *Legislative history.* Retrieved from http://www.ssa.gov/history/tally65.html

SPSS. (2011). Retrieved from http://www.spss.com/

Stankovic, A. K., & DeLauro, E. (2010). Quality improvements in the preanalytical phase: Focus on the urine specimen flow. *MLO: Medical Laboratory Observer, 42*(3), 22, 24–27.

URAC (2014). *Case management accreditation.* Washington, DC: Author. Retrieved from https://www.urac.org/accreditation-and-measurement/accreditation-programs/all-programs/case-management/

Weinstein, L. C., LaNoue, M., Collins, E., Henwood, B. F., & Drake, R. E. (2013). Health care integration for formerly homeless people with serious mental illness. *Journal of Dual Diagnosis, 9*(1), 72–77.

Whiting, A., & Donthu, N. (2009). Closing the gap between perceived and actual waiting times in a call center: Results from a field study. *Journal of Services Marketing, 23*, 279–288.

Womack, J. P., & Jones, D. T. (2003). *Lean thinking.* New York, NY: Free Press.

Wübker, A. (2007). Measuring the quality of healthcare: The connection between structure, process and outcomes of care, using the example of myocardial infarction treatment in Germany. *Disease Management and Health Outcomes, 15*, 225–238.

Yap, C., Siu, E., Baker, G. R., Brown, A. D., & Lowi-Young, M. P. (2005). A comparison of systemwide and hospital-specific performance measurement tools. *Journal of Healthcare Management, 50*, 251–263.

Yun, E. K., & Chun, K. M. (2008). Critical to quality in telemedicine service management: Application of DFSS (design for six sigma) and SERVQUAL. *Nursing Economic$, 26*, 384–388.

Building Relationships and Engaging Communities Through Collaboration

Barbara A. Benjamin

One silver bracelet does not make much jingle.

—African proverb

Let us consider this adage when we think community health assessment (CHA). The primary purpose of building relationships and engaging communities through collaboration is to facilitate a dialog to aid in the assessment, planning, action, and evaluation of challenging care-based issues through program design and development. By working with the community, healthcare professionals have the opportunity to collaborate on issues relevant to the community to ensure sustainability and long-term success of community-based programs. This type of collaboration fosters bidirectional communication, understanding, and knowledge in the quest to ensure compassionate, quality, and culturally sensitive interventions.

MATRIX FOR COMMUNITY PRACTICE

Four determinants are especially relevant to this chapter. They are the American Association of Colleges of Nursing (AACN), the Affordable Care Act (ACA), community-based advanced practice registered nurse (APRN) competencies, and the Quad Council Practice Competencies for Public Health Nurses.

American Association of Colleges of Nursing

Elizabeth Lenz (2005), in an article "The Practice Doctorate in Nursing: An Idea Whose Time Has Come," includes management of care for individuals and populations, administration of nursing and healthcare organizations, and

213

health policy formulation and evaluation in her definition of doctoral-level advanced practice nursing. The practice-focused doctorate is an important alternative to research-focused doctorates in nursing. The choice to use a second approach was based, in part, on a long-standing conceptualization of nursing practice as having two related domains: the direct and the indirect, with the latter defined as activities that are carried out in support of the provision of direct care. Furthermore, Lenz felt that the decision to define nursing practice more inclusively than hands-on care is based on the recognition of the authority and responsibility to make decisions that influence nursing and healthcare. In addition, ultimately, patient outcomes often reside at the system level (e.g., with nursing administrators and policy makers). According to Lenz, there is an increasing need for insightful and visionary nursing leadership in practice; there must be a place at the decision-making table for the nurse. To paraphrase Lenz, the ability to make decisions at the community level requires that the APRN who works in the community (prepared at the doctoral level) be part of the higher level of care management and policy decision making in concert with the community-based consortium of healthcare policy makers. Lenz (2005) states, "It [doctor of nursing practice degree] is increasingly the credential that is needed for credibility in leadership positions" (para. 24).

The AACN (2006) published "The Essentials of Doctoral Education for Advanced Practice Nurses." According to this document, doctoral programs prepare experts in specialized advanced nursing practice and focus heavily on practice that is innovative and evidenced based. AACN defines *advanced nursing practice* as "any form of nursing intervention that influences healthcare outcomes for individuals or populations, including the direct care of individual patients, management of care for individuals and populations, administration of nursing and healthcare organizations and the development and implementation of health policy" (AACN, 2006, p. 3). Building relationships and engaging communities through collaborations address these AACN criteria as they incorporate many of the principles suggested by this definition. AACN further states that the Doctor of Nursing Practice (DNP) program prepares the graduate to "[c]onduct a comprehensive and systematic assessment of health and illness parameters in complex situations, incorporating diverse and culturally sensitive approaches" (AACN, 2006, p. 16).

Darlyne Bailey (1992) defines a community-based consortium as "a partnership of organizations and individuals representing consumers, service providers, and local agencies or groups who identify themselves with a particular community, neighborhood, or locale and who unite in an effort to collectively apply their resources to the implementation of a common strategy for the achievement of a common goal within that community" (p. 72). It is necessary for community-based APRNs to know the community and to work with its leaders toward a common healthcare goal when making healthcare decisions at the community level.

In order for the APRN to practice at the level inclusive of all of the particulars described by Lenz, that nurse must know the community. The CHA is the most effective and efficient method used to develop that knowledge. Shuster and Goeppinger (2008) state that "[c]ommunity assessment is one of the three core functions of public health nursing" (p. 351). The objective of a CHA is to determine the healthcare needs of the community and to address those needs by developing a comprehensive plan for the community. The Affordable Care Act includes a mandate for many hospitals to conduct CHAs.

The Affordable Care Act

The Affordable Care Act was passed by Congress and then signed into law by President Barack Obama on March 23, 2010. The purpose of this act is to provide quality, affordable care to all Americans. It reduces what families will have to pay for healthcare by capping out-of-pocket expenses and requiring preventive care to be fully covered without any out-of-pocket expense. Americans without insurance coverage are able to choose the insurance coverage that works best for them (U.S. Department of Health and Human Services, [HHS], 2014a).

The ACA created several additional requirements, one of which is that organizations that operate one or more hospitals seeking to maintain or achieve 501(c)(3) tax-exempt status regularly perform a community needs health assessment. Note: A 501(c)(3) hospital is one that qualifies for exemption from federal income tax as it is organized and operated exclusively as a charitable organization (National Association of County and City Health Officials, 2014).

The Internal Revenue Service (IRS) is responsible for the tax provisions of the ACA that are implemented. The IRS published *New Requirements for 501(c)(3) Hospitals Under the Affordable Care Act*. IRS Section 501(r)(3) of the *New Requirements for 501(c)(3) Hospitals Under the Affordable Care Act* requires that hospital organizations conduct a community health needs assessment (CHNA) every 3 years and adopt and implement strategies to meet the community health needs identified through the assessment. The CHNA must take into account input from persons who represent the broad interests of the community/communities served by healthcare facilities, including those with special knowledge of, or expertise in, public health. This document further defines persons who represent the broad interests of the community/communities as (a) persons with special knowledge of or expertise in public health; (b) federal, tribal, regional, state, or local health or other departments or agencies, with current data or other information relevant to the health needs of the community served by the hospital facility; and (c) leaders, representatives, or medically underserved, low-income, and minority populations, and populations with chronic disease needs, in the community served by the hospital facility (Internal Revenue Service, 2014).

Compliance With the Affordable Care Act

In many states, nonprofit hospitals have joined with local health departments to fulfill their requirement to conduct a CHA because health departments are also required to conduct community assessments on a regular basis and have the expertise to do so. In Wake County, North Carolina, the Wake County Health Department (WCHD) joined with WakeMed, Rex, and Duke Raleigh hospitals to comply with the ACA. Involved parties included the resources of the various hospitals, the United Way, the WCHD, Community Care of North Carolina (CCNC), and the local federally qualified health center (FQHC).

FQHCs include all organizations receiving grants under Section 330 of the Public Health Service (PHS) Act. FQHCs qualify for enhanced reimbursement from Medicare and Medicaid, as well as other benefits. FQHCs must serve an underserved area or population, offer a sliding-fee scale, provide comprehensive services, have an ongoing quality-assurance program, and have a governing board of directors (U.S. Department of Health and Human Services, Health Resources and Services Administration, 2014b). The WCHD led the process as they had experience doing CHAs. Data were gathered using focus groups and surveys. A full report was generated and a priority list of care needs of the community was generated. Sue Lynn Ledford, division director of WCHD stated, "We cannot treat the patient until we have the chart; so, as the community is the patient, we must triage the issues of concern that are bleeding out first in order to treat the community" (S. L. Ledford, personal communication, June 2014).

Often, in more rural areas the assessment is regional. In one such instance in western North Carolina, a regional collaboration was involved in an area assessment. The Western North Carolina Network (WNCN) collaborated with the local not-for-profit hospitals to do an area wide assessment, thereby pooling resources for the assessment. A steering committee that included the WNCN and the hospitals was formed to determine strategies for working together and methodologies for data collection. The data were collected using a random sample telephone survey across the counties. Health issues requiring intervention by both the hospitals and the WNCN were prioritized and addressed (H. K. Gates, personal communication, July 2014).

Health departments and hospital professionals have the opportunity to collaborate on health issues relevant to the community to ensure sustainability and long-term success of both hospital- and community-based programs. This type of collaboration fosters building relationships and engaging communities through collaborations, thus ensuring relevant, quality, and culturally sensitive interventions. Collaboration also facilitates compliance with the IRS New Requirements for 501(c)(3) hospitals under the Affordable Care Act.

Competencies Related to APRN Practice in Public/Community Health

The National Clinical Nurse Specialist Competency Task Force met at the American Nurses Association (ANA) headquarters in May 2008. Their charge was to develop a set of competencies for the clinical nurse specialist (CNS) on identified and valued behaviors. By the end of the meeting, the task force achieved the final listing of eight core competencies and the behaviors needed to accomplish each competency; these competencies and their behaviors were accepted and published. The eight competencies are (a) direct care, (b) consultation, (c) systems leadership, (d) collaboration, (e) coaching, (f) research, (g) evaluation of clinical practice, and (h) ethical decision making. Each competency contains a clarification and behavior statements (National Association of Clinical Nurse Specialists, National CNS Competency Task Force, 2013).

APRNs utilize every competency in this list; however, the collaboration competency is especially valuable. This competency provides a matrix for the establishment of relationships within and across all aspects of the CHA, including data collection, planning, delivery of care, and outcomes evaluation. One of the behavioral statements is "Provides leadership in promoting interdisciplinary collaboration to implement outcome-focused patient care programs meeting the clinical needs of patents, families, groups, and communities" (National Association of Clinical Nurse Specialists, National CNS Competency Task Force, 2013, C.6). Within the community we can conceptualize collegiality to include hospitals, health departments, religious congregations, community leaders, strategic services, focus groups, and any other aggregate group within the community.

Another competency that has especially strong meaning to the APRN within the community is the research competency. According to Bruce Leonard (2010), participatory research is one way to empower communities. He suggests that this approach can be carried out through collaboration between healthcare professionals and community leaders; thus, these two competencies are especially relevant to the CHA.

Quad Council of Public Health Nursing Organizations Practice Competencies for Public Health Nurses

Although the CNS core competencies are relevant to all APRNs, they are especially relevant to the APRN practicing in the community (K. Qureshi, personal communication, July 2014). The Quad Council of Public Health Nursing Organizations (Quad Council) is a coalition of four nursing organizations with a focus on public health nursing. Its competencies are based on a set of competencies developed by the Council on Linkages for public health professionals that were developed in 2011. The goal of the council was to ensure that public health nursing fits into the domain of public health science and practice (Quad Council of Public Health Nursing Organizations, 2011).

The Quad Council competencies are defined as observable and measurable knowledge and performance indicators that contribute to improving population health. These competencies ensure that public health practitioners achieve a certain level of competence in their practice to both safeguard the public and enhance practitioners' effectiveness at achieving optimal population health outcomes (The Quad Council of Public Health Nursing Organizations, 2011).

The Quad Council lists eight practice domains for public health nursing: (a) analytic and assessment skills, (b) policy development/program planning skills, (c) communication skills, (d) cultural competency skills, (e) community dimensions of practice skills, (f) public health science skills, (g) financial management and planning skills, and (h) leadership and systems thinking skills. Each domain has multiple applications attached that interpret the domain. These domains are divided into tiers; each tier has implications for a level of practice in public health nursing. Tier 1 applies to the generalist, and tier 2 applies to the APRN with an array of responsibilities such as supervisory or program implementation. Tier 3 applies to PHNs (public health nurses) at an executive or leadership position in public health organizations (The Quad Council of Public Health Nursing Organizations, 2011). A copy of the competencies can be found on the Quad Council's website (quadcouncilphn.org/).

The work of the AACN, National CNS Competency Task Force, and Quad Council provides a comprehensive foundation for APRN practice in population-based nursing. In order to build relationships with communities and to be successful in population health endeavors, APRNs require skills in leadership, management, research, and policy making. Through interdisciplinary teamwork and by collaborating with community leaders and other aggregate groups within the community, APRNs can engage communities in activities to improve health outcomes.

IDENTIFYING COMMUNITY NEEDS

Why Assess the Community?

Community assessment and analysis is a cornerstone of effective care and is the first step in community practice. There is an essential incentive for conducting a community assessment. A thorough assessment should identify the community needs by recognizing the diversity of the community and understanding the community's goals and listening to its priorities. Assessment can help to identify what works and what does not work and can help to address perceived advantages and disadvantages by both parties, thus meeting the needs of that community.

Any plan to meet the needs of the community that is derived from a CHA may truly be considered an evidence-based practice plan. According to the Centers for Disease Control and Prevention (CDC), addressing health improvement is a shared responsibility of federal, state, and local governments, policy makers, business, healthcare providers, professionals, educators, community leaders, and the American public (Centers for Disease Control and Prevention, 2014a). Therefore, if health improvement is the goal, all segments of the community must be involved in a CHS. It must be a collaborative effort.

A CHA may focus on a community as defined by its geopolitical boundaries (e.g., towns, cities, counties) or on a defined population or an aggregate of a community. Aggregates are subpopulations within the larger population, a collection of individuals having one or more characteristics in common (Stanhope & Lancaster, 2013). CHAs are most often conducted for geographical communities. These assessments can be used to identify populations that need more intensive study of specific problems that require an aggregate assessment. A comprehensive community assessment addresses the characteristics of the community's physical environment, infrastructure, and population characteristics. It is through this type of assessment that the APRN can begin to identify the strengths and weaknesses of a community. This information will be required when the time comes to work with community members to achieve mutually agreed-upon goals for improvement in targeted outcomes.

Conducting the Assessment

The APRN who works in the community in collaboration with the principal players in the healthcare environment of the community has many options when deciding what method is best to use for the community that is being assessed. Assessment can be done by any number of methodologies and can include assessment tools, surveys, focus groups, and windshield surveys.

FIGURE 9.1 • Symphony Used to Achieve a Comprehensive Community Assessment

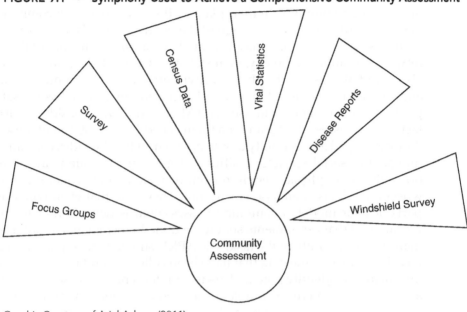

Graphic Courtesy of Ariel Adams (2011).

Information found in online databases and on websites (an excellent way to begin is by accessing county and municipal home pages on the Internet) is an invaluable resource for every community-based APRN. Online databases can provide a plethora of information, including, but not limited to, the following:

- Geographical composition of the community
- Vital statistics such as births, deaths
- Morbidity, mortality, communicable diseases
- Housing, migration, population density
- Education, employment
- Marriages, divorces, adoptions
- Health services provided
- Insurance companies, accidents, police, and fire reports

The experienced APRN will use a combination of methods to conduct an evidence-based CHA. Using research from online resources, as well as a combination of quantitative methods (e.g., searching databases), or qualitative methods (e.g., focus groups and surveys), the APRN can accomplish a fuller, richer, more powerful CHA (see Figure 9.1) (Hanchett, 1988).

No one should attempt to assess a community alone. The APRN should involve many people in the assessment because all stakeholders within a community have something to offer. The APRN who can mobilize an inter-disciplinary team of administrators, policy makers, and members in public service, such as police and fire departments, educational facilities, and health departments, will have diverse resources of knowledge to access for a CHA. And by working together on the assessment, the initial steps taken toward an early collaboration will improve the chances of achieving targeted outcomes (AACN, Task Force on the Clinical Doctorate, 2004).

The APRN might decide to customize an assessment tool to suit the needs of a specific community. In their plan for the assessment of a community Anderson and McFarlane (2014) suggest that many essentials need to be included in the assessment. Among these essential factors are the history of the community, demographics, ethnicity, vital statistics, values, beliefs, and religion. It is also essential to assess the physical environment of the community, the health and social services provided within that community, as well as the safety and political environments. Anderson and McFarlane (2014) considered all of these factors in an assessment plan for a town called Rosemont. Using these factors, they developed a community assessment wheel that includes communication, human and social services, politics and government, safety and transportation, education, physical environment, recreation, and economics. From that wheel they devised an assessment tool. They note that even when using all parts of their model, a community assessment is never complete, and they recommend that assessments should be done in increments in order to better manage the enormity of the task. The APRN should stop at predetermined intervals, synthesize the data that have been collected, and use the accumulated information to identify potential areas for intervention. These authors feel that although no CHA is ever complete, their model provides a framework for success and the basis for creating a plan for successful intervention.

During the analysis and evaluation phase of the assessment data, the APRN may discover that further information is needed. The scope of the data collected may be large but certain parts may be missing. For example, if the APRN is interested in childhood obesity and needs more information on the scope of the problem in the community, it may be essential to assemble a group of parents within the community to better assess the problem. This subgroup of the population can meet using an open discussion methodology, in which the parents discuss their concerns about childhood obesity in their own community. Qualitative information derived from community members can be as valuable as, or in some cases more valuable than, quantitative information. An additional benefit is by allowing parents to derive their own conclusions about the root of the problem, this may yield a significant amount of insight into this community's values and needs. This may also lead parents to consider solutions that work best for their own family and communities, which is more likely to ensure long-term buy in and success.

Assessment Tools

Most community health textbooks contain examples of CHA tools. Angeline Bushy, in her textbook *Orientation to Nursing in the Rural Community* (2000), details a comprehensive plan for a CHA, inclusive of phases of assessment with objectives and activities for completion of the assessment. Bushy's community assessment design emphasizes the importance of forming community partnerships and using and understanding community data as well as evaluating the outcomes of the community health plan.

For the process phase, she lists the types of assessment as well as primary and secondary sources. She stresses the importance of engaging partners in the CHA process and having the community take responsibility for planning, implementing, and evaluating the action plans that are developed to deal with the community's health-related concerns. For Bushy, the CHA goes well beyond collecting data. Importance is placed on bringing communities together to solve local problems (Bushy, 2000).

For three decades, the Healthy People initiative has provided a comprehensive set of national 10-year health-promotion and disease prevention objectives aimed at improving the health of all Americans (see Chapter 2 for more background). It is grounded on the notion that establishing objectives and providing benchmarks to track and monitor progress over time can motivate, guide, and focus action. Healthy People 2020 will continue in the tradition of its predecessors to define the vision and strategy for building a healthier nation with a focus on reducing disparities. According to Healthy People 2020, the determinants of health are individual biology and behavior, physical and social environments, policies and interventions, and access to quality healthcare. These determinants have a profound effect on the health of individuals, communities, and the nation. An evaluation of these determinants is an important part of developing any strategy to improve health (U.S. Department of Health and Human Services, 2008).

In their text *Public Health Nursing: Practicing Population-Based Care* (2012), Truglio-Londrigan and Lewenson used a systematic approach to design the Public Health Nurse Assessment Tool (PHNAT). The PHNAT is thorough and inclusive. The authors feel that their tool provides a systematic method for community assessment and "offers a kaleidoscope way to view the individual, family, community system and population." The authors further suggest that the use of the online versions of their tool "further facilitates the use of this tool because it can be more easily manipulated and implemented in that format" (Truglio-Londrigan & Lewenson, 2012, p. 56).

Healthy People 2020 updates this concept to include "a feedback loop of intervention, assessment, and dissemination of evidence and best practices that would enable achievement of Healthy People 2020 goals" (U.S. Department of Health and Human Services, 2008, p. 7). This updated model adds monitoring and evaluation to the graphic. *Assessment* is considered by both the nursing profession and Healthy People 2020 to be the cornerstone of effective care. Collaboration was also considered invaluable in the development of this action model (Figure 9.2) "The Healthy People process is inclusive; and its strength is directly tied to collaboration" (CDC, 2014b, Strength in Collaboration section, para. 1). This assessment tool, similar to the others mentioned earlier, stresses community collaboration as necessary for a successful community assessment.

ASSESSMENT METHODOLOGIES

Focus Groups

CHA can be enhanced through the use of focus groups. Through the focus-group format, community members can provide inputs about what they feel their community needs. Sometimes, specific stakeholders in a community, such as members of government, designees from police or fire departments, clergy, and representatives from senior or youth groups, form the focus group. More

FIGURE 9.2 • Action Model to Achieve Healthy People 2020. Overarching Goals

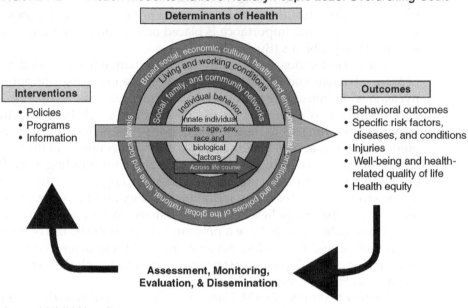

Source: HHS (2008, p. 7).

often the focus groups are open meetings to which all members of a community are invited. Several community destinations, such as churches or public libraries, provide appropriate settings, and a variety of meeting times optimize the opportunities for community members to participate.

A focus group should have a well-prepared moderator to lead the group. The moderator should guide the group so that it does not stray from the issues or topics being addressed, and the moderator should ask explicit questions that are specifically worded to elicit public input. Without an experienced moderator, focus can be lost and the discussion may become tangential and too diffuse to extract useful information. An experienced moderator can actually prompt or cue the members in a way that elicits innovative and constructive ideas with creative solutions. It may be helpful to record meetings to avoid missing any thoughts and ideas or nuances from the discussion. During focus-group discussions, it can sometimes become apparent that the project that has been targeted by the APRN may not be important to, or a high priority for, the community; this often leads to a change in project focus, which should not be considered a negative outcome of a focus group but a success, as it is important for the community to buy into the project in order to have long-term sustainability. It is appropriate for community members to prioritize their needs.

Butler, Dephelps, and Howell (1995) suggest that selective community members who have relevant knowledge can provide the needed information through a focus-group approach. Focus-group leaders should be selected from the community. Often pastors of community churches, members of service groups, such as the Rotary Club or the Elks, or local politicians are asked to lead focus groups as they have some experience leading groups and can relate to community members. These leaders can be schooled in the topic of the focus group, and the outcomes of the discussions will be productive.

A school nurse intervention program for inner-city Mexican American children was planned by Cowell, McNaughton, and Ailey (2000) using data obtained from focus groups. The focus groups, conducted in Spanish, focused on mothers of Mexican American children attending a local elementary school. The mothers were asked to discuss what nursing services they would like and where these services should be located. The problems these mothers identified included discipline, domestic violence, substance abuse, and unemployment. The mothers also discussed their problems with American culture. As a result of the focus groups, home visits by nurses were planned, with interventions designed to address the identified problems. It is important to note that the needs of the community were assessed and addressed by the focus group. This led to a mutually agreed-upon solution with a good chance for success because participants felt that they were heard. Programs designed with inputs from focus groups that include community members have a better chance of addressing a community's needs and wants and a higher likelihood of success than programs developed without community input.

Surveys

Surveys form an excellent matrix for the collection of information about a population. In a CHA survey, questions are usually asked of a sample of the community's population, and the responses generate information that is either numeric (quantitative) or written (qualitative) about the topics under examination. Surveys can be distributed to community members via face-to-face interaction, e-mail, telephone, and/or mail. They can also be distributed through schools and churches, and in some cases through the local newspaper. An excellent site for survey development is SurveyMonkey (*www.surveymonkey.com*).

Lundy and Janes (2009), in their text *Community Health Nursing: Caring for the Public's Health*, discuss the use of a survey to discover the rates of drug use among long-haul truck drivers and the influence of the drugs on truck accidents and fatigue. Thirty-five truck drivers were surveyed at truck stops and loading facilities across cities and towns in Queensland, Australia. Truck drivers reported high rates of usage of prescription medications, over-the-counter drugs, and amphetamines. They also reported that they were motivated to use drugs because of peer pressure, socialization, and the need for relaxation, in addition to wanting to fit the image of a truck driver. The data collected through the survey identified those social factors that must be considered when developing drug prevention and treatment programs for truck drivers. This is an example of how surveys can be useful for describing the characteristics of a population. Surveys, however, are not useful when trying to establish a cause-and-effect relationship. In this case, there are three potential variables—peer pressure, socialization, and the need for relaxation—that cannot be easily controlled. If an APRN wants to explore how these variables may be related to drug usage among truck drivers, a literature review may be performed. If no relationship is evident in the literature, additional studies may need to be designed to establish the impact of these variables on drug usage among truck drivers. Regardless, the use of surveys can establish a pattern of behaviors and attitudes that may need to be addressed in the assessment phase. By carefully reviewing the literature and history of similar population-based interventions, the experienced APRN can approach this problem with evidence-based solutions or establish new solutions using the information obtained in the assessment.

Windshield Survey

A windshield survey refers to that information that can be obtained about a community by driving through it. It is an excellent tool for getting an overall feel or impression of a community. The APRN can use a windshield survey to view the amount of open space, the number and types of retail stores and commercial developments, and the type and condition of housing in a community. Walking through the community can yield similar results (Stanhope & Lancaster, 2013). The PHNAT tool of Truglio-Londrigan and Lewenson (2012) is useful when conducting a windshield survey as it provides a comprehensive matrix for describing the physical environment of the community.

One CHA windshield survey that undergraduate students conducted in a small industrial town revealed a large number of taverns. On visiting the taverns, the students discovered that many of the men who patronized them smoked cigarettes. They learned that it was the usual custom for the men in this community to stop at these places on their way home after work in the local industries to enjoy some socialization. A review of local health department data also revealed a high incidence of oral cancer in this town. This is an example of how a windshield survey, combined with health-related data, can be used to identify potential areas for intervention in a community. The interventions that ensued included an oral screening clinic and a smoking-cessation program that targeted the tavern patrons.

Internet Sites

The CHA is further enhanced when data are collected from a variety of sources. Essential #3 of the AACN *Position Statement on the Practice Doctorate in Nursing* (2004) states that graduates of DNP programs should be able to use information technology and research methods to collect appropriate and accurate data to generate evidence for nursing. A comprehensive discussion for locating population data is presented in Chapter 2 of this text.

Census Data

As required by the U.S. Constitution, the U.S. Census Bureau conducts a census of the entire population every 10 years. Although basic data are collected on everyone, a selected sample of the population is surveyed in greater detail using the "long form." This extensive form gathers more detailed information about the population such as income, housing, employment, language spoken, ancestry, education, poverty, monthly rent/mortgage, commute to work, and so on. The census data provide a plethora of community characteristics (e.g., age, sex, race, education, employment, income) and better describe the makeup of communities. The information gathered is compiled and analyzed and reported to the nation. It should be noted that low-income and migratory populations are often underrepresented in the data. Ervin (2001) writes that the importance of census data as a source of information is invaluable. She notes that the census is a rich source of information and can provide details that will help identify important community characteristics (e.g., culture, socioeconomic characteristics). Census information is available at www.census.gov.

Health Department Vital Statistics

Vital statistics are an excellent source of information about a community and are easily obtainable. Although considered "dry" by many community assessors, data on births, deaths, marriages, and divorces are vital statistics within a community and are collected on an ongoing basis. There is also a wide spectrum of quantitative information on populations available on the Internet. Information from health departments, in combination with information gleaned from other sources such as surveys or focus groups, provides solid data for the development of specific interventions (e.g., high mortality rates due to breast cancer in a community might suggest the need for an increase in breast screening and improved access to mammography) (Ervin, 2001). This information is also useful for comparing data before and after interventions to determine whether a community intervention is successful (Ervin, 2001). As described in an earlier example, college students combined data from a windshield survey, discussions with residents, and morbidity statistics. By combining quantitative data from databases with more personal and qualitative CHA methods, the students were able to capture a more comprehensive view of the community and able to better identify community needs.

Disease Reports

The CDC publishes the *Morbidity and Mortality Weekly Report* (www.cdc.gov). The APRN may want to subscribe to this free publication. The data within these reports are often not available elsewhere and can be invaluable sources of health information. Morbidity and mortality data are also available from the HHS and CDC websites. Information on notifiable diseases and specific topics, such as registries, adverse drug reactions, injury surveillance, occupational health, and birth defects, is available from these two government agencies. Most of this information is useful for an APRN's community assessment and is provided at little or no cost. It can also help the APRN generate new and innovative ideas in survey design or development of a focus-group questionnaire.

BUILDING RELATIONSHIPS

Collaboration: Community Partnership

Although one musical note may have no meaning, add a few notes and then a few more and it becomes a melody that can be sung and enjoyed. A community is made of many people, and the APRN must have a comprehensive understanding of those people in order to build a trusting relationship. Understanding a community's culture is essential to program success.

Traditionally, a "community" has been defined as a group of interacting people living in a common location. The word is often used to refer to a group that is organized around common values and is attributed with social cohesion within a shared geographical location, generally in social units larger than a household. The word *community* is derived from the Old French *communite*, which is derived from the Latin *communitas* (*cum*, "with/together" + *munus*, "gift"), a broad term for fellowship or organized society (Editors of The American Heritage Dictionaries, 2002); For more information on defining populations and subgroups, refer to Chapter 1.

Community involvement is the foundation of a successful CHA. The members of the community, including the people, the government, the health department, the churches, the local businesses, to name a few, all need to be involved. Who are the leaders in the community? Who are the people who are respected and trusted and can engage community members? This is not always a political leader but can be a church member, a parent, a community advocate, and so on. Many communities do not have an inherent trust in "outsiders" who come into their community. There may be a history of people who have started programs only to leave without providing community members with the tools (financial or otherwise) to sustain programs after they are gone. The APRN will have the most success in building programs by working with and being guided by a trusted member of the community than by starting programs without first seeking the input and trust of the community.

It is also imperative that communities are not viewed as having a "problem" that needs to be fixed. Communities want to feel they are productive and cohesive and do not want someone to tell them how to fix their problems. They want partnership and understanding of who they are and what they stand for. When approaching a community, it is essential that you identify the community's strengths and weaknesses. By knowing the strengths, you can establish more trust from community members because they do not want to be defined only by their problems. This mutual understanding can build trust and cooperation. It requires listening by both parties and should provide the community and its members with the tools to sustain programs on their own. A sense of independence and self-sufficiency is important for long-term success. This is the ultimate form of involvement. Education and learning should be bidirectional. APRN partnerships should be built on trust, cooperation, and communication. Methodologies for using data to improve healthcare in the community are presented in Chapters 6, 7, and 10.

Building Relationships and Engaging Communities Through Collaboration: An Example

The concept of community collaboration can be illustrated by using an example taken from Lee County, North Carolina. As has been discussed earlier, there are many methods for creating a community profile. In Lee County, a CHA was implemented using a survey. First, a general overview of the community was ascertained by using a combination of geographical information and vital statistics. Lee County is located in the geographical center of the state, covering 259 square miles, and it is one of the smallest counties in North Carolina. The county comprises eight townships and has had a population increase of 13.2% since April 2000. It continues to grow at a steady rate. According to the U.S. Census, the 2005 population of Lee County was 55,704. The per capita income, although slightly lower than the North Carolina average, has been increasing since 2000. Lee County has maintained an unemployment rate slightly higher than the rest of the state since 2000. Employment opportunities are a concern among all groups, especially Hispanics. This collection of vital statistics from the U.S. Census provided a snapshot of the strengths of the community, as well as some areas that could be targeted for intervention. To create a truly comprehensive CHA (a variety of methodologies were needed to fully assess and address the community's needs), a task force was created.

The CHA Task Force

The lead in this CHA was a task force composed of the members of the Health Department, the supervisor of school nurses for Lee County, and the members of the Healthy Carolinians Partnership in Lee County, known as the Community Action Network (LeeCAN). The LeeCAN is a partnership with representation from government agencies, civic groups, citizen groups, and members from the faith-based communities. The mission of the LeeCAN is "to increase awareness and resources to effectively address health and safety issues in Lee County through a collaborative community effort" (S. Oates, personal communication, September 2010).

Lee County

To ensure adequate community participation, primary data for the CHA were collected using a community survey that was distributed and made available in a variety of modalities: online, paper/pencil, local newspaper, and through "open house" and "community forum"-type events. Local churches, volunteer fire departments, and local businesses also distributed information about the survey.

Members of the CHA team first looked for an appropriate instrument for collecting information. A CHA should measure the variables of interest consistently, dependably, and accurately. The survey selected was originally used in three other North Carolina counties—Montgomery, Moore, and Richmond—as the tool for their CHA. The survey was validated for use as a health assessment data-collection tool. It included a total of 28 questions. Demographic questions included age, gender, race/ethnicity, zip code of residence, marital status, number of people living in the household, number of children in the home aged 18 years or younger, education levels, and employment status. In addition to demographic questions, the survey also included questions that ask respondents their perceptions about community problems or issues, specific health-related issues, access to healthcare and insurance, and prevalence of diseases and disability.

Based on the innovative model of the Northeastern NC Partnership for Public Health, the North Carolina Public Health Incubator Collaboratives (NC

PHICs) is a collaborative of local health departments working together voluntarily to address pressing public health issues (The North Carolina Public Health Incubator Collaboratives, 2014). The state is divided into several geographical incubator groups. Lee, Montgomery, Moore, and Richmond Counties are all located in the south central incubator group and data are compared within incubator groups.

Lee County Community Health Opinion Survey

"This survey is in the public domain. Community health assessment is the process of learning about the health status of our community. We use this information to identify needs/concerns about our community and then develop ways to address those needs" (see Exhibit 9.1) (S. Oates, personal communication, September 2010).

Survey results

The data were analyzed and reviewed by an advisory team from Lee County Public Health Department and members of the LeeCAN. Health-related concerns in Lee County were identified during this process. According to Oates (personal communication, September 2010), the survey respondents believed the most prevalent health-related problems for the county were the following:

- Access to mental health services
- Access to dental care
- Teen pregnancy
- Crime
- Poverty
- Migrant children whose parents are no longer in seasonal migrant jobs

The top five diseases identified by the CHA as a "major problem" in Lee County were as follows:

1. High blood pressure
2. Adult obesity
3. Diabetes
4. Childhood obesity
5. Heart disease

The CHA was used as a tool to identify areas that need improvement and to prioritize health issues of Lee County residents. It engaged community members by having them identify their needs and, in doing so, raised their awareness of areas that needed improvement. The information garnered from the CHA also assisted community agencies in planning their program goals and objectives and in determining priority health issues. A further benefit has been its usefulness in identifying community resources (Lee County Public Health Assessment Team & LeeCAN, 2006).

The information that has been collected through the CHA has been of great value. It identified the priorities of community participants and, in doing so, helped members of the collaborative identify those areas in the community

EXHIBIT 9.1 • Lee County, North Carolina, Community Survey

1. Thinking about your community, what kind of place is it to live? (Check only one.)

_____ Excellent _____ Good _____ Fair _____ Poor

2. In your opinion, does your community have a problem with any of these issues listed? (Please check whether you think it is no problem, a minor problem, a major problem, or I do not know.)

Living in Our Community	No Problem	Minor Problem	Major Problem	I Do Not Know	Priority
Traffic safety					
Affordable, safe housing					
Employment opportunities					
Recreational programs and facilities					
Education and training for adults					
Water supply and quality					
Racial/ethnic discrimination					
Legal services					
Crime					
Air quality					
Animal control					
Public transportation					
Food safety					
Solid waste disposal					
Terrorism (biological, chemical)					
Quality education (K–12)					

3. Now, out of this list, please rank your top five concerns with "1" having the highest priority, "2" being next, and so on.

4. How long have you lived in Lee County?

_____ less than 1 year _____ 1 to 5 years _____ 6 to 10 years
_____ more than 10 years _____ my whole life

5. In your opinion, are these issues a problem in your community?

Living in Our Community	No Problem	Minor Problem	Major Problem	I Do Not Know
Alcohol abuse				
Illegal drug use/substance abuse				
Tobacco use				
Driving/riding without seat belts				
Homelessness				

(continued)

EXHIBIT 9.1 • Lee County, North Carolina, Community Survey (*continued*)

Sexually transmitted diseases				
Poor eating habits				
No physical activity/exercise				
Family violence				
Child abuse				
Juvenile delinquency				
Suicide				
Work safety				
Youth access and use of weapons				
Teen pregnancy				
Men's health				

6. In your opinion, do people in your community have a problem finding/using these services?

Health and Human Services	No Problem	Minor Problem	Major Problem	I Do Not Know
Routine healthcare				
Hospital services				
Dental care				
Mental healthcare/counseling				
Emergency medical care				
Pharmacy/drug stores				
Drug and alcohol treatment				
Health education programs				
Transportation to healthcare				
Health insurance coverage				
Enrolling in Medicaid/Medicare				
Food assistance ($ or food)				
Housing assistance				
Electricity, fuel, or water bills				
911 emergency services				
Long-term care facilities				
Care for pregnant women				
Childhood immunizations				
After-school care				
Child care for infants/preschoolers				
Car seats for infants and children				
Home healthcare				
Parenting skills education				
Adult day care/respite care				
Nutrition help				
Medical equipment				

(continued)

EXHIBIT 9.1 • Lee County, North Carolina, Community Survey (*continued*)

7. Why do you think people may not use the services in question 6? Please give us your opinion by checking the appropriate answer.

Health and Human Services	No Problem	Minor Problem	Major Problem	I Do Not Know
Person's dislike of the provider				
Cost of services				
No information about services				
Lack of transportation				
Inconvenient times				
Lack of child care				
Inconvenient locations				
Language barriers				
Wait too long for service				
Concerns about confidentiality				
Quality of service				
Prior bad experience				
People were not friendly				
Lack of handicap access				
Reluctance to go for help				
Racial/ethnic discrimination				

8. In the past year, have there been any health-related services you or a member of your household have needed but have not been able to find in your community?

Yes/No

If you answered "yes" to this question, list those services on the line given here.

_____

9. Are you covered by a health insurance plan? Yes/No

If "yes," what type of coverage do you have? (Please check all that apply.)

_____ Medicare (includes supplemental policy) _____ Medicaid

_____ Private insurance _____ Other

Does everyone living in your household have health insurance?

Yes/No

10. If you have private insurance, who pays the premium cost? (Please check all that apply.)

_____ My employer pays the majority of the cost.

_____ I (or my family) pay the majority of the cost.

_____ Employer and I (or my family) each pay about half.

11. Where do you go for routine healthcare when you are sick? (Please check all that apply.)

_____ Doctor's office _____ Hospital emergency room _____ Free clinic

(continued)

EXHIBIT 9.1 • Lee County, North Carolina, Community Survey (*continued*)

_____ Health department _____ Chiropractor _____ Other _____

_____ Urgent care _____ I do not seek healthcare

12. Where do you get most of your health-related information about your health? (Please check all that apply.)

_____ Friends and family _____ Doctor/nurse/pharmacist

_____ Newspaper/magazine/TV _____ Help lines (telephone)

_____ Health department _____ Church _____ School _____ Internet

_____ Hospital _____ Free clinic _____ Other _____

13. In your opinion, does your community have a problem with any of these diseases or disabilities?

Diseases and Disabilities	No Problem	Minor Problem	Major Problem	I Do Not Know
Lead poisoning				
Breast cancer				
Lung cancer				
Prostate cancer				
Other cancers				
Diabetes				
Heart disease				
High blood pressure				
HIV/AIDS				
Pneumonia/flu				
Stroke				
Mental health problems				
Dental problems (adult)				
Dental problems (child)				
Learning and developmental disabilities				
Bulimia/anorexia				
Adult asthma				
Childhood asthma				
Adult obesity				
Childhood obesity				
Depression				
Diseases people get from animals (rabies, West Nile)				
Arthritis				

In order to understand the results of this survey, we need to know more about you.

The answers to these questions will be kept strictly confidential. We do not ask for your name on this survey.

(continued)

EXHIBIT 9.1 • Lee County, North Carolina, Community Survey (*Continued*)

14. What is your zip code? _____

15. What is your age? (Please check one.)
_____ 0–17 _____ 18–34 _____ 35–54 _____ 55–64 _____ 65–74
_____ 75 or older

16. Are you male or female? (Please circle.)

17. What is your current marital status? (Please check one.)
_____ Single, never married _____ Married _____ Separated
_____ Divorced _____ Widowed

18. What is your race/ethnicity? (Please check.)
_____ White _____ Black _____ Native American _____ Asian/Pacific Islander
_____ Hispanic/Latino _____ Other _____

19. How many people live in your household? _____
How many children living in your home are 18 years old or younger? _____
How many adults are 65 and older? _____

20. What was your household income last year? (Please check one.)
_____ Less than $10,000 _____ $10,000 to $19,999
_____ $20,000 to $29,999 _____ $30,000 to $49,999
_____ $50,000 to $74,999 _____ $75,000 or more

21. What is the highest level of schooling you have completed?
_____ Less than 12th grade _____ High school graduate or equivalent
_____ Vocational training
_____ Associate degree in college _____ 4-year college degree (bachelor's)
_____ Advanced degree in college (master's, doctorate)

22. Are you a member of a faith organization? Yes/No

23. What is your employment status?
_____ Employed full time _____ Employed part time _____ Retired
_____ Unemployed _____ Disabled _____ Student _____ Homemaker

24. What is your job field?
_____ Agricultural (farming, ranching)
_____ Business and industry (banking, retailer, plumber, attorney, factory)
_____ Government (city manager, county officer, police)
_____ Education (teacher, principal, professor)
_____ Health (physician, nurse, administrator)
_____ Student
_____ Homemaker
_____ Other _____

that must be addressed. The process of collecting the information was invaluable as it built relationships and engaged the community in the process. The data obtained were useful for writing grant proposals. Additionally, data were used to leverage an increase in funding to address specific county priority issues (S. Oates, personal communication, September 2010).

Lee County Reassessment

After reviewing the results of the survey, it was noted that certain areas of Lee County had a poor rate of survey returns. Lee County has only two incorporated areas: the city of Sanford and the town of Broadway. The town of Broadway has just over 1,000 residents. Lemon Springs is a small community outside of these two areas; however, it is not incorporated into a town. Very few surveys (less than 10) were received from Broadway and Lemon Springs. Several factors were cited as possible barriers to returning surveys:

- Some community members are not able to read English or are illiterate (language barriers)
- Anything that comes from the health department or the government is viewed with suspicion by some members of these communities (trust issues)
- Complacency of community members (S. Oates, personal communication, February 2011)

Focus Groups

Because of the small number of surveys from Lemon Springs and Broadway, the assessment team felt another method was needed to gain input from those communities; a qualitative approach, using focus groups, was employed. Focus groups were held in each of the areas. Community leaders were identified and invited to attend. Topics were preselected from the surveys, and a moderator familiar with the CHA process and not actively involved in the data collection was chosen. The meetings were held on a weekday in a central location during midday; food was provided. No record of attendees was kept in order to maintain anonymity. Some of the population came for intrinsic reasons. The population that responded to the focus group meetings needed some incentive to do so as this might be the only way to get the responses; door prizes and refreshments were provided (S. Oates, personal communication, February 2011).

Focus Group Results

The focus groups unearthed valuable information. Common themes were as follows: affordability of health insurance, lack of specialty care in Lee County, and the need to educate residents about public health services. Specific concerns of the focus groups were drugs and the subsequent negative impact on their communities. In addition, more activities or community facilities were requested to cater to older adults and children. The focus group participants generally felt their community was a good place to live. However, there were concerns in the community about drugs, fear of criminal activity, and funding for community services, such as law enforcement, mental health services, fire department, and assistance for the disabled. Participants stated that the local hospital had a very long emergency room wait time, and that they could go to another hospital in a nearby county and get better and faster service. Participants offered concerns regarding a lack of mental health services, especially services for drug addiction. Focus-group participants felt services were needed to "help the ones who need help," because most drug addicts are "good people who have gotten in a bad place." They stated more training was needed for local clergy on how to counsel addicts and how to refer them to available services. Participants stated that they wanted to know how to teach children about avoiding drug use and to provide parents who have problems with help. They also commented about the need for the unemployed to have access to training that matches available employment in the area. Additionally, transportation was noted as "always an issue." Focus-group members stated that more public transportation was needed to access healthcare services in the community.

The qualitative data collected from the focus groups provided rich information that confirmed and built on results from the completed surveys. This combination of information obtained from surveys and focus groups was used to develop action plans to target the issues identified by community members. The CHA survey and the focus groups were helpful in revealing residents' perceptions about health and quality-of-life issues in Lee County. To validate the survey findings and to fill gaps in information, secondary data sources were also used. Data were pulled from reports and queries from the North Carolina State Center for Health Statistics and the North Carolina Department of Health and Human Services.

Additional resources were used to obtain relevant data about Lee County (Lee County Public Health Assessment Team & LeeCAN, 2006):

- Statistical data from the North Carolina State Center for Health Statistics
- North Carolina Department of Health and Human Services
- North Carolina Division of Public Health: Office of Minority Health and Health Disparities
- North Carolina Department of Public Instructions
- 2000 Census Data
- Sanford/Lee County Strategic Services
- Center for Health Services Research, University of North Carolina
- Community Level Information of Kids: Annie E. Casey Foundation
- Employment Security Commission of North Carolina
- North Carolina Office of the Governor
- North Carolina Child Advocacy Institute
- North Carolina Crime Statistics: North Carolina State Bureau of Investigation

The value of focus groups cannot be understated. In this example of a CHA, the survey response was not adequate alone to capture the needs of the community. By reaching out to those communities that had a poor survey return, a better assessment of community values was obtained using multiple approaches. Participant bias can skew the results of an assessment; so it is important to reach out to those communities using multiple modalities. This allows for a better assessment of community values and needs.

SUMMARY

The CHA process extends beyond collecting community data; it includes establishing rapport among partners and is a continuous process. Community programs are most successful when community members participate in the planning, implementation, and evaluation of programs that address local health concerns (Bushy, 2000). The Lee County experience described at the end of this chapter provides the APRN with an example of a successful collaboration. Another example of a successful community collaboration is demonstrated in Case Study 9.1. This example illustrates the relationship between a university and its surrounding community.

Building relationships and engaging communities through collaboration is a rewarding experience for the APRN. The CHA must be totally inclusive and reflect the collaboration necessary to create an accurate and comprehensive depiction of the community. It is also a dynamic process and should incorporate multiple methods to assess and address a community's needs.

The CHA should be readdressed at regular intervals to identify changing needs. With the information obtained through a well-designed CHA, the APRN has the data needed to develop evidence-based projects that meet the needs of the community. Working with community leaders is critical for success, especially in engaging community members in the process. Only then can

CASE STUDY 9.1

A university had a contractual relationship to provide healthcare services for an underserved urban community, physically located near its catchment area. The school of nursing (SON) intended to engage the community with the goals of providing health-promotion services, health education, and primary care to improve the health of the community, as well as to provide a site for student clinical education. Beyond the high-level agreements that were in place, a relationship had to be forged among SON faculty, administrators, students, and community members in order to realize the goals of the SON. Mutual goal setting was needed in order to fully develop a partnership that would be "real" and "realistic," not just an agreement on paper. SON held meetings with various community groups interested in engagement as part of the assessment process. Elements of the assessment process can be related to the Action Model to Achieve Healthy People 2020 goals (The Secretary's Advisory Committee on National Health Promotion and Disease Prevention Objectives for 2020, 2008). In the assessment phase, conversations between the SON and multiple community partners centered on the organizational culture, timing of services, need for health services, and feasibility. Some of the organizations that the SON had conversations with had health services needs that were far beyond what undergraduate and graduate nursing students could provide; others proved to have a different culture. A collaborative learning model was sought, one in which community members and students could learn from each other. Multiple projects were anticipated, with different characteristics and service provisions.

One relationship that developed was between the SON and a church nurse group. During the assessment and initial collaboration stage, several common

(continued)

CASE STUDY 9.1 • (continued)

elements were found. First, a major purpose of the church nurse group was health promotion and education, mirroring the community health and primary care focus of the nursing curriculum. Members of the church nurse group were not professional nurses; by and large, they were caring individuals who were called to care for the sick and address health concerns in their church community. Second, timing was important. Classes for the SON and church nurse meetings were held at night. The timing fit well into students' schedules, and as a result, no class rotations had to be rearranged. The services of health promotion and education were handled by the undergraduate students; concomitantly, graduate nurse practitioner students rotated through a clinic setting to provide direct primary care-related services under the auspices of the university's nursing care center. A small foundation grant was secured to offset some of the anticipated costs associated with the program—church suppers, educational material, supplies, and advertising. Thus, the feasibility of the partnership was assured.

A premise of the collaboration was that addressing individual behaviors would impact the health of the community at large. This premise was held by both the church members and the SON faculty and students. The relationship between the two groups deepened as discussions were held on what health behaviors the two groups would address. The format of the program was to include education sessions in a church-supper format and health fairs, and referrals to clinics for acute care problems. The SON faculty and students proposed a curriculum based on health disparities addressed in Healthy People 2010. The church nurse group proposed topics that they felt were the most pressing concerns in the community. Discussion shifted away from the federal guidelines to the real issues of health in the community.

The church nurses identified uncontrolled diabetes as a problem and wanted to host a health fair and were able to tailor a health program to the needs of the community. They implemented a diabetes screening program and performed mass finger sticks to identify persons with high blood glucose levels. This strategy is not in the health-promotion guidelines, but was adapted for a successful health fair. Community members came to the health fair, and church nurses provided information on where to get low-cost or free diabetic supplies in the community. Additionally, they had some supplies on hand and urged people to "keep their sugar under control." Student nurses provided one-on-one counseling for people with a known diagnosis of diabetes, answering questions about medication, diet, and exercise. The mass screening of 100 community members yielded four people with blood glucose levels well over 500 mg/dL, and they were referred to the nursing center for immediate follow-up. Student nurses worked to ensure individual privacy, whereas the community members saw the screening as a "family affair," with each person responsible for his or her neighbor's health. This unorthodox approach to health promotion education and screening caused a buzz in the community and paved the way for a multiyear health-promotion project and ongoing relationships.

Evaluation of the program occurred at individual, group, and community levels. The success of the relationship was evident in the personal relationships that developed among students, faculty, and community members.

Adapted from Kotecki (2002a, 2002b).

community programs be developed and integrated into a successful health-care plan for the community. To paraphrase the old African saying, "Many silver bracelets do make much jingle."

EXERCISES AND DISCUSSION QUESTIONS

Exercise 9.1 Using a professional journal, the newspaper, or the web, locate an article that describes the development of a community partnership. Select a partnership that focuses on health and has at least three partners, if possible.

- Using case study 9.1 as an example, identify what strategies may have been implemented during the community assessment phase by the partners in the article that you selected.
- Identify any assessment tools described in the case study that were used or should have been used in the selected article.
- What databases would be appropriate to access and to use to demonstrate the need for the partnership?
- If the partnership focuses on health disparities, what epidemiologic studies should have been conducted? What would suggest that the partnership was based on evidence, relationship, or politics?
- Apply the Action Model to Achieve Healthy People 2020 goals to the partnership from the selected article. What elements of the model can you identify?

REFERENCES

American Association of Colleges of Nursing. (2006). *The essentials of doctoral education for advanced nursing practice.* Washington, DC: Author. Retrieved from http://www.aacn.nche.edu/publications/position/DNPpositionstatement.pdf

American Association of Colleges of Nursing, Task Force on the Clinical Doctorate. (2004). *AACN position statement on the practice doctorate in nursing.* Washington, DC: AACN. Retrieved from http://www.aacn.nche.edu/publications/position/DNPposition-statement.pdf

Anderson, E. T., & McFarlane, J. (2014). *Community as partner: Theory and practice in nursing* (7th ed.). Philadelphia, PA: Wolters Kluwer Health.

Bailey, D. (1992). Using participatory research in community consortia development and evaluation: Lessons from the beginning of a story. *American Sociologist, 23*(4), 71–82.

Bushy, A. (2000). *Orientation to nursing in the rural community.* Thousand Oaks, CA: Sage.

Butler, L. M., Dephelps, C., & Howell, P. E. (1995). *Focus groups: A tool for understanding community perceptions and experiences. Community ventures: Partnerships in education and research series.* Retrieved from http://wrdc.usu.edu/files/publications/publication/pub__1158330.pdf

Centers for Disease Control and Prevention (CDC). (2014a). Healthy People 2020. Retrieved from http://www.cdc.gov/nchs/healthy_people/hp2020.htm

Centers for Disease Control and Prevention (CDC). (2014b). *Strength in collaboration.* Retrieved from http://www.cdc.gov/news/2008/03/HealthyPeople2020.html

Cowell, J. M., McNaughton, D. B., & Ailey, S. (2000). Development and evaluation of a Mexican immigrant family support program. *Journal of School Nursing, 16*, 4–7.

Editors of the American Heritage Dictionaries. (2002). *The American Heritage Dictionary of the English Language* (4th ed.). Community. Boston, MA: Houghton Mifflin.

Ervin, N. E. (2001). *Advanced community health nursing practice.* Upper Saddle River, NJ: Prentice Hall.

Hanchett, E. S. (1988). *Nursing frameworks and community as client: Bridging the gap.* Norwalk, CT: Appleton & Lange.

Internal Revenue Service. (2014). *New requirements for 501(c)(3) hospitals under the Affordable Care Act.* Retrieved from http://www.irs.gov/Charities-%26-Non-Profits/Charitable-Organizations/New-Requirements-for-501(c)(3)-Hospitals-Under-the-Affordable-Care-Act

Kotecki, C. N. (2002a). A health promotion curriculum for faith-based communities. *Holistic Nursing Practice, 16,* 61–69.

Kotecki, C. N. (2002b). Incorporating faith based partnerships into the curriculum. *Nurse Educator, 27*(1), 13–15.

Lee County Public Health Assessment Team & LeeCAN. (2006). *Lee County community health assessment,* Sanford, NC. Retrieved from http://publichealth.nc.gov/lhd/cha/resources.htm

Lenz, E. R. (2005). The practice doctorate in nursing: An idea whose time has come. *Online Journal of Issues in Nursing, 10*(3), Manuscript 1. Retrieved from http://www.nursingworld.org/MainMenuCategories/ANAMarketplace/ANAPeriodicals/OJIN/TableofContents/Volume102005/No3sept05/tpc28_116025.aspx

Leonard, B. (2010). Community empowerment and healing. In E. T. Anderson & J. McFarland (Eds.), *Community as partner theory and practice in nursing* (6th ed., pp. 91–110). Philadelphia, PA: Lippincott Williams & Wilkins.

Lundy, K. S., & Janes, S. (2009). *Community health nursing: Caring for the public's health.* Boston, MA: Jones and Bartlett.

National Association of Clinical Nurse Specialists, National CNS Competency Task Force. (2013). *CNS core competencies.* Retrieved from http://www.nacns.org/docs/CNSCoreCompetenciesBroch.pdf

National Association of County and City Health Officials. (2014). *Public health infrastructure and systems.* Retrieved from http://www.naccho.org/topics/infrastructure/mapp/chahealthreform.cfm

The North Carolina Public Health Incubator Collaboratives (NC PHICs). (2014). Retrieved from http://nciph.sph.unc.edu/incubator/

The Quad Council of Public Health Nursing Organizations. (2011). *Quad Council competencies for public health nurses.* Retrieved from http://www.achne.org/files/Quad%20Council/QuadCouncilCompetenciesforPublicHealthNurses.pdf

The Secretary's Advisory Committee on National Health Promotion and Disease Prevention Objectives for 2020. (2008). *Recommendations for the framework and format of Healthy People 2020.* Retrieved from https://www.healthypeople.gov/sites/default/files/PhaseI_0.pdf

Shuster, G. F., & Goeppinger, J. (2008). Community as client: Assessment and analysis. In M. Stanhope & J. Lancaster (Eds.), *Public health nursing: Population-centered health care in the community* (7th ed., pp. 339–372). St Louis, MO: Mosby Elsevier.

Stanhope, M., & Lancaster, J. (2013). *Public health nursing: Population-centered health care in the community* (8th ed.). St Louis, MO: Mosby Elsevier.

Truglio-Londrigan, M., & Lewenson, S. B. (2012). *Public health nursing: Practicing population-based care.* Boston, MA: Jones & Bartlett Publishers.

U.S. Department of Health and Human Services (HHS). (2008). *The Secretary's Advisory Committee on National Health Promotion and Disease Prevention Objectives for 2020. Phase I report. Recommendations for the framework and format of Healthy People 2020.* Retrieved from http://www.healthypeople.gov/sites/default/files/PhaseI_0.pdf

U.S. Department of Health and Human *Services* (HHS). (2014). *How the health care law benefits you.* Retrieved from http://www.hhs.gov/health care/facts/bystate/Making-a-Difference-National.html

U.S. Department of Health and Human Services (HHS), Health Resources and Services Administration. (2014). *What are federally qualified health centers (FQHCs)?* Retrieved from http://www.hrsa.gov/healthit/toolbox/RuralHealthITtoolbox/Introduction/qualified.html

Challenges in Program Implementation

Janna L. Dieckmann

The role of the nurse in healing includes compassionate and quality care not only for the individual but also for the family and the community. Advanced practice registered nurses (APRNs) seek to improve the circumstances that contribute to poor population health by working with community members to modify or change the behaviors that may contribute to poor health outcomes. This type of collaboration has the potential to make or facilitate changes that improve health and reduce morbidity and mortality.

The APRN should approach communities with an open mind and a focus on a comprehensive community health assessment (CHA; see Chapter 9). A CHA helps the APRN to gain an understanding of the community, its residents, their diversity, their goals, their aspirations for healthier lives, and the barriers to achieving these goals. People want a better life. They want to be healthier and they want to live longer, happier, and more productive lives. The challenge lies in changing the behaviors and attitudes of individuals and communities. For many, change is uncomfortable or difficult, but is a necessary process for communities that want to make improvements. But a process of change is unlikely to be smooth if community members do not buy into this change and are not willing to take a risk or make a sacrifice for the unknown.

LEWIN'S STAGES OF CHANGE

Lewin's Three-Stage Model of Change provides a brief but profound approach to change at the aggregate or community level (Allender, Rector, & Warner, 2013). In the role of a change agent, the APRN begins by destabilizing the group or community by asking questions to generate hope and visions of something different, something possibly better. Perhaps the group or community is already experiencing a desire for something different. Disequilibrium in the current moment underscores the relevance and potential of change and of moving out of the current comfort zone.

Unfreezing

The first stage of change is *unfreezing*, and may arise from the community's own self-assessment or it may be activated by the APRN through motivation, health education, advocacy, or other strategies (Allender et al., 2013; Connelly, 2014). An APRN may initiate unfreezing during the course of usual practice. For example, as part of a primary care practice, an APRN may find that many adult patients want to increase their physical activity, but the lack of designated walking or biking trails is a barrier that prevents this change. The APRN initiates a conversation with the head of the local farmers' cooperative and with the director of the county's agricultural extension office. A community meeting is planned, with broad attendance by local residents and representatives of other community organizations. Many express interest in increased physical activity, but doubt their ability to make changes to their community that will make it more "walker friendly." This meeting is the first of many opportunities to present the problem to the community and address possible solutions, and begin to build a bridge of confidence between the community and the healthcare provider. Focus groups (see Chapter 9) can also further this goal and provide more individual attention to potential barriers while proposing possible solutions to address those concerns.

Changing, Moving, or Transition

The second stage in Lewin's model reflects an understanding that change is not a timed event but an ongoing process that can be facilitated by the actions of the APRN. This stage is known variously as *changing*, *moving*, or *transition* (Allender et al., 2013; Connelly, 2014). Community members begin as individuals and as a group to transition to new attitudes and behaviors as they acquire new skills and perspectives.

The combination of destabilizing the present state and the challenge of questioning the status quo of behaviors and attitudes can make the second stage the most difficult. The support role of the APRN is very important, as the nurse must accept the community's attempts at change against the risk of early failures. The APRN cannot necessarily direct community change, as community residents benefit from developing their own new patterns of behavior as these emerge from who they are and their past experiences. The APRN can motivate and guide community members and help them build on their experiences to make the changes necessary for success. Using the earlier example, the APRN should provide encouragement about the value of change (e.g., an improvement in residents' physical activity levels leads to improved health and less need for medications), implement strategies to reduce fears (e.g., educate residents about other successful programs), develop skills to unlock new behaviors (e.g., encourage residents to work together as peer support), provide prompts underscoring the importance of change attempts (e.g., use simple outcome measures for residents [i.e., step counters] to track progress and set goals), and remind residents about the benefits of the community's goal (e.g., a healthier community is a more productive community) (Allender et al., 2013; Connelly, 2014). As a result of regular community meetings, the rural community raises funds and constructs new walking trails on public land. A park with a picnic shelter is also built to provide families and groups a place to gather after walking.

Refreezing

The third stage of change is *refreezing* (or *freezing*), which reflects the restabilization of the community that follows after making change. This stage can require a period of time, as the change or transition that community members experience can lead to a change in their relationships and in their daily lives as they internalize what is now different. The system adapts to the impact of the change, and the community integrates the change into a newly stable and rebalanced present state. For example, the walking trails that were once seen as improbable are now embraced and accepted by the community. The APRN can provide the community with additional tools to stabilize the change and to reinforce and maintain new community behaviors. Families are encouraged to try out the new walking trail and to use the new picnic area for a healthy meal. Neighborhood events can center on the use of the park so as to introduce other community members to the benefits of the community space. Periodic reminders to area residents about the walking trails can be included in local print and visual media.

The success of the change process can lead to an enhanced partnership between the nurse and the community with the potential for further collaboration. Ideally, over time, the rural community will increase its physical activity and may seek additional consultation, for example, on how to select and prepare nutritional meals. Two-way communication can identify and address resistance or barriers to change. The APRN needs to identify potential problems or doubts and reinforce the benefits and values of the changed behaviors. The emergence of a new equilibrium signals a potential exit point for the APRN's engagement with the community (Allender et al., 2013; Connelly, 2014).

COMMUNITY ENGAGEMENT

Engagement

APRNs are more likely to succeed in addressing community concerns when communities are prepared to engage in the process of change. *Engagement* is different from wishing or acknowledging that "something" needs to change in order to improve. According to the CDC (Centers for Disease Control and Prevention), community engagement is "the process of working collaboratively with and through groups of people affiliated by geographic proximity, special interest, or similar situations to address issues affecting the well-being of those people" (McCloskey et al., 2011, p. 7). Before beginning a community engagement effort, the APRN must carefully consider the target community/population. What are the results of the CHA, and what is known about the community? What has been the history of this community during and following previous change and engagement efforts? How are the community and its various groups likely to perceive the APRN, and what is the potential for a successful engagement of community members (Centers for Disease Control and Prevention/Agency for Toxic Substances and Diseases Registry [CDC/ATSDR] Committee on Community Engagement, 1997)? Is the community prepared to engage in change? Would the community's social or physical environment facilitate or impede change? During this assessment and initial contact, the APRN needs to recognize the core principle of community self-determination and the limits of professional action. It is critical that the APRN clearly recognize the principle that "[n]o external entity should assume it can bestow to a community the power to act in its own self-interest" (CDC/ATSDR Committee, 1997, Principle 4). Community members will find their own power when they seek it in themselves and take action for themselves, their families, and their community.

Involving the community is a second important and necessary step in assessing the potential for engagement. The APRN needs to establish relationships and build trust through contacts with community leaders and community organizations. As mentioned in earlier chapters, the community leaders are not always the political leaders, but rather can include leaders in the church, schools, charitable foundations, or any member of the community who is trusted as a leader. The successful engagement with the community will depend on developing relationships with these community leaders. Each community is distinctively unique; engaging with a community will require acknowledgment and inclusion of the cultures and diversity of that community in all steps of the engagement. Only by taking these steps can the APRN fully identify and mobilize community assets and resources and lay the groundwork for building long-term change in the community. With that said, healthcare professionals must recognize the limits of professional control and the need and/or cost of making a long-term commitment with the community and its residents (CDC/ATSDR, 2011; Table 10.1).

Gaining the Trust of the Community

When working with a community, population, or aggregate, the APRN must include strategies to initiate, develop, and sustain trust among the APRN and community leaders, community members, and stakeholders. Trust requires mutual intention and is characterized by reciprocity (Lynn-McHale & Deatrick, 2000). As a key element in social interaction, trust facilitates communication and mutual understanding. Trust is a basis for change, a constant connection that provides support when the change process destabilizes a known situation in favor of an unknown outcome. A focus on developing trust begins with the initial contact with community members (Macali, Galanowsky, Wagner, & Truglio-Londrigan, 2011). The resulting nurse–community relationship is a critical prerequisite to population intervention. Through a trusting relationship, the community member gains the security of the APRN's stable presence as a prerequisite to risking the unknown.

Four categories of trust have been described: calculative, competence, relational, and integrated. In *calculative trust*, potential members of the community initiative estimate the balance of benefits and costs to be derived from

TABLE 10.1 • Principles of Community Engagement

Before starting a community engagement effort:
- Be clear about the purposes or goals of the engagement effort and the populations and/or communities you want to engage.
- Become knowledgeable about the community in terms of its economic conditions, political structures, norms and values, demographic trends, history, and experience with engagement efforts. Learn about the community's perceptions of those initiating the engagement activities.

For engagement to occur, it is necessary to:
- Go into the community, establish relationships, build trust, work with the formal and informal leadership, and seek commitment from community organizations and leaders to create processes for mobilizing the community.
- Remember and accept that community self-determination is the responsibility and right of all people who constitute a community. No external entity should assume it can bestow to a community the power to act in its own self-interest.

For engagement to succeed:
- Partnering with the community is necessary to create change and improve health.
- All aspects of community engagement must recognize and respect community diversity. Awareness of the various cultures and other factors of diversity must be paramount in designing and implementing community engagement approaches.
- Community engagement can only be sustained by identifying and mobilizing community assets and by developing capacities and resources for community health decisions and actions.
- An engaging organization or individual change agent must be prepared to release control of actions or interventions to the community and be flexible enough to meet the changing needs of the community.
- Community collaboration requires long-term commitment by the engaging organization and its partners.

Source: Centers for Disease Control and Prevention/Agency for Toxic Substances and Diseases Registry Committee on Community Engagement. National Institutes of Health (2011).

a potential collaboration as well as each member's assets and linkages. *Competence trust* hinges on whether group members are capable of doing what they commit to do; this type of trust also underlies the development of mutual respect among the participants. *Relational trust* reflects the personal relationships that quickly arise among members of any group. Members may express the value of mutual exchanges and develop a sense of commitment to mutual goals. Taken together, these three categories of trust constitute *integrated trust*, the foundation of an ongoing partnership (Logan, Davis, & Parker, 2010).

Initiating trust is an essential first step in building a bond between the nurse and the community. The nurse's *presence* in the community is qualitative evidence of the intent to develop a professional relationship with the community and its members. The community's willingness to view this presence positively will hinge on the APRN's clear communication of his or her role with the community. The APRN should seek to frame his or her presence within the broader outlines of the consensus needs or goals of the community, to the extent that these are known.

On the basis of knowledge obtained from a CHA, the APRN should interact appropriately with community members, for example, in relation to personal demeanor, communication patterns, cultural sensitivity, expressions of interest, and communication of knowledge about the community. Being "liked" by community members can be indefinable in its intent or as a goal, but either way it is nearly essential in practice. The APRN should always review and consider what the community needs or wants first. The nurse's expressions of interest in the community and its members are concrete indications of commitment and, to a certain extent, obligate the APRN to the community and to assisting with the community members' priorities. If there is a specified time frame or funding for the program, the APRN needs to share this limitation with the community and provide the community with the tools needed to sustain or build the program on its own.

Processes of Developing and Sustaining Trust

The process of developing trust between the APRN and the community will likely emerge from early collaborative efforts. In most cases, selecting small, achievable goals that can be met swiftly is recommended. The success of early visible outcomes enhances the nurse's credibility and increases the community's willingness and openness to trust. Increasing the breadth and depth of community participation with these goals will also increase the proportion of community members who have had contact with the APRN and will be an advantage as the nurse–community collaboration continues. It is likely that the community will embark on testing or probing the nurse's knowledge, behavior, and character for the sake of better understanding and will withhold open trust until the community's needs begin to be met. As the nature of the nurse–community relationship is constructed and evolves during this period of role negotiation, the APRN must maintain commitment to the initial shared goals, demonstrate professional openness to engagement with the community, and continue visible and concrete participation in the community. As APRNs share a community presence with the public health nurse, it is relevant to consider that "[t]he less experience people have with trusting relationships and the less sense of personal power and control they have, the more time public health nurses must spend developing trust and strength" (Zerwekh, 1993, p. 1676).

Sustaining the community's trust is built on a record of commitment and ongoing interaction with the community and its members. The nurse's continuing presence within the community establishes a sort of continuity that is reinforced by reliable actions. Decisions by APRNs that become predictable to the community build the community's independence in self-management. When community members can predict "what the nurse would do," they are well on their way to independent decision making for their health. As community members gain independence, the importance of the APRN's leadership becomes less necessary. With increased community competence, the APRN may face new challenges in sustaining the community's trust, and the APRN's role as a leader will change. As a community gains self-efficacy and confidence in self-determination and in its individual perspectives, conflicts become more likely. Mutual participation in thoughtful resolution is essential.

Sustaining the community's continued trust will depend on the APRN's personal and professional skills and willingness to modify relationships with the community and its members and accept a new role as defined by a strengthened community.

Building Partnerships

If trust is an essential prerequisite for change, then partnerships are the essential underpinning for negotiating, planning, and implementing change. The long-lasting relationships that characterize some partnerships build on existing strengths even as new capacities are forged and developed. Themes of engagement, autonomy, and self-determination have shaped contemporary ideas of partnership since the mid-20th century. The Alma-Ata Declaration (1978) proposed a social model of health that underscored the need for "citizen's greater self-reliance and decisional control over their own health" (Gallant, Beaulieu, & Carnevale, 2002, p. 152), and alerted national health systems to more formally involve citizens in healthcare decisions (Gallant, Beaulieu, & Carnevale, 2002). This is even more salient when addressing 21st-century healthcare demands that require individual and community initiatives to address and improve health promotion and disease prevention (Courtney, Ballard, Fauver, Gariota, & Holland, 1996).

Agency–Academic Partnerships

One long-standing approach to partnership is the bridging of health agencies and academic institutions through joint ventures. An early example occurred in Ohio in which the University Public Health Nursing District (in Cleveland, Ohio, 1917–1962) linked local schools of nursing with an independent nursing agency that provided clinic services, public health services, and nurse home visiting (Farnham, 1964). Nursing students were assigned to the district for their public health nursing experiences. Assignments for diploma school students tended more to observation of activities during a brief few weeks, compared to collegiate nursing students, who became fully engaged over a semester in the breadth of public health nursing work. The key structural element was the public health nursing staff of the district, who served as clinical educators for students as well as direct care providers.

As effective and contributory as such programs are, the agency–academic partnership model of collaboration between a health agency or primary care practice and an academic institution has a limited impact when community residents and the wider service-resource network remain uninvolved, and when services are delivered outside of a collaborative planning process that includes community participants at the table from the beginning. Agency–academic partnership programs that focus on delivering services and improving health, but do not address the critical underlying barriers to improving health, are too limited in scope. Changes in the community—both change that benefits community members and change that transforms the community's health—are more likely to occur successfully with the participation of community representatives, both community members and leaders. One promising approach for successful academic–community partnerships uses the community-oriented primary care model to address the structural inequalities underpinning these challenges by placing a community-based organization in the central coordinating role for the partnership (Cherry & Shefner, 2004). An example of one such partnership is the one between Rush University and a community located in Chicago. The Rush University Colleges of Nursing, Medicine, and Health Sciences formed an academic partnership with Marillac House, an existing and trusted social service agency. The goal of the partnership was to provide interdisciplinary and primary healthcare services to a medically underserved neighborhood in Chicago. This partnership benefits both the community and the university as it provides much needed medical services to community residents, and the university uses the clinical site for its students, who gain valuable experience working with a diverse and underserved population (McCann, 2010). The university fostered engagement with the community by partnering with an established agency within the neighborhood and working with community members.

This discussion of agency–academic partnerships highlights the contrast between the APRN as advocate or as catalyst when engaging with a community for health changes. In both the advocate and catalyst roles, the APRN respects the community and its self-determination as a basis for developing strategies to assist or complement the community's efforts for improved health. The *advocate* understands "the world view, life circumstances, and priorities of those requesting or receiving care and exploring the possible options with them in light of their preferences" (Walker, 2011, p. 75). While recognizing the community partner's individuality and self-determination, the nurse advocate takes action on behalf of a community to raise awareness in community members or make change in policy, economic, or social systems affecting the community (Walker, 2011). This advocate approach is closest to the APRN role in the agency–academic partnership. In contrast, the APRN as *catalyst* understands the community as containing "all the necessary qualities and resources for change" and focuses on providing "the spark that will initiate change, as desired by the community and on its terms" (Walker, 2011, p. 75). The "nurse as advocate" role provides the framework for APRN practice in sustainable partnerships and coalitions.

Sustainable Partnerships

Developing long-term relationships between the APRN and community representatives and organizations is a necessary component for preparing communities for long-term change. Sustainable partnerships are characterized by a relationship process through which the nurse and partners "work and interact together" (Gallant et al., 2002, p. 153). Power is shared in a "power-with" approach "emphasizing the positive force created between partners and how this force sustains and propels a relationship forward" (Gallant et al., 2002, p. 154). Win–win negotiation models are recommended in the clinical nursing context (Roberts & Krouse, 1990), and have value in the APRN's collaborations with community leaders and members. Not only are all parties' views heard and valued, but also the power to make decisions is shared, leading to "a sense of responsibility and power" (Roberts & Krouse, 1990, p. 33). This is particularly important when establishing a context for the emergence of an empowered community.

Sustainable partnerships are supported by public participation that enhances decision making by reflecting the interests and concerns of partnership members and by highlighting the underlying values guiding partnership operation. The community that is affected by a decision should be able to participate in influencing the decision and should be included in a way that enables their full participation. Including community members in decision-making committees is an important part of community engagement. Decisions are likely to be more sustainable when the needs, concerns, and interests of all parties are communicated. Communication strategies themselves should be open and negotiated to accommodate representative styles and approaches. Finally, feedback must be provided to all participants and the public about how the decision was made and the role of their input in making the decision (International Association for Public Participation, 2014; Rippke, Briske, Keller, & Strohschein, 2001).

Partnerships can only be characterized as such when certain conditions exist: Each partner must be recognized as having his or her own power and legitimacy, own purpose and goals, and own connection to that locale or community. At the same time, the work of the partnership itself must be or become more than any one partner's own goals. This is reflected in clear partnership objectives and mutual expectations. Regular patterns of feedback from and among all parties should be planned and shared. And finally, all partners should strive for open-mindedness, patience, and respect for others' views (Labonte, 2012).

Working With Community Leaders and Members: Building Coalitions

A coalition-building strategy can establish the groundwork and/or initiate intra-community relationships that contribute to an effective, sustained effort to identify and respond to community challenges and needs. Coalition building "promotes and develops alliances among organizations or constituencies for a common purpose. It builds linkages, solves problems, and/or enhances local leadership to address health concerns" (Keller, Strohschein, & Briske, 2008, p. 204). Coalitions bridge sectors, organizations, and constituencies to provide a benefit to the wider community.

Coalitions are used widely in community interventions because of their flexibility and their "democratic appeal" (Parker et al., 1999, p. 182). For example, Healthy People coalitions at the county or city level study their community and develop several health-promotion or disease prevention objectives. As these coalitions include health and social service professionals, business people, and religious and social organizations, they contain the expertise and connections that have an impact on a community's health. Coalitions are useful for many reasons. First, involving a broad range of community groups provides a diverse basis to address local problems and change community expectations.

Second, health professionals believe that coalitions develop the capacity of local organizations; skills gained in one effort lead to organizational abilities that will later be applied to solve other problems. Third, coalitions can improve service coordination among community agencies, resulting in less duplication and more effective use of resources (Parker et al., 1999). For example, when organizations exchange information as part of the coalition's work, organizational leaders may identify overlapping programs. The cost of duplicate efforts can then be reduced through cooperation across agencies or consolidation at one host agency. Coalitions can also provide a springboard for community empowerment, "an enabling process through which individuals and communities take control of their lives and their environment" (Rippke et al., 2001, p. 212).

The APRN should consider the use of a coalition as it can bring diverse resources together and assist in the community's recognition and response to health concerns. Even though coalitions have many important characteristics, the APRN should consider whether devoting existing resources (such as time, energy, and commitment) to coalition building will lead to the best outcome. The decision also depends on the availability and willingness of the right members for the coalition. Candidate members for the coalition should represent an organization or constituency, and they should have access to the members and resources of the groups they represent. Coalitions can include 12 to 18 members, but smaller groups are able to address more specialized interests or more easily gain sufficient trust to permit mutual collaboration (Rippke et al., 2001). Many coalitions may need to add additional members as the coalition's focus broadens. Depending on the coalition's program, additional groups may need to be added and additional resources may need to be requested from new partners. For example, a coalition meeting to address head injuries among children might refine its focus to promote safety-helmet usage in activities such as bicycling and skateboarding. This coalition might add the expertise of emergency department representatives and the resources of local store owners who sell bicycles or safety helmets.

The intent of a coalition is to assemble around a common interest in which each coalition member has a stake in the outcomes. As in any organization, coalitions require both structure and resources to achieve goals. As coalitions incorporate representatives of diverse organizations who hold diverse perspectives, it is important to facilitate good interpersonal dynamics and to develop reliable group processes for decision making (Rippke et al., 2001). A community coalition should be able to work together on a broad vision of what needs to be accomplished. A mission statement can be useful in providing formal guidance to the coalition effort, especially when a variety or range of perspectives exist among members. When developed collaboratively, this "common vision" can assist with formalization of the next steps (Wald, 2011).

The Process of Establishing Community Priorities

Most community leaders and members can easily identify a wide range of concerns or issues that reflect their wants or needs to improve their community's health. In strained economic times, such lists are likely to become even longer. During prioritization, the available data and community information are reviewed by the coalition and community members to decide what to address and where resources should be targeted (Issel, 2013). The process of setting priorities includes selecting the most important concerns for attention by the coalition. Making this selection can be difficult or frustrating, because in many cases there are multiple problems that need to be addressed in the community. Some community leaders and members will approach this by advocating critical priorities affecting the community, whereas other coalition members will advocate their own personal priorities. Identifying a consensus priority will facilitate the coalition's purpose of finding a common vision or goal.

When considering what actions should receive high-priority attention, how can *wants* and *needs* be differentiated? Needs reflect an objective assessment or conform to a set of expected requirements, as compared to wants, which may be personal wishes or aspirations that fail to rise to the level of necessity. But it may be that the dividing line between wants and needs has more to do with *who* sorts wants from needs, rather than *how* the sorting is done. Wishes and needs for the same target community may differ based on the perspective of the viewer: Insiders and outsiders to the community may propose quite different lists. Rather than asking how to separate needs and wants, the better question may be: Should needs and wants be separated? Perhaps it is more constructive to view both as important and critical to address. For example, a group of health professionals concluded that the priority intervention for a neighborhood in a small, rural community in North Carolina should be to reduce infant mortality, based on significant epidemiological evidence. However, when neighborhood residents heard about the professionals' proposal, they insisted that their priority was a safe playground for their children—and it was built. This should not be considered a failure but rather a success. Although one priority solution was sought, another priority was identified and addressed, leading to a positive outcome for the community.

The practice of priority setting is not purely quantitative; the highest ranking items do not have to be selected over lower ranked items. The process of decision making is interactive, perhaps even political. For example, an APRN may believe that funding and personnel resources should be directed toward the most common diseases in a community. But what if the most frequent disease in a community is sinusitis? Should sinusitis receive attention above all other chronic diseases? Perhaps severity of illness should be an additional criterion. How should duration of illness be factored in? What about considering the possibility of recovery or rehabilitation as a criterion? And what about the actual cost of illness care? Perhaps immunizations are cost-effective because they prevent morbidity and mortality at a very low price. Through questions such as these and related community and partnership discussions, priority-setting discussions reveal much about the values and beliefs of the community and the coalition members.

Ordinarily, several priorities are selected by a coalition. Several of the selected priorities may require different resources, and some priorities may separately seek external grant funding. Priority setting can be helpful in suggesting which items should be addressed first and which should be discarded from the list because of lack of coalition interest or lack of confidence that the problem is solvable given existing resources (Blum, 1981). On the other hand, the availability of external resources or funding may justify selecting a priority, as it is most likely to be viable. In practice, the availability of funding often guides program decisions.

If a coalition priority requires financial support that is not immediately available, the coalition could make a decision (a) to wait for a specified period of time until a funding source is willing to provide financial support, (b) to raise local funding specifically to support the coalition priority, or (c) to downsize the magnitude of the coalition's planned program by implementing a small pilot program or by initially implementing only a portion of the program. For example, if a community seeks to address the low immunization rates among preschool children, then the coalition's priority might be to improve access to and parental education on immunizations for all preschool children in their community. However, no funding is available for their larger goal. Because the coalition has some resources, they decide to develop a pilot program that focuses on improving MMR (measles, mumps, and rubella) immunization rates in preschoolers. The coalition can begin their program immediately, which reinforces the success of the coalition's common goals and actions. The coalition will also gain a lot of information, as well as organizing and technical skills through implementing the pilot program. Additionally, information on cost savings and health benefit should be obtained to further justify continuing and/or expanding the program. In some cases, coalitions can work with insurance providers to fund programs such as these to prevent or reduce costs incurred with emergency and hospital admissions for preventable diseases. This skill acquisition, as well as the pilot program experiences and outcomes, will provide a strong foundation and justification when applying to fund a broader program to improve childhood immunizations rates.

Priority-Setting Approaches

The process of setting priorities is best conducted through a combination of qualitative and quantitative methods. Statistics about the frequency, duration, severity, disability, and mortality of certain health problems tell one story. Social understandings of health concerns and qualitative estimations of these health problems tell a different story. By making the community aware of the current state of health in their community, discussions can commence and goals for the community can be set. Priority setting allows for open discussion about perceptions, judgments, and understandings that can be the most valuable part of conducting a priority-setting session. When the coalition discusses the community and its priorities, this furthers the coalition's work.

Criteria that are used to rate priorities can vary. A coalition's discussion is best served if it first decides which criteria are important to the group, and, second, applies these criteria to rank the community's issues and concerns. Coalition members will learn much about each other's preferences from both the first and second parts of the discussion, and subsequent decision making will be enhanced. Community members' viewpoints should also be incorporated; community forums or focus groups can be an effective means for involving community members. Those unable to attend a forum because of family obligations, work-shift timing, or disability can be contacted directly and their perspectives and opinions can still be included as input. For example, Dallas County, Texas, initiatives directed by Parkland Hospital's Community-Oriented Primary Care program employed a community prioritization approach that focused on "(1) leadership forums and (2) community advisory boards associated with each health center" (Pickens, Boumbulian, Anderson, Ross, & Phillips, 2002, p. 1729).

Priority Chart

As mentioned earlier, several priority-setting approaches use a combination of quantitative and qualitative methods to provide comparative rankings that can highlight community concerns and issues that should receive attention. Tarimo (1991) includes a priority chart that incorporates several variables in a brief format suitable for discussion by nonprofessionals. Small groups are formed to evaluate the health problems (preferably no more than seven) or risk factors of concern in a population. The problems or factors are then listed and should relate to a single target population. Ranking is simplified when the list includes either health problems (heart disease, asthma, arthritis, adolescent pregnancy, etc.) or risk factors (tobacco use, high-fat diets, sedentary lifestyles, poor access to birth control methods, etc.). Small-group members discuss and rank each health problem or risk factor using the following variables: frequency in the population, mortality in years of potential life lost, morbidity in years of reduced health, costs of solutions, and effectiveness of solutions (Tarimo, 1991, pp. 20–21). The priorities selected by the small groups are reported back to the larger group, tallied, and discussed. This approach can be powerful and instructive in the priority-setting process.

Problem Priority Criteria

Shuster and Goeppinger (2004) propose a more complex, mathematical system that shares some of Tarimo's Priority Chart assumptions. Their *Problem Priority Criteria* include the following: "(1) community awareness of the problem, (2) community motivation to resolve or better manage the problem, (3) nurse's ability to influence problem solution, (4) availability of expertise to solve the problem, (5) severity of the outcomes if the problems are unresolved, and (6) speed with which the problem can be solved" (p. 362). Each criterion is independently rated on a 1 (low) to 10 (high) scale based on two questions: (a) How important is the criterion to problem solution? (b) Does the partnership have the ability to resolve the problem? In addition, a rationale for rating each parameter is documented. The two resulting numeric ratings (for problem importance and for ability to resolve) are multiplied to yield a problem-ranking number (variable from 0 to 600). These steps are repeated for each separate problem that the group seeks to address (Shuster & Goeppinger, 2004). The community problems are then ranked from highest to lowest score. As this system requires detailed knowledge about each separate problem, it works best if those involved are very familiar with the issues or concerns being prioritized, such as coalition leaders.

A "Skilled Planner" Approach

For setting priorities, Green and Kreuter (2004) recommend a series of key questions for use by "skilled planners" in "a process that balances the perceptions of stakeholder [sic] with objectively constructed descriptions of prevailing health problems and how these are distributed in the target population" (p. 99). Green and Kreuter's key questions reflect many of the themes of the two previous priority approaches, including comparison of relative mortality, morbidity, costs, and ease of solution. For example, one key question asks: "Which problems are most amendable to intervention?" (p. 99). Added themes include a concern for higher risk subpopulations (such as children, mothers, or ethnic minorities), and the disproportionate burden of the problem on the focus community compared to other communities. For example, a key question here is: "Which problem is not being addressed by other organizations in the community?" (Green & Kreuter, 2004, p. 99). This approach works well when professionals (the "skilled planners") conduct prioritization comparisons. Although this approach is less helpful in the APRN's work with community coalitions, the "key questions" have the potential to add to or help guide discussions or reflections by coalition members or community residents.

The Hanlon Method and PEARL

The *Hanlon Method*, also referred to as the *Basic Priority Rating System* (Pickett & Hanlon, 1990, pp. 226–228; School of Public Health, University of Illinois at Chicago, 2004), is structured "to allow decision makers to identify explicit factors to be considered in setting priorities, to organize the factors into groups that are weighted relative to each other, and to allow the factors to be modified as needed and scored individually" (School of Public Health, University of Illinois at Chicago, 2004, p. 1). Three main components are independently rated on a scale for each candidate priority: (a) size of the problem, (b) seriousness of the problem, and (c) estimated effectiveness of the solution. The numeric results for each of the three variables are placed into an equation, and the results multiplied by the *PEARL factor* score to obtain the comparative rating (School of Public Health, University of Illinois at Chicago, 2004).

The PEARL factors are interpreted as strongly influencing whether or not a particular goal can be addressed in a specific community, even though the factors are not directly related to the health problem. The PEARL factors are broken down as follows: *Propriety* (P) asks whether a proposed problem or program is consistent with the overall mission of the sponsoring organization. *Economic feasibility* (E) balances the costs of intervening or not intervening, including the economic outcomes of not intervening. *Acceptability* (A) addresses whether the community or program recipients will accept any intervention to address the goal. *Resources* (R) are assessed to determine whether sufficient resources are available to address this goal. And last, *Legality* (L) poses the question of whether current laws will permit addressing this goal (School of Public Health, University of Illinois at Chicago, 2004).

The PEARL factors are scored individually as "possible" or "not possible" (e.g., each is rated as "one" or "zero" respectively); given the mathematical formula, if even one of these qualifying factors is rated as "not possible" (e.g., as zero), then the Basic Priority Rating is zero, which indicates that the particular candidate priority should not be considered. When this occurs, a planning coalition may decide that their first step is to modify the PEARL factor that is rated as "not possible." For example, if an intervention is currently not *acceptable* to the population, steps might be taken to educate the population on the potential benefits of the intervention. If population opinion shifts and becomes more accepting of the intervention, it could be reconsidered and implemented (School of Public Health, University of Illinois at Chicago, 2004). Incorporating the PEARL factors into priority setting provides a stronger and more comprehensive perspective, as part of the process is deciding which goal or program to select. The PEARL factors may also lead to additional analyses in combination with any priority-setting approach, especially as it addresses each individual component (e.g., PEARL) of a proposed need or program.

Selecting Goals to Address Prioritized Issues and Concerns

As a result of the priority-setting process, the community coalition identifies a ranked group of issues and concerns. The next question is: Should the coalition focus on a single goal or on multiple goals? Single goals do have an appeal of simplicity and require fewer resources. When a coalition focuses on multiple linked goals, it has more of an impact on the underlying causes of the problem and more opportunity to draw community members into understanding these linkages. In the earlier example of creating walking trails, the combination of increasing physical activity and improving healthy food choices both address achieving an appropriate weight to prevent chronic disease. By linking two disease prevention behaviors through the walking trails intervention, the need for community members to combine several related actions to reduce the risk of poor health outcomes is underscored.

In fact, most community health issues and concerns are complex, multifaceted, and challenging to address. Based on the multicausation model (see Chapters 3 and 4), multilevel planning models underscore the numerous sources of health problems. The *Multilevel Approach to Community Health* (MATCH) suggests that health problems will be resolved only when they are addressed simultaneously at the individual/family, organization, community, and government levels. This allows for a more effective modification of policy, practice, and behavior. Although this approach requires a potentially vast skill set, it can offer more efficient use of resources at a faster speed (Simons-Morton, Greene, & Gottlieb, 1995; Simons-Morton, Simons-Morton, Parcel, & Bunker, 1988). For example, it is not sufficient for the APRN to convince a patient and his family that his sodium intake should be reduced. A broader approach should be taken to address the barriers in the community that make it difficult for an individual to make long-term changes. As in this case, the best patient teaching cannot easily overcome the barriers if local food stores carry only high-sodium food choices. The APRN could participate in a community coalition to advocate local food stores to stock healthier, low-sodium foods. County or state policy changes could persuade food stores that stocking low-sodium foods is to their advantage if, for example, they received a tax credit for the amount of healthier foods they carried and sold. Multilevel approaches provide more effective and sustainable changes, as these modify the underlying causes of current health problems and address the issues at a community and policy level.

The *Transtheoretical Model of Change* suggests that in any given population, individuals are at different points or stages in considering or implementing personal change. Ten stages are included in this model. The first five are experimental stages and begin with consciousness raising (increasing awareness), and the last five are behavioral, ending with self-liberation (committing Prochaska, Redding, & Evers, 2008). This model suggests that patients prescribed a lower sodium diet will undergo a personal change process in deciding and acting on reducing dietary sodium. When a community coalition plans to modify personal health choices among community members, it should consider designing interventions that simultaneously target residents at each of the stages of change. The intervention design will also support individuals and families in moving stepwise through the stages of change and in assisting backsliders to recommit to engaging in change.

In the Diffusion of Innovations model, the members of a population adopt new behaviors, new technologies, and so on, at predictable but very different rates and for very different reasons (Oldenburg & Glanz, 2008). In this case, to reach all members of the community, the coalition should target strategies at early, middle, and late points in the campaign to reduce dietary sodium. Those who are early adopters of the innovation respond to different approaches than those who are late adopters, and specific targeted approaches are employed based on their ability to change and the stage of change.

Both *Lewin's 3-Stage Model of Change* and the Diffusion of Innovations models underscore the importance of using multiple methods in modifying health-promoting behaviors among diverse community members. As with many learning theories, APRNs must recognize that individuals learn differently and change their behaviors at different rates. By recognizing this early on in the change process, more success is likely to occur and sustainable success is also more likely as approaches are adaptable and targeted. As a means to understand these complex relationships and to identify possible interventions, *The Community Guide* provides intensive, highly developed recommendations for community-targeted health promotion and disease prevention programs (Community Preventive Services Task Force, 2014). Given the complex nature of contemporary health promotion and disease prevention, theoretical and evidence-based approaches are critical in properly addressing individual and community issues and concerns. For example, if an APRN is planning a program to reduce dietary fat, the *Nutrition Guidelines for Americans, 2010* (U.S. Department of Agriculture & U.S. Department of Health and Human Services, 2010) is a useful and evidence-based resource to assist in guiding this process.

Sustaining New Programs: Identifying Barriers in the Program-Planning and Implementation Process

One challenge to sustaining new programs is not addressing existing or potential problems at the time the goal or program was selected as a focus by the coalition. Thorough, objective assessment of proposed community goals/

programs will often yield doubts about implementation of a program or whether the implementation effort risks serious obstacles. The APRN and the coalition's intervention team must be both carefully analytic and thoroughly honest. When potential problems are revealed, they must be acknowledged and addressed because a "wait-and-see" approach is not effective. Barriers to program success can also emerge during implementation. Symptoms of potential problems include the following: delays in the implementation timeline, waning resources, disaffected partnerships, or recurring communication difficulties during coalition meetings. These challenges can be detected early by conducting an ongoing program review or formative evaluation. Both symptoms of problems and problems detected during program evaluation require the community intervention team to be honest about the presence of and need to address the barriers, and the importance of taking prompt action to address threats to the coalition's work. The APRN brings problem-solving experience to these situations and should remind the coalition of the normative nature of the challenges to implementing a health-promotion/disease prevention program.

Regardless of when in the process a barrier is identified, the characteristics of barriers can be grouped as follows: (a) characteristics of the goal/program; (b) characteristics of needed resources; (c) characteristics of community members, coalition members, and coalition leadership; (d) characteristics of the APRN; or (e) a mismatch between community or coalition partners and the APRN.

Barriers Caused by Program Characteristics

Certain types of programs or goals may not be feasible to study in certain communities. Some goals may receive community support and have the weight of evidence behind their use, but are a violation of law (or illegal). For example, needle-exchange programs are effective in preventing the spread of blood-borne pathogens, but are illegal in some areas (Benjamin, O'Brien, & Trotter, 2002). In another case, the timeline necessary to achieve the stated program or goal may not match community expectations. For example, would the community's support wane before program goals are achieved? Will the community demand program outcomes immediately, but lack the means or resources to quickly achieve the goals? Air quality is an important quality-of-life issue, and poor air quality is a short- and long-term health problem; however, modifying the sources of air pollution is time-consuming and challenging (Yip, Pearcy, Garbe, & Truman, 2011). The community might not have patience to wait for change during successive law suits and environmental policy interventions over a prolonged period of time.

Barriers Due to Unavailable Resources

Another barrier that is commonly encountered occurs when goals/programs lack sufficient resources to succeed, perhaps because of inadequate financing or because of insufficient, inadequate, or poorly trained leadership. Some groups may proceed to develop programs or goals even after the lack of resources has been recognized in the hope that sufficient personnel or financial resources will be secured. Not only are such programs initiated on unstable foundations, but existing resources that could be dedicated to program development are instead lost to failed attempts to explore and acquire needed resources.

Barriers Due to Human Factors

The leadership involved in the coalition can often be a barrier to its success. Community or coalition partners, who participate in the development of community goals, may be unenthusiastic or disaffected in relation to the focus that was actually selected for implementation. Community partners may simply lack interest in the current priority and may wish to terminate their involvement in the coalition. Partners can also become disengaged or separated from coalition communications; they may disengage in working meetings or miss meetings altogether. Given the contrasting possibilities, the APRN and other coalition members need to assess the reasons these coalition members appear to be disaffected.

Partners can also become distracted by what is to them a more salient goal or concern, leaving little time and attention for coalition priorities. Reassessment of the goal or program should be carried out if it is deemed unlikely that these partners will change their minds. If they do change their minds, then one of the coalition's interventions should address recruitment and community awareness about program/goal benefits.

Apparent disinterest in coalition activities may also quietly signal that two or more subgroups in the coalition are unable to collaborate, even though both are necessary to the project's success. The APRN and other coalition leadership should reach out to these subgroups to have a more complete picture of the difficulties and to support and counsel reinclusion of the subgroups. In this serious situation, negotiation among the conflicted subgroups may be possible, but the APRN must be extremely diplomatic to avoid the appearance of siding with one group and further damaging the potential for collaboration.

The APRN may also experience a lack of sustained interest in the program focus, perhaps because the selected program is only indirectly related to health concerns. Similar to community members or other coalition partners, the APRN may find another goal more salient. It is difficult to consider, but important to acknowledge, if the nurse has become disengaged from the community and the coalition, whether because of circumstances in the nurse's personal life or because working with the community and/or the coalition has become difficult, that the APRN may find herself/himself overwhelmed with responsibilities that compete with other obligations. It may be difficult for the nurse to agree to a realistic timeline for goal or program implementation if it appears that there may be a prolonged timeline or the potential for a significant time commitment. The APRN should acknowledge these personal challenges and seek support from within the coalition, or from elsewhere, to identify the barriers to participation and make a plan to reconstruct linkages with the coalition, or to make a decision to acknowledge the barriers and formally withdraw.

Barriers Due to the Nurse–Coalition Interface

Last, it may emerge that the community/coalition lacks the skills to partner with the APRN. One appropriate step is to delay immediate programmatic work and focus efforts on skill building. This challenge is more likely to be revealed and addressed early if program implementation begins in an incremental way that permits skill and confidence building. In fact, incorporating these necessary elements as a first, planned stage of a larger program implementation is advantageous.

Preventing Problems in Collaborative Efforts

In the midst of hard work and complex organizing, some would suggest that some of these barriers could *not* have been anticipated or prevented. But on the whole, these problems should be foreseen by the coalition leadership and actions taken to prevent a negative impact on developing collaborative efforts. Three steps must be included in any initiative: First, during the planning stage, a coalition should dedicate time to honest refection, anticipation, and identification of potential problems and barriers to any identified goals. Are coalition members genuinely "buying into" group plans? Is the coalition's road map realistic in its timeline and requirements for community participation? Second, every coalition should periodically reassess its goals and plans. Depending on the nature and composition of the coalition, this reassessment can be conducted by the leadership (in its broadest, most representative, and diverse sense). In addition, a community meeting will generate an even better understanding of the current status of the coalition's efforts. The community meeting provides a forum for recognizing and acknowledging successes and failures to date, celebrating the successes and focusing/refocusing on next steps. Honest reflection on symptoms and suggestions of problems should lead to specific strategies to further understand and address the issues and concerns to minimize negative consequences on the larger coalition and the initiative itself. Third, if issues and concerns are revealed, the coalition leadership should make a judgment about the nature and process of the initiative. Should the initiative continue as currently planned, or should changes be made? Would it be better to modify or eliminate a goal, or would this lead to a coalition member dropping out? Coalition leaders might decide to face a conflict and openly discuss the challenge and its many facets, and by identifying a solution, strengthen the overall initiative and the coalition itself.

In sum, "side-stepping" the problems means that the APRN and the coalition can and should be alert to potential challenges. Regular reassessment of the program and early awareness of potential problems are essential for success, as is finding a prompt solution. Early success in any effort builds the collaborative and spurs efforts forward. Conflicts and confusion that drain energy from the coalition partners should be prevented if possible or at least minimized. Facing confusion and/or conflicts can strengthen collaborative work and model problem-solving strategies that can result in increasing community capacity to address future challenges.

Developing Outcomes for Coalition Work

The priority-setting discussions should identify at least one issue or concern, but likely several, for the APRN and the coalition's project. The next step is to develop outcomes and related means to achieve these outcomes, based on the selected priorities. Identifying outcomes is essential to later work, including program evaluation. The process of defining outcomes or even revising outcomes can be daunting (see Chapter 2). This process can be a critical step in program development and can lay the groundwork for successful and sustainable programs. Even when all of the constituencies in the coalition have previously agreed on the priorities for the community's health, establishing outcomes for these priorities can lead to unforeseen barriers. First, traditional academic/professional configuration of outcomes may be unfamiliar to community members within the partnership; consideration of alternative means to present these ideas, steps to achievement, and a related timeline can facilitate the process. Outcomes should remain in a contextual format that is appropriate for the target community for the duration of the project. Second, well-defined outcomes that are clearly stated may be the first indication to coalition partners of the extensive work ahead. Presenting the outcomes with a clear timeline and delineation of the steps needed to achieve these goals are a way to demonstrate a well-thought-out plan that addresses the process that is necessary to achieve these outcomes. It can also facilitate a sense of community efficacy, as it sets up the framework to show that these goals are achievable. In addition, having well-defined outcomes can also demonstrate long-term feasibility and potential reduction in healthcare costs, which can assist in securing long-term funding.

When the APRN and coalition members have agreed on the stated outcomes, the next step is to commit to work toward improving these outcomes. As coalition members represent their constituencies, these members should take responsibility for communicating with their organizations or neighborhoods about the coalition's plans. The APRN can assist coalition members to design campaigns to involve their constituencies (see Chapter 7). These campaigns can assist coalition members to facilitate adoption of both the outcomes and the steps to achieve the outcomes among their constituents. Focused organizational or neighborhood meetings/gatherings are useful in accomplishing this. The overall goal is to achieve a "buy-in" and commitment to work on the goals among the constituents and the coalition partners.

To support the coalition members, the APRN and the coalition as a whole should set a "launch date" for the planned program and have a celebration to develop energy and reflect the commitment of the diversity of coalition partners. Coalition efforts to recruit and retain the dedication and interest of constituency members will also validate the leadership role of each constituency's representative within the coalition. This results in strengthening the leader roles of coalition representatives in their community. APRN activities in coalitions can often include leadership development of the coalition members.

Continued work toward achieving the planned outcomes will likely have both periods of accomplishment and periods of minimal progress. The APRN can remind the coalition of the previously identified interim markers of progress toward the selected coalition outcomes. Achievement of each significant step should be recognized and celebrated. Pictures that are posted in fund-raising campaigns that show increases in donations using an oversized thermometer posted in a visible location are a good example of a way to mark progress. Visible indicators or a giant "checklist" can convey to community members the status and growing impact of the coalition's efforts. Small rewards or giveaways, such as a celebratory balloon or a coalition-emblazoned key chain, can also be used to signal progress toward outcomes.

The APRN and the coalition members should plan periodic formative evaluations of the progress in attaining outcomes, as well as summative evaluations of those elements of the overall plan that have been completed. Marking success and progress is important for the coalition efforts as well, and offers possibilities for events that build the coalition team and the interpersonal relationships among coalition representatives. When the APRN breaks down the program into doable steps, the efficacy of community members and retention of coalition partners is enhanced.

Sustaining Programs and Initiatives

As programs and initiatives gain strength and the coalition members see their planning lead to better health outcomes in the community, the APRN should consider ways to keep the work going and to establish it as a permanent element of that community. To do this, the APRN and the coalition must take steps to institutionalize the initiative. These plans will ensure the continuity of the work and, with increased duration of the program, will increase the potential for achieving the identified outcomes. The APRN should introduce and guide the coalition first through a careful strategic plan for institutionalization. This will focus the coalition on what is needed. In fact, consideration of sustaining or institutionalizing an initiative should begin when it is first conceptualized, or at least when clear outcomes have been identified and are beginning to be implemented (Community Toolbox, 2011a). The importance of the institutionalization plan underscores the APRN's key role in guiding program development and in guiding the team to an understanding about what steps are necessary at which phase in the program planning and implementation.

Planning for Institutionalization

How should the APRN guide the coalition in planning for institutionalization? A first step is to acknowledge that what it does is important and that the coalition's program is worth continuing. In that light, it will make sense to ensure that the program's mission, staffing, and resources are adequate. Given continued confidence in its planned outcomes, noting program accomplishments will provide the coalition with motivation to continue to build. Publicizing the coalition's successes will solidify both the coalition and its constituencies and, more important, can draw the public into the coalition's mission and work. Community members are key players in long-term sustainability and can assist in the institutionalization process. When programs involve more people, their staying power increases (Community Toolbox, 2011b). Perhaps a nearby community would like to develop a similar program? Perhaps outsiders would like to learn about how the program operates and how it achieves its goals? Enhancing the connections and respect for the program and spreading the coalition's programs to new neighborhoods improve how others see the program, and this translates into more support for the program.

Funding: A Major Barrier to Sustainability

The major barrier to sustainability and to institutionalization is adequate financing. For many organizations, sustained financial support is an ongoing challenge to accomplishing the planned outcomes. As with other factors that support sustainability, planning for future financial security is best addressed from the start of program inception. A place to begin is to market the organization by letting others know what the coalition's program has accomplished. It can also be helpful to show financers what other similar programs have accomplished using similar models in different communities. Additionally, presenting the potential cost savings in the long term can also secure financial support, as funders can see the long-term benefits of financial investment in such programs. The APRN and coalition members can build their image and community relations, develop members and friends, and actively deliver the coalition's message for health and personal/community change.

Existing financial resources may go further if staff positions are shared with another compatible organization. Or the coalition's program may become so successful that a larger organization would like to support it, or perhaps even assume responsibility for the coalition, its identified outcomes, and its programs in operation. Grants, fund-raising functions, third-party funding, public funding, a fee schedule, and in-kind support may also assist with financing (Community Toolbox, 2011c). Community health programs can be particularly attractive to academic partners, such as nursing, public health, medical schools, and universities, which the APRN can assist in recruiting or in facilitating relationship building. Personnel resources may be available in the form of educational or training programs in nursing, medicine, social work, public health, and other professions.

Stabilization and Reassessment

The role of the APRN with the coalition and the change process is very active, but this role draws to an end during the step in Lewin's 3-Stage Model of Change known as *refreezing*. During this step, reassessment and stabilization are typical and expected, and this focuses "the change agent's and actor's attention and energy on progress and continuity for the change" (Kettner, Daley, & Nichols, 1985, p. 288). The APRN may or may not continue with the community coalition. But even when the APRN continues, the role of change agent is less necessary and begins to fade as the change is institutionalized or stabilized. But rather than immediately separating from a successful coalition program, the APRN should emphasize the autonomous functioning and continued survival of the program (Kettner et al., 1985).

The APRN should initiate a reassessment of the change process and the coalition's work. Input is sought from all participants about whether the impact of the coalition's changes is meeting their needs. Members of the community coalition itself give feedback, as do a sample of their constituents who are recruited to reflect on the practical consequences and the meaning of the change effort. To what extent has the change been accepted, approved, and adopted among coalition members, their constituents, stakeholders, and other community members? A careful review of whether the community coalition's goals were met should be included. Although perhaps challenging to anticipate, this step will be easier if early in the project the APRN guides the community coalition to accompany specification of goal outcomes with clear descriptors for outcome achievement.

The APRN will also assist and explore with the community coalition appropriate ways to share their experiences with a wider audience through oral presentations; visual and audio media publicity; and articles for publication in magazines, journals, community newspapers, and online postings. The APRN and coalition members may offer assistance to other community groups that are in the early stages of planning similar efforts. Coalition members may take the strengths of this coalition experience, with their new skills and abilities, and apply what they have gained to other issues in support of their own communities.

SUMMARY

The APRN's ability to employ the change process is an essential component of reaching beyond the clinical encounter to address the community context and conditions that lead to poor health in individuals and families. The community encounter engages the APRN and community partners in an ongoing process of increased understanding and skill/ability development.

The APRN who sets out to engage communities in change requires many skills. Foremost is the ability to strategically and successfully introduce the need for change to improve population health. At any time, the APRN may be called on to moderate a focus group, diplomatically defuse a situation, collect data in order to identify targets for intervention and to measure change, and help in the identification and construction of achievable outcomes. Although the initial role of the APRN is leader, he or she must also be prepared to step aside and allow members of the community to identify priorities for change. It is paramount that the APRN understands that it is community members who make final decisions about health priorities. An important role of the APRN is helping community members to acquire the necessary skills to make changes and to create a sustainable environment. It requires a true partnership between the APRN and the community to create meaningful changes, and by helping communities to sustain those changes and by becoming leaders themselves that those changes will become embedded in the community.

Extending APRN practice into the community improves clinical outcomes directly because, as community problems are identified and managed, this complements the APRN's efforts to reduce individual and family health problems. Sustaining the coalitions and programs that develop as a result of the APRN's partnership with community members has the potential to achieve far-reaching improvements in population health.

EXERCISES AND DISCUSSION QUESTIONS

Exercise 10.1 What ethical principles apply when working with communities? Conduct a personal skills inventory. Of the ethical principles that you have identified, which ones do you have sufficient skills in to be able to work effectively with a community coalition? Are there areas in which you would like to develop stronger abilities? How would you go about developing the skills and knowledge to do so?

Exercise 10.2 Consider a community known to you. If you were working with a partnership group to set priorities for community collaboration, which priority-setting criteria would you recommend for use by your group?

Exercise 10.3 What factors would you consider before you made an implicit/explicit commitment to engage with a community or neighborhood to improve residents' health status? How would you specifically engage with the community to negotiate your role?

Exercise 10.4 Consider a community known to you. You wish to take initial steps to build a partnership with the community. What data and information should you analyze and consider before you contact community leaders/members/organizations? Which area leaders/members/organizations would you contact initially, to introduce the idea of a partnership?

Exercise 10.5 Obtain a copy of the Tarimo (1991) Priority Chart (see the reference list). Break into groups and select six or seven community issues or concerns and rank these using the tool. What did your group agree about? Disagree about? In what ways would your group consider modifying the tool?

REFERENCES

Allender, J. A., Rector, C., & Warner, K. (2013). *Community health nursing: Promoting and protecting the public's health* (8th ed.). Philadelphia, PA: Wolters Kluwer/Lippincott Williams & Wilkins.

Benjamin, G., O'Brien, D. J., & Trotter, D. (2002). Do we need a new law or regulation? The public health decision process. *Journal of Law, Medicine & Ethics, 30*(3), 45–47.

Blum, H. L. (1981). *Planning for health: Genetics for the eighties* (2nd ed.). New York, NY: Human Sciences Press.

Centers for Disease Control and Prevention/Agency for Toxic Substances and Diseases Registry Committee on Community Engagement, National Institutes of Health. (2011). *Principles of community engagement: Applying principles to the community engagement process.* Retrieved from www.cdc.gov/phppo/pce/part3.htm

Cherry, D. J., & Shefner, J. (2004). Addressing barriers to university-community collaboration: Organizing by experts or organizing the experts? *Journal of Community Practice, 12*(3), 219–233. doi:10.1300/J125v12n03_13

Community Preventative Services Task Force. (2014). *The community guide.* Retrieved from Community Guide website: http://www.thecommunityguide.org/

Community Toolbox. (2011a). *Our model of practice: Building capacity for community and system change.* Retrieved from Kansas University website: http://ctb.ku.edu/en/

table-of-contents/overview/model-for-community-change-and-improvement/building-capacity/main

Community Toolbox. (2011b). *Strategies for the long-term institutionalization of an initiative: An overview.* Retrieved from Kansas University website: http://ctb.ku.edu/en/table-of-contents/sustain/long-term-institutionalization/overview/main

Community Toolbox. (2011c). *Strategies for sustaining the initiative.* Retrieved from Kansas University website: http://ctb.ku.edu/en/table-of-contents/sustain/long-term-institutionalization/sustainability-strategies/main

Connelly, M. (2014). *The Kurt Lewin change management model.* Retrieved from http://www.change-management-coach.com/kurt_lewin.html

Courtney, R., Ballard, E., Fauver, S., Gariota, M., & Holland, L. (1996). The partnership model: Working with individuals, families, and communities toward a new vision of health. *Public Health Nursing, 13,* 177–186.

Farnham, E. (1964). *Pioneering in public health nursing education: The history of the University Public Health Nursing District, 1917–1962.* Cleveland, OH: Press of Western Reserve University.

Gallant, M. H., Beaulieu, M. C., & Carnevale, F. A. (2002). Partnership: An analysis of the concept within the nurse-client relationship. *Journal of Advanced Nursing, 40,* 149–157.

Green, L. W., & Kreuter, M. W. (2004). *Health program planning: An educational and ecological approach* (4th ed.). Boston, MA: McGraw-Hill.

International Association for Public Participation. (2014). *IAP2 core values for the practice of public participation.* Retrieved from http://www.iap2.org/?page=A4

Issel, L. M. (2013). *Health program planning and evaluation: A practical, systematic approach for community health* (3rd ed.). Burlington, MA: Jones & Bartlett Learning.

Keller, L. O., Strohschein, S., & Briske, L. (2008). Population-based public health nursing practice: The intervention wheel. In M. Stanhope & J. Lancaster (Eds.), *Public health nursing: Population-centered health care in the community* (7th ed., pp. 187–214). St. Louis, MO: Mosby Elsevier.

Kettner, P. M., Daley, J. M., & Nichols, A. W. (1985). *Initiating change in organizations and communities: A macro practice model.* Monterey, CA: Brooks/Cole.

Labonte, R. (2012). Community, community development, and the forming of authentic partnerships: Some critical reflections. In M. Minkler (Ed.), *Community organizing and community building for health* (3rd ed., pp. 95–109). New Brunswick, NJ: Rutgers University Press.

Logan, B. N., Davis, L., & Parker, V. G. (2010). An interinstitutional academic collaborative partnership to end health disparities. *Health Education and Behavior, 37,* 580–592. doi:10.1177/1090198110363378

Lynn-McHale, D. J., & Deatrick, J. A. (2000). Trust between family and health care provider. *Journal of Family Nursing, 6,* 210–230.

Macali, M., Galanowsky, K., Wagner, M., & Truglio-Londrigan. (2011). Hitting the pavement: Intervention of case finding. In M. Truglio-Londrigan & S. B. Lewenson (Eds.), *Public health nursing: Practicing population-based care* (pp. 185–219). Sudbury, MA: Jones & Bartlett.

McCann, E. (2010). Building a community-academic partnership to improve health outcomes in an underserved community. *Public Health Nursing, 27*(1), 32–40. doi:10.1111/j.1525-1446.2009.00824.x

McCloskey, D. J., McDonald, M. A., Cook, J., Heurtin-Roberts, S., Updegrove, S., Sampson, D., Gutter, S., & Eder, M. (2011). Community engagement: Definitions and organizing concepts from the literature. In *National Institutes of Health* (NIH Publication No. 11-7782). Retrieved from http://www.atsdr.cdc.gov/communityengagement/pdf/PCE_Report_Chapter_1_SHEF.pdf

Oldenburg, B., & Glanz, K. (2008). Diffusion of innovations. In K. Glanz, B. K. Rimer, & K. Viswanath (Eds.), *Health behavior and health education: Theory, research, and practice* (4th ed., pp. 313–333). San Francisco, CA: Jossey-Bass.

Parker, E. A., Eng, E., Laraia, B., Ammerman, A., Dodds, J., Margolis, L., & Cross, A. (1999). Coalition building for prevention. In R. C. Brownson, E. A. Baker, & L. F. Novick (Eds.), *Community-based prevention: Programs that work* (pp. 182–198). Gaithersburg, MD: Aspen.

Pickens, S., Boumbulian, P., Anderson, R. J., Ross, S., & Phillips, S. (2002). Community-oriented primary care in action: A Dallas story. *American Journal of Public Health, 92,* 1728–1732.

Pickett, G., & Hanlon, J. J. (1990). *Public health: Administration and practice* (9th ed.). St. Louis, MO: Times Mirror/Mosby College Publishing.

Prochaska, J. O., Redding, C. A., & Evers, K. E. (2008). The transtheoretical model and stages of change. In K. Glanz, B. K. Rimer, & K. Viswanath (Eds.), *Health behavior and health education: Theory, research, and practice* (4th ed., pp. 97–121). San Francisco, CA: Jossey-Bass.

Rippke, M., Briske, L., Keller, L. O., & Strohschein, S. (2001). *Public health interventions: Applications for public health nursing practice.* St. Paul, MN: Minnesota Department of Health.

Roberts, S. J., & Krouse, H. J. (1990). Negotiation as a strategy to empower self-care. *Holistic Nursing Practice, 4*(2), 30–36.

School of Public Health, University of Illinois at Chicago. (2004). *Guide for establishing public health priorities* (Rev. ed.). Retrieved from http://www.uic.edu/sph/prepare/courses/ph440/mods/bpr.htm

Shuster, G. F., & Goeppinger, J. (2004). Community as client: Assessment and analysis. In M. Stanhope & J. Lancaster (Eds.), *Community and public health nursing* (6th ed., pp. 342–373). St. Louis, MO: Mosby.

Simons-Morton, B. G., Greene, W. H., & Gottlieb, N. H. (1995). *An introduction to health education and health promotion* (2nd ed.). Prospect Heights, IL: Waveland Press.

Simons-Morton, D. G., Simons-Morton, B. G., Parcel, G. S., & Bunker, J. F. (1988). Influencing personal and environmental conditions for community health: A multilevel intervention model. *Family and Community Health, 11*(2), 25–35.

Tarimo, E. (1991). *Towards a healthy district.* Geneva, Switzerland: World Health Organization. Retrieved (in pdf) from http://apps.who.int/iris/bitstream/10665/40785/1/9241544120.pdf?ua=1

U.S. Department of Agriculture & U.S. Department of Health and Human Services (HHS). (2010). *Dietary guidelines for Americans 2010* (7th ed.). Washington, DC: United States Government Printing Office. Retrieved from http://health.gov/dietaryguidelines/dga2010/dietaryguidelines2010.pdf

Wald, A. (2011). Working together: Collaboration, coalition building, and community organizing. In M. Truglio-Londrigan & S. B. Lewenson (Eds.), *Public health nursing: Practicing population-based care* (pp. 267–283). Sudbury, MA: Jones & Bartlett.

Walker, S. S. (2011). Ethical quandaries in community health nursing. In E. T. Anderson & J. McFarlane (Eds.), *Community as partner: Theory and practice in nursing* (6th ed., pp. 73–85). Philadelphia, PA: Wolters Kluwer/Lippincott Williams & Wilkins.

Yip, F. Y., Pearcy, J. N., Garbe, P. L., & Truman, B. I. (2011). Unhealthy air quality—United States, 2006–2009. *Morbidity and Mortality Weekly Report (MMWR), 60*(1). Retrieved from http://www.cdc.gov/mmwr/preview/mmwrhtml/su6001a5.htm?s_cid=su6001a5_w

Zerwekh, J. V. (1993). Commentary: Going to the people—Public health nursing today and tomorrow. *American Journal of Public Health, 83,* 1676–1678.

Implications of Global Health in Population-Based Nursing

Irina McKeehan Campbell and Gloria J. McNeal

CORE COMPETENCIES IN GLOBAL HEALTH

The American Association of Colleges of Nursing (AACN) 2005 Task Force on the Essentials of Nursing Education for the doctorate of nursing practice (DNP) has outlined the requirements of DNP practice. Throughout this book, these essentials and core competencies are addressed for multiple advance practice registered nurse (APRN) roles. Particularly relevant to global health issues are Essential V (healthcare policy for advocacy in healthcare), Essential VI (interprofessional collaboration for improving patient and population health outcomes), and Essential VII (clinical prevention and population health for improving the nation's health). The AACN has formed an interdisciplinary collaboration with the Association of Schools of Public Health (ASPH) to develop global health competencies. There are seven core domains in the public health Global Health Model with concomitant competencies within each skill domain. Domains 1 and 2 concern community engagement, domains 3, 4, and 6 address ethical practice and social justice, and domains 5 and 7 are related to program operation (Association of Schools of Public Health [ASPH], 2011).

Exhibit 11.1 demonstrates how ASPH global health domains 1 to 4 and 6 complement AACN DNP Essentials V to VII. Healthcare delivery to individuals and populations often involves working with programs that cross political and national borders. Global health is an extension of population health. In terms of geographic scale, diseases can affect people across geographic boundaries and specific population aggregates, such as mothers and children or those who have hepatitis or are HIV positive. APRNs who implement the global health domains in practice can play a focal role in developing the models that

EXHIBIT 11.1 • ASPH Global Health Competency Model

DOMAIN 1: Capacity Strengthening

Capacity strengthening is the broad sharing of knowledge, skills, and resources for enhancement of global public health programs, infrastructure, and workforce to address current and future global public health needs.

1.1 Design sustainable workforce development strategies for resource-limited settings.

1.2 Identify methods for assuring health program sustainability.

1.3 Assist host entity in assessing existing capacity.

1.4 Develop strategies that strengthen community capabilities for overcoming barriers to health and well-being.

DOMAIN 2: Collaborating and Partnering

Collaborating and partnering is the ability to select, recruit, and work with a diverse range of global health stakeholders to advance research, policy, and practice goals, and to foster open dialogue and effective communication.

2.1 Develop procedures for managing health partnerships.

2.2 Promote inclusion of representatives of diverse constituencies in partnerships.

2.3 Value commitment to building trust in partnerships.

2.4 Use diplomacy and conflict-resolution strategies with partners.

2.5 Communicate lessons learned to community partners and global constituencies.

2.6 Exhibit interpersonal communication skills that demonstrate respect for other perspectives and cultures.

DOMAIN 3: Ethical Reasoning and Professional Practice

Ethical reasoning and professional practice is the ability to identify and respond with integrity to ethical issues in diverse economic, political, and cultural contexts, and promote accountability for the impact of policy decisions on public health practice at local, national, and international levels.

3.1 Apply the fundamental principles of international standards for the protection of human subjects in diverse cultural settings.

3.2 Analyze ethical and professional issues that arise in responding to public health emergencies.

3.3 Explain the mechanisms used to hold international organizations accountable for public health practice standards.

3.4 Promote integrity in professional practice.

DOMAIN 4: Health Equity and Social Justice

Health equity and social justice is the framework for the analysis of strategies to address health disparities across socially, demographically, or geographically defined populations.

4.1 Apply social justice and human rights principles in public health policies and programs.

4.2 Implement strategies to engage marginalized and vulnerable populations in making decisions that affect their health and well-being.

4.3 Critique policies with respect to impact on health equity and social justice.

4.4 Analyze distribution of resources to meet the health needs of marginalized and vulnerable groups.

(continued)

EXHIBIT 11.1 • ASPH Global Health Competency Model (*continued*)

DOMAIN 5: Program Management

Program management is the ability to design, implement, and evaluate global health programs to maximize contributions to effective policy, enhanced practice, and improved and sustainable health outcomes.

5.1 Conduct formative research.

5.2 Apply scientific evidence throughout program planning, implementation, and evaluation.

5.3 Design program work plans based on logic models.

5.4 Develop proposals to secure donor and stakeholder support.

5.5 Plan evidence-based interventions to meet internationally established health targets.

5.6 Develop monitoring and evaluation frameworks to assess programs.

5.7 Utilize project management techniques throughout program planning, implementation, and evaluation.

5.8 Develop context-specific implementation strategies for scaling up best-practice interventions.

DOMAIN 6: Sociocultural and Political Awareness

Sociocultural and political awareness is the conceptual basis with which to work effectively within diverse cultural settings and across local, regional, national, and international political landscapes.

6.1 Describe the roles and relationships of the entities influencing global health.

6.2 Analyze the impact of transnational movements on population health.

6.3 Analyze context-specific policy-making processes that impact health.

6.4 Design health advocacy strategies.

6.5 Describe multiagency policy making in response to complex health emergencies.

6.6 Describe the interrelationship of foreign policy and health diplomacy.

DOMAIN 7: Strategic Analysis

Strategic analysis is the ability to use systems thinking to analyze a diverse range of complex and interrelated factors shaping health trends to formulate programs at the local, national, and international levels.

7.1 Conduct a situation analysis across a range of cultural, economic, and health contexts.

7.2 Identify the relationships among patterns of morbidity, mortality, and disability with demographic and other factors in shaping the circumstances of the population of a specified community, country, or region.

7.3 Implement a community health needs assessment.

7.4 Conduct comparative analyses of health systems.

7.5 Explain economic analyses drawn from socioeconomic and health data.

7.6 Design context-specific health interventions based on situation analysis.

are proposed by the Global Health Initiative (GHI), Centers for Disease Control and Prevention (CDC), and the World Health Organization (WHO), as a means for linking population health with health policy, the containment of infectious diseases, and the elimination of health disparities. The core competencies in global health complement GHI projects in domestic and international programs by promoting the following strategies: capacity strengthening, collaborating and partnering, ethical reasoning and professional practice, health equity and social justice, program management, sociocultural and political awareness, and strategic analysis.

This chapter explores the implications, benefits, and barriers of practicing global health for the APRN. The following areas are discussed:

- How geography, climate, and demographic factors influence the causes, transmission, and outcomes of communicable and noncommunicable diseases
- Global health competencies developed by the ASPH and AACN
- Effects of multilevel contexts of global health, population, and individual health
- Relationships between global health competencies and interdisciplinary collaboration
- Health initiatives of pivotal international agencies, such as the United Nations (UN) and the WHO
- Global health educational opportunities that exist for APRNs and doctorally prepared practitioners.

Changing American Demographic Landscape

The demographic landscape of the American population has become more culturally diversified and mobile as immigrants, migrants, and refugees seeking a higher quality of life enter the United States. The number of corporate, business, student, and academic exchanges has also increased in recent decades. The APRN, working on the front lines of primary and preventive care, will increasingly encounter people from other countries. These new arrivals have an increased likelihood of having been exposed to infectious diseases, may lack vaccinations, and may be at high risk for chronic diseases. APRNs, guided by the core competencies, can work with existing stakeholders and international programs to provide optimal health services to both citizens and noncitizens in the United States.

The United States admitted over 600,000 refugees between 2000 and 2011. The United States Immigration and Nationality Act (INA), derived from the post-World War II UN 1951 Convention, defines a refugee as "someone who: is located outside of the United States; is of special humanitarian concern to the United States; demonstrates that they were persecuted or fear persecution due to race, religion, nationality, political opinion, or membership in a particular social group" (Immigration and Nationality Act, 1965). In 2009, there were more than 13 million refugees globally, these refugees live predominantly in the Middle East; Africa; Syria; South, East, and Central Asia; the Americas, and Europe (American Immigration Council, 2014). Many will seek entry into the United States.

The Immigration and Naturalization Act has regulated immigration into the United States with a systematization of various laws since 1921. The act was amended in 1965 as the Hart–Celler Act. This act made changes to the immigration quota system based on country and nationality. It was designed to maintain the same ethnic proportion in the United States as was reflected in the 1920 Census. Asians were excluded from immigration by amendments in the 1924 Act. The 1965 immigration criteria replaced nationality or country-of-origin quotas with requirements for employable skills and reuniting families with connections in the United States. Before 1965, immigrants accounted for 10% of the American population. This changed to 30% in 2000 and 37% in 2010. The distribution of the census-designated Hispanic White population increased from 25% in 1990 to 37% in 2011 (Immigration in America, n.d.).

The 2012 Census revealed that out of nearly 308 million Americans, 40 million were foreign born, including 22 million noncitizens. Of these, 1.4 million were unemployed and nearly 5.5 million lived below the federal poverty level (U.S. Census, 2012). The 2007 American Community Survey enumerates the non-English languages spoken in the United States and the level of proficiency in English. This survey identified that 55.4 million people, 5 years of age and older, spoke a language other than English at home, and 4.5 million did not speak English at all (Kominski, Shin, & US Census Bureau 2010). Such diversity in the population, with an increased rate of mobility across international borders, presents challenges for the APRN.

In 2009, U.S. immigration agents detained over 3,000 children at the Southwest border, and in 2011, 6,000 children crossed the southern U.S. border illegally. There were estimates that nearly 90,000 children would enter without permission in 2014 (Hirsen, 2014). Government services provided to undocumented immigrants include housing, public education, emergency and other healthcare. New York taxpayers paid over $147 million, Texas $78 million, and California $64 million for educational school programs for undocumented children (Federation for American Immigration Reform [FAIR], 2014). As of March 2012, nearly 12 million unauthorized immigrants were living in the United States, and state health programs have funded approximately $2 billion/year for emergency treatment of undocumented immigrants, although federal law prohibits undocumented immigrants from receiving Medicaid (Kaiser Health News, 2013; Pew Research Center's Hispanic Trends, n.d.).

APRNs need to be familiar with federal policies that bar hospitals from asking about citizenship before providing services. The 1986 Emergency Medical Treatment and Active Labor Act (EMTALA), which is part of the Consolidated Omnibus Budget Reconciliation Act (COBRA), stipulates that hospitals deliver emergency healthcare to everyone, regardless of national origin, legal status, or ability to pay (42 U.S.C., n.d.). Such care is uncompensated at the hospital and state level, unless Medicaid funds are appropriated for various population health programs to cover charity care.

Twenty-first-century advances in communication, trade, transportation technologies, and scientific exchanges bring health issues from other continents to the threshold of the American urban and community hospital. These advances are accompanied by national security concerns, as was acutely evident with the 2014 Ebola outbreak in West Africa. APRN population-based practice has daily relevance as people bring their national, environmental, socioeconomic, and cultural contexts with them whenever they visit their healthcare provider. APRNs, who encounter individuals from other countries, need to understand and become familiar with programs or policies addressing the complex global factors influencing the context of individual and population health.

Health as an International Phenomenon

Individual health is embedded in the larger socio-ecological context of the global community. Not only does each individual's health status affect others, but also the health of one group in a society can influence the welfare of other groups, as was evident in the 2014 Ebola outbreak. The importance of maintaining health in populations was also exemplified in the measles outbreak of 2014 to 2015. The spread of preventable disease again revealed the importance of vaccination not only nationwide but worldwide. This led to an increasing need for reinforced education regarding the evidence behind vaccination. The diffusion of medical technology and evidence-based practice can positively affect a nation's health, much as the spread of infectious diseases can affect it adversely. The reform of international health systems to better address these issues was facilitated by the recognition of healthcare as a universal human right after World War II.

Article 25 of the Universal Declaration of Human Rights (UDHR) stipulates that all people have the right to a standard of living that guarantees health. This article was adopted by the UN Charter of 1948. In 1960, the UDHR further specified health as the highest attainable standard of physical, social, and mental well-being rather than as solely the absence of disease. Health, according to the UDHR, is achievable through the promotion of maternal and child health, reduction of mortality and morbidity, improvements in environmental sanitation, and the provision of adequate medical services (United Nations, n.d.). The UN reaffirmed health as an intrinsically valuable end by emphasizing that poor health is caused primarily by poverty and environmental conditions. A 1978 WHO conference held in Alma-Ata, Kazakhstan, a republic of the now former Soviet Union, supported the global issue of equity through accessibility to health for all, by recommending the implementation of primary healthcare and disease prevention strategies in national policies (Campbell, 1995).

The human rights movement in health, which raised the issue of equity in health status, tied universal access to comprehensive medical and health services for different social groups. Universal access implies the availability of services to all individuals and groups. Evaluating the distinctions between individual medical care and public healthcare becomes important as a means of monitoring health status, measured by indicators of equity and quality of care. Equity in access does not automatically lead to equity in health status. Equity in health status among social groups is constrained by the macro social process of the delivery of healthcare, as well as by the sociocultural, economic, and political arrangements of the community in which the delivery system functions. Global health programs have initiated various strategies to resolve these social determinants of health, increase access to basic health services, and achieve equity in outcomes.

Social Determinants of Health

The WHO conceptual framework for social determinants of health identifies five multifactorial components of population health that impact health outcomes: biology and genetics, individual behavior, social environment, physical environment, and health services. This framework accounts for the interrelationships among the determinants of health interactions; their influence on inequities; and the sociopolitical and economic influences on structural, social, and intermediary constructs affecting health and well-being (Solar & Irwin, 2010). The status of the health of a nation is an international phenomenon that is embedded within the larger socio-ecological, cultural, and political context of the global community. Arguably, the United States is the most technologically advanced country in the world, with internationally renowned medical centers and cutting-edge treatment modalities that are grounded in the tenets of Western medical scientific research. Yet among civilized nations, its healthcare outcomes, especially for preventable diseases and access to health services, lag far behind those in its counterparts with regard to multiple indicators, including infant mortality (ranked 25th) and life expectancy (ranked 23rd; Marmot & Bell, 2011).

Multilevel Model of Global Health

The growth of population-based nursing not only illustrates the need for further documentation of ethnocultural variation in health outcomes but provides an equally important mandate to translate clinical research into culturally competent programs. Population health is an emerging paradigm, differentiated from global health not only by scope but also by a focus on which groups are susceptible or at greater risk for specific diseases. Global health, on the other hand, provides a broader perspective on the extent to which the complex relations of macro structural factors of health determine the distribution of population-level and individual-level health outcomes. Macrofactors of salience explain how the environment, education policy, information technology, ethnic diversity and health disparity, geographic, socioeconomic factors, and inequities affect disease transmission and the delivery of health services across national borders.

To promote a greater understanding of the links among individual health, population health, and global health, the U.S. government has developed programs that address such relationships, domestically and abroad. The best practices and lessons learned from global health programs, such as the GHI, have demonstrated that the more acute issues visible in global environments are also relevant in the domestic context. Since GHI was legislated as a national priority in 2009, government agencies have sought to address global health challenges that may compromise well-being at home and around the world. The GHI seeks to align national security interests through collaboration with global partners to strengthen aid effectiveness. However, effectiveness in health promotion and disease prevention depends on aligning the dominant models of health, from individual clinical assessment to accessing primary care, and from population attributable risk assessment to ecological and multilevel models of health.

Figure 11.1 Micro- and Macrofactors in Obesity as Health Outcomes

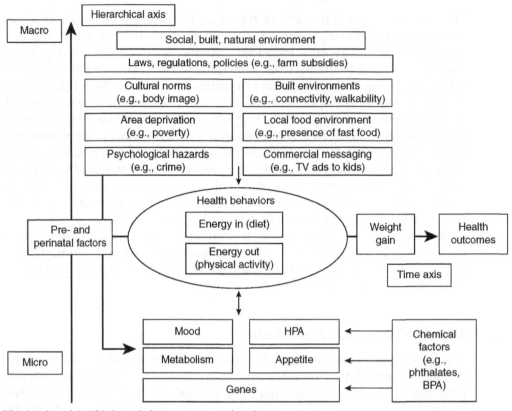

BPA: bisphenol A; HPA: hypothalamic–pituitary–adrenal axis.

Note: The life span is horizontal; factors are depicted hierarchically, individual level at the bottom of the figure to community level at top of the figure.

Source: National Research Council and Institute of Medicine (2013).

Multilevel models of global health (Figure 11.1) take into account the emergent properties of social structure, such as cultural norms, poverty, social policies, and distribution of primary care physicians, in conjunction with microlevel properties, such as genetics, gender, ethnicity, educational level, and individual health behaviors. Context or emergent properties of structure at each level refer to those characteristics that exemplify aspects of the whole unit of analysis and not the separate components of that unit. Whole units, such as population groups or health systems, have distinct properties other than the sum of their individual parts. Contextual analysis can explain the influences that a unit has within a hierarchy, and multilevel analysis can focus on multiple hierarchies of units within the same model. The individual is part of a family, ethnic group, social network, community, political group, geographic area, and country. It is a central objective in the population health perspective of healthcare to assess the context in which macro- and microunits change, given the complex nesting of individuals within social groups and cultures (Campbell, 2004, 2006; McKeehan, 2000).

Effective population health strategies aim at identifying groups at risk and specific risk factors causing poor health. Emergent properties of social structure are often not considered as determinants of health by medical practitioners. Health-promotion policies may develop two distinct intervention strategies by which health risks can be reduced for vulnerable groups as well as for the general population: (a) high-risk interventions, such as tertiary care (e.g., specialized consultative care; medical technology or surgery), which reduce high risks for a small number of individuals; and (b) population risk interventions, such as primary prevention (e.g., prohibiting lead in consumer paints, seat belt requirements), which reduce pervasive low risks for large sectors of a population (Primer on Public Health Population, n.d.).

Application of both intervention strategies is necessary to avert the "prevention paradox"; that is, individual-level interventions affect community health minimally, whereas community-level interventions have limited impact on high-risk individuals. The "prevention paradox" is paralleled by the "risk intervention paradox"; that is, the mass exposure of a large number of individuals to low levels of negligible risks, such as trans fats, may produce a larger number of disease cases than a small number of individuals exposed to high risks, such as BMI (body mass index) >35. Treating only very sick individuals leaves scarcely sick populations with minimal health treatment.

Preventing disease by shifting the population distribution of specific disease risks may be more productive than treatments directed only toward high-risk individuals. "For instance, estimates suggest that in North America a 14% decrease in the number of cerebrovascular accidents could be achieved either by decreasing the average blood pressure by 2 mmHg or by successfully treating everyone with a diastolic pressure of 95 mmHg or greater" (Association of Faculties of Medicine of Canada, n.d., para 2). Mass prevention reduces negligible risk a little for many and not at all for some, whereas most derive at least minimal benefits.

The prevention paradox proposes the concept that population health policies are developed for sick populations rather than for sick individuals, a cost borne by the "healthier" community. Global health intervention differs from medical intervention foremost in its emphasis on the socio-environmental context of individual health status. Second, global health recognizes that a continuous distribution in health status, such as blood pressure, characterizes populations. Third, global health programs are not restricted by focusing solely on the clinical designation of individuals, as potential cases for treatment, with or without disease.

A clearer understanding of global health identifies the differences in individual health, while retaining the ethnocultural context experienced by people. The multilevel model of population and global health enables the identification of health differences between individuals and between social groups. It also identifies specific structural conditions in the community that affect the health of people living there. Last, it separates the structural and ethnocultural determinants of health from the effects of individual psychosocial and health behaviors on health outcomes. For example, health disparity is part of the community context within which people live: country of origin, ethnicity, and cultural values are group characteristics. But ethnocultural factors are almost always measured at the individual level, a misspecification of the research model. The domain of preventive strategies in community health is the at-risk population as a whole and that of clinical medicine is the at-risk individual.

A multilevel evaluation of global health, therefore, gauges negligible and high-risk factors at both the population level and the individual level. As abundant research has shown, individual lifestyle behaviors, given a specific level of socioeconomic development, account for a majority of the risk factors for general well-being. A major issue is to determine which risk factors are amenable to policy interventions. Mass levels of low exposure require a mass level of intervention even if the impact is negligible, because the community will benefit as a whole, and subsequently individual members will benefit. The risk factors, which affect individual health, are not the same at the community level. Population health policy, therefore, needs multilevel research strategies that include the sui generis properties of communities and their attendant risk factors. These community properties cannot be reduced to a collective aggregate of its individual members. Access to health systems and geocultural environments may be designated as structural properties of communities rather than of individuals, and as such are the community context in which individuals live. GHIs tend to emphasize structural community factors to improve health outcomes, as is discussed in the section on the UN Millennium Development Goals.

Improvements in the quality of life depend in large part on the development of a model of health that puts the individual back into the community context. Personal risks to health under control of the individual (amount of daily sugar or salt intake) and social risks to health not directly controllable by the individual (a clean water supply) are embedded in a larger community context. Effective global programs sift through such causal complexity, expanding the biomedical model of disease to an ecological multilevel model of health.

Global health programs promote information initiatives to connect systems capable of supporting a broad range of public health functions: disease detection, surveillance, analysis, interpretation, alerting, and interventions. For example, in the WHO Health Report, "the term 'health services' is used to include promotion, prevention, treatment and rehabilitation. It includes services aimed at individuals (e.g., childhood immunization or treatment for tuberculosis) and services aimed at populations (e.g., mass media anti-smoking campaigns)" (WHO, 2007, p. 11).

Evaluating public health risk factors at multiple levels is even more relevant in global health in which community and cultural contexts vary significantly across geographic regions. Modifiable community factors have a direct effect on health, separately and independently from the effects of nonmodifiable individual factors and modifiable individual lifestyle practices. Individual behavioral solutions may be sought for population-level issues, when attributing or generalizing individual characteristics to the group. In designing or implementing large-scale health programs, the APRN should be aware that both individual and community contextual factors, including geographic locators, should be systematically included in public health education and research, to design effective programs (Campbell, 1995).

An effective APRN-administered population health program considers several factors:

- Community context has a direct effect on individual health outcomes, controlling for individual demographic factors.

- The relative ranking of geographic areas by healthcare access, environmental quality, and socioeconomic factors are characteristics of the area and a contextual determinant of individual health, controlling for individual demographic characteristics.
- Living in areas ranked as having better healthcare access, better environmental quality, residential land use, and less poverty has a positive effect on individual health outcomes.
- Beneficial community context has a moderating effect on the individual health outcome of individuals from disadvantaged or vulnerable demographic subgroups.
- Living in higher quality-ranked areas has a greater positive effect on individual health outcomes for minority individuals than for individuals who are not characterized as being from disadvantaged or vulnerable demographic subgroups.

As part of planning a population-based program, APRNs should assess which modifiable community factors have a direct effect on health, separately and independently from the effects of modifiable individual lifestyle behaviors and nonmodifiable individual demographic factors.

National Global Health Initiatives

The U.S. administration has spent over $60 billion to increase access to health services in global programs and to ensure national security since 2009. The Obama GHI prioritizes a three-pronged health strategy to contain infectious diseases and foster national security. This includes initiatives to protect communities from infectious diseases, eliminate AIDS in the new generation, and prevent child and maternal mortality (U.S. Government Interagency Website, 2014). Although infectious diseases still abound and new outbreaks of such diseases as Ebola, SARS (severe acute respiratory syndrome), and H1N1 threaten national security, vaccine-preventable diseases have been nearly eliminated in the United States. At the time of this publication, however, measles infections have reached their highest numbers (since the resurgence of 1989–1991) in the United States because of unvaccinated immigrants entering the United States and, more recently, because of inconsistent vaccination practices and parental refusal of vaccines altogether. APRNs have a role in shaping public opinion and have many opportunities to improve population health through health promotion, education, and research (see www.cdc.gov/vaccines/pubs/pinkbook/meas.html for more details about measles). Public health programs and health education, for example, have successfully contained the HIV epidemic, and many preventative programs in the United States focus on chronic diseases. Until the 20th century, communicable diseases were the singular cause of mortality, but chronic diseases now top the list. The smallpox vaccine was responsible for preventing nearly 2 million annual deaths around the world by 1980. In the 1950s, polio crippled about 35,000 children in the United States annually, but was largely eradicated through vaccination by 1979. However, several other countries, such as Afghanistan, Nigeria, and Pakistan, with absent or low vaccination rates, continue to experience high polio rates. Polio is currently spreading in the war-torn countries of Syria, Djibouti, Eritrea, Ethiopia, and Somalia (Centers for Disease Control and Prevention, n.d.-b). Another example of a preventable infectious disease is meningitis A. Although largely controlled in the United States, over 100,000 people died of meningitis A in the 1990s across Africa, spurring the CDC, the U.S. Agency for International Development (USAID), and the National Institutes of Health (NIH) to develop an affordable vaccine, MenAfriVac, for distribution. More recently, millions of dollars have been invested in a critical search for a safe Ebola vaccine. Phase-I clinical trials were successful in November 2014 (National Institutes of Health, n.d.). Such quick collaboration among national groups underscores the critical role that the United States plays in global health, as well as the interconnections between national security and public health.

Healthy People 2010 outlined national health goals for America but did not include global health as an issue. Following the 2003 SARS epidemic and 2009 H1N1 flu outbreak, Healthy People 2020 added a new global health goal "to improve public health and strengthen U.S. national security through global disease detection, response, prevention, and control strategies" (Healthy People 2020, n.d.). The 2014 Ebola outbreak demonstrates how the Healthy People 2020 connections between American health status and global developments are relevant. Diseases prevented with vaccinations are the cause of one of every five deaths among children younger than 5 years in underdeveloped countries. For example, measles was largely eradicated by 2000 in the United States, but in 2013 there were 175 cases, almost entirely because of people bringing the disease with them into the United States, where an increased number of families are choosing not to vaccinate their children, reducing the strength of herd immunity (CDC, 2014). Healthy People 2020 and the Institutes of Medicine (IOM) advocate a focal role for the United States in increasing the global capacity for establishing an infectious disease surveillance system to protect U.S. national security and to prevent the cross-border spread of diseases.

Many U.S. government agencies provide funding, human resources, and technical support to international health agencies and initiatives, including UN's *Millennium Development Goals* (MDGs); WHO *Global Polio Eradication Initiative; President's Emergency Plan for AIDS Relief* (PEPFAR); and CDC programs to address *malaria*, neglected tropical diseases (such as Ebola), and tobacco use. The U.S. administration's health strategy in 2014 recognizes noncommunicable diseases as a leading cause of mortality globally and the second major problem faced by the United States in health-promotion and disease prevention projects. Africa is an exception, because it must still address infectious diseases as a health priority. The GHI invested $63 billion over 6 years to help partner countries improve health outcomes through strengthened health systems, with a particular focus on improving the health of women, newborns, and children. In addition, by November 2014, there was a $6.2-billion appropriations request before Congress to fight Ebola in West Africa (Senate Appropriations Committee, n.d.), and the CDC funded $2.7 million for personal protective equipment (PPE) kits to help American hospitals and to augment the Strategic National Stockpile. The Department of Homeland Security (DHS) issued travel restrictions in October 2014 on flights to the United States from Liberia, Sierra Leone, and Guinea. All flights from these three West African

countries were directed to fly to one of only five airports with screening protocols in place: New York's JFK, Chicago's O'Hare, Atlanta's Hartsfield-Jackson,
Newark's Liberty, and Washington's Dulles. Although the WHO continues to
issue alerts for changing incidence and mortality rates attributed to Ebola by
country, the U.S. Department of Health and Human Services (HHS) instituted
new travel regulations to the United States, restricting entry to anyone either
sick or exposed to Ebola from Guinea, Liberia, or Sierra Leone on November
12, 2014 (National Association of EMS Physicians, 2014). The CDC and professional associations have also invested in developing education programs for
health practitioners to ensure the safety of clinicians by updating protocols
on patient treatment and monitoring of Ebola patients as well as developing
nationwide hospital and outpatient clinic surveillance systems (AACN, 2014;
American Medical Association, n.d.). The U.S. military was deployed to West
Africa as part of humanitarian aid to deliver supplies and equipment and to
build temporary hospitals, developing the health infrastructure required to
contain the Ebola crisis (The White House, 2014).

United States and the Global Health Gap

Mortality differences among nations have been associated with various theories of health disparities between populations and countries, some of which
are dependent on policy. This is an extensive list that includes socioeconomic
transformation, environmental pollution, lack of an adequate social safety
net, relative poverty, socioeconomic deprivation, historical and generational
effects of a political heritage, regional disparities, and psychosocial stress.
Other perspectives emphasize individual lifestyle such as poor health practices and violent behavior. The United States has the highest standard of living
in the world, yet health indicators lag behind those of European and other
high-income members of the Organization of Economic Cooperation and
Development (OECD). OECD member countries control 80% of global trade
and investments. The Organization for European Economic Cooperation was
formed after World War II to support the reconstruction of Europe. Canada
and the United States joined in 1960, establishing the OECD in 1961. Japan
joined in 1964. As of 2014, there were 40 OECD countries, which participate in
discussing solutions to world economic and health problems (OECD, n.d.-b).

The relationship between average income, whether gross domestic product (GDP) or per capita, and life expectancy is attenuated after a certain standard of living is achieved, as has been the case in market economies in OECD
countries. Average income is weakly related to mortality within wealthier
countries, such as the United States. However, the relative distribution of income, rather than average income, is more strongly associated with differences
in death rates within wealthy countries. This is due to the relative deprivation
of some population sectors and not others because of an uneven distribution
and concentration of resources (Campbell McKeehan, 2000).

Figure 11.2 illustrates that life expectancy is higher in countries with
more egalitarian distributions of income, such as those of Scandinavia, where
relative deprivation is less pronounced. The effect of average income on the
life expectancy of men and women in Western economies of OECD countries
is consistent with a relationship between wealth and health. Health disparities

FIGURE 11.2 • Total Expenditure on Health as a Percentage of the Gross Domestic Product, 2012

Legend:
≤3.0
3.0 - 5.0
5.1 - 8.0
8.1 - 10.0
10.1 - 13.0
>13.0
Data not available
Not applicable * Based on data updated in April 2014.

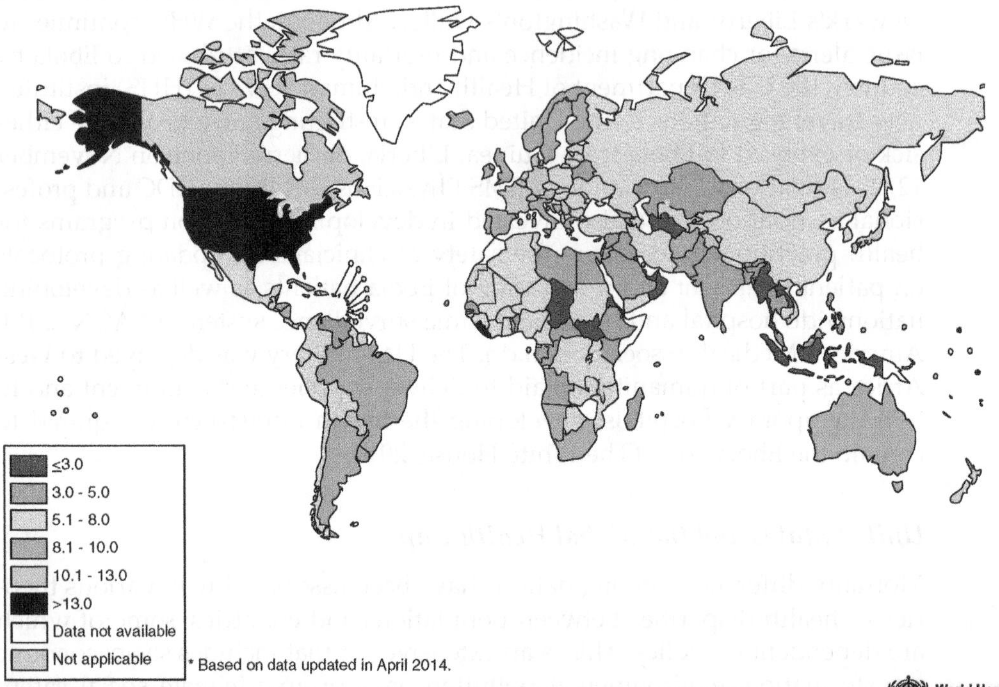

The boundaries and names shown and the designations used on this map do not imply the expression of any opinion whatsoever on the part of the World Health Organization concerning the legal status of any country territory, city or area or of its authorities, or ceoncerning the delimitation of its frontiers or boundaries. Dotted and dashed lines on maps represent approximate border lines for which there may not yet be full agreement.

Data Source: Global Health Observatory, WHO
Map Production: Health Statistics and Information Systems (HSI)
World Health Organization

World Health Organization

Reproduced, with the permission of the publisher, from the Global Health Observatory, WHO Map Production: Health Statistics and Information Systems, (HIS). WHO (2014). *Total expenditure on health as a percentage of the gross domestic product, 2012.* Retrieved from http://gamapserver.who.int/mapLibrary/Files/Maps/TotPercentGDP_2012.png, accessed December 2014.

increase with comparative income disparities relative to various groups having different income levels (OECD, n.d.-a). Health outcomes appear to be more closely related to how national health systems are organized than to the size of health expenditures, which are inflated by multiple private for-profit interests. In the United States, the growth in the cost of health services is not related to a concomitant growth in better health status of the population (Frenk, 2010). A study of hospital administrative costs in eight countries found that the United States has the highest costs, with 25% of U.S. hospital spending going to salaries for staff responsible for coding and billing, among other administrative costs. The Netherlands was second highest, spending 20% on administrative costs, followed by England at 16%, and Canada at 12% (Himmelstein, Jun, Busse et al., 2014).

OECD (2013) statistics indicate that the total health expenditure of the United States in 2011 was 16.9% of the GDP and $7,662 per capita, as compared to total OECD expenditures of 9.3% of the GDP and $2,867 per capita. The United States had double the expenditure per capita ($885) for pharmaceuticals of all the OECD countries ($414) in 2011. Nonetheless, the life expectancy at birth in the United States was 78.7 years versus 80.1 years in the OECD. In 2011, life expectancy at birth for U.S. men was 76.3 and for men in OECD countries was 77.3. Although the difference in life expectancy between the United States and other OECD countries is less than 2 years, health expenditures are almost double in the United States. Recent economic research (Lorenzoni, Belloni, & Sassi, 2014) indicates that most of the growth in differences of health expenditure between the United States and OECD was due to private health sector prices, particularly pharmaceuticals, and not due to growth in provider health delivery or performance (OECD, 2013).

Health sector costs are the most important component of U.S. health expenditure growth. The authors note that the "staggering levels of expenditure" in the United States cannot be fully explained by higher wealth levels, the age structure of the U.S. population, or the larger prevalence of risk factors such as obesity. Instead, "high health sector prices are due to intense use of health-related technologies, low productivity, decentralized price negotiations, fragmentation in the insurance market, and a high level of provider concentration, as the main explanations for high spending" (Center Lorenzoni, Belloni, & Sassi, 2014, p. 84; OCED, n.d., para 7). A positive relationship between health sector prices and better health outcomes (Figure 11.3) has not been established for the United States, as comparative global health indicators demonstrate (Lorenzoni et al., 2014; OECD, 2015.).

An international comparison of U.S. health status with those of other high-income countries (National Research Council & Institute of Medicine, 2013) demonstrates that the United States had lower health outcomes on at least nine indicators: infant mortality and low birth weight, injuries and homicides, adolescent pregnancy and sexually transmitted infections, HIV and AIDS, drug-related deaths, obesity and diabetes, heart disease, chronic lung disease, and disability. These poorer health outcomes in America are attributed to several lifestyle and health system factors: a large uninsured population, barriers to accessing primary care, likelihood of having a BMI >29, and physical inactivity. The lack of primary care practitioners in the United States is notable, given that most chronic diseases are preventable (Figure 11.4). An international OECD survey found that the United States had the lowest ratio of general practitioners out of all physicians in 2009, when compared to 15 other high-income countries. The United States also has a large sector of the population living below the federal poverty level and significant income inequality, both related to poor health status.

American National Security and Global Health

Although Americans have a comparatively poorer health status than peer countries, federal initiatives, such as Healthy People 2020, try to address these health disparities. Healthy People 2020 includes the global health goal of strengthening U.S. national security by detecting, preventing, and controlling global diseases. The U.S. government, through the USAID and the CDC, actively collaborates with global health agencies and participates in global, regional, and country-specific public health programs. The two focal organizations are the UN and the WHO. The mission of the USAID is to work with governmental and nongovernmental agencies, as well as the military, providing foreign assistance to resolve and prevent instability or active conflicts around the world. The USAID works to ensure domestic security by investing in health systems, democratic institutions, and agricultural advances (U.S. Agency for International Development, n.d.-a).

FIGURE 11.3 • Deaths from noncommunicable diseases and all causes (deaths per 100,000 age adjusted), 2008.

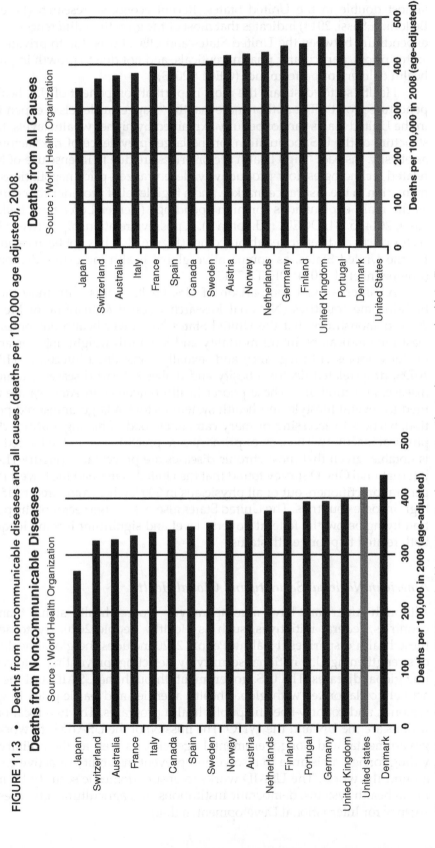

Deaths from Noncommunicable Diseases

Source : World Health Organization

Deaths from All Causes

Source : World Health Organization

Source: The National Academies. (2013). U.S. health in international perspective: Shorter lives, poorer health (p. 5).

FIGURE 11.4 • General practitioners as a proportion of total doctors in 15 peer countries, 2009.

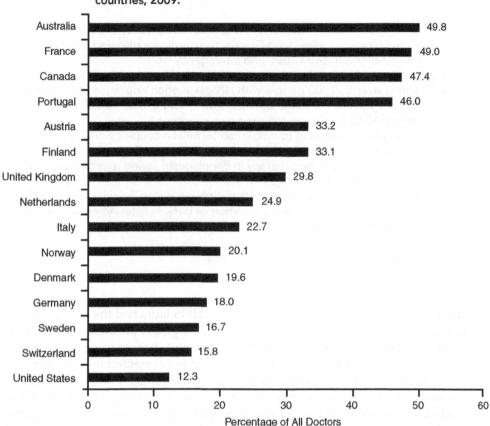

Source: National Research Council and Institute of Medicine. (2013). *General practitioners as a proportion of total doctors in 15 peer countries, 2009.* In S.H. Woolf & L. Aron (Eds.), *U.S. health in international perspective: Shorter lives, poorer health* (p. 116). Washington, DC: The National Academies Press. Retrieved from http://www.nap.edu/openbook.php?record_id=13497

The Foreign Assistance Act of 1961, supported by President Kennedy, formed the USAID from several post-World War II foreign assistance programs. The USAID was responsible for promoting development by administering aid to other countries. Recently, the USAID has focused primarily on preventing hunger, promoting women's education and health, and population planning around the world as a means to curtail political conflicts. These efforts have also entailed supporting free market economic growth, nongovernmental organizations (NGOs), and antipoverty programs. The USAID, as the main government agency tasked with ending extreme poverty and building democracy abroad, was responsible for helping to rebuild Afghanistan and Iraq by building social safety nets with healthcare and education programs in the region (USAID, n.d.-b).

The USAID has spearheaded U.S. technical and financial aid to increase health and economic self-sufficiency in the developing world through polio eradication, family planning, and maternal and child health programs. The U.S. President's Emergency Plan for AIDS Relief and President's Malaria Initiative are successful programs that have significantly impacted the incidence

EXHIBIT 11.2 • USAID Global Health Program Outcomes

- Activating a Disaster Assistance Response Team (DART) staffed by the CDC, in Monrovia, Liberia, and Guinea, to coordinate planning, operations, logistics, administrative issues, and interagency work
- Saving more than 3 million lives with immunization programs
- Reaching over 850,000 people with HIV-prevention education after establishing programs in 32 countries since 1987; training over 40,000 people to support HIV/AIDS programs in their own countries
- Providing family planning to more than 50 million couples worldwide
- Training 21,000 Honduran farm families to prevent soil erosion
- Providing oral rehydration therapy in Bangladesh; saving tens of millions of lives worldwide with this program
- Providing loans and operating costs to Bolivian Banco Solidario (BancoSol), which is the first self-sustaining commercial bank in Latin America to focus on microbusiness (small business loans averaging $200 each)

Source: U.S. Agency for International Development. (n.d.-d).

and prevalence of these infectious diseases. HHS launched the GHI in 2009 to integrate multiple government programs with global partners, as well as to cooperate with the WHO in health-promotion and disease prevention efforts.

Former Secretary of State Hillary Clinton implemented policy reforms in global health with GHI funding, including establishing a new agenda "USAID Forward." Included in the new agenda are strategies that seek to establish evidence for what works and what does not work in global health programs. Exhibit 11.2 enumerates the successful results the USAID has obtained with global health investments.

WHO

USAID works with WHO to promote and protect health as an essential element for human welfare, economic, and social development (WHO, n.d.-a). The WHO was created in 1946, as part of the UN, to find solutions for post-World War II Europe. Any member country of the UN can be a member of the WHO. The WHO, recognizing that international collaboration could control infectious diseases better than any single country, spearheaded the establishment of International Health Regulations (IHR; formulated in 1969, revised in 2005, in force 2007), which delineates the legal framework for global public health security (Prentice, T., Reinders, L. T., & World Health Report Team, 2007). The WHO states that "global public health security minimizes vulnerability to acute public health events that endanger the collective health of populations living across geographical regions and international boundaries, and includes the impact on economic, political stability, trade, tourism, access to goods and services, and demographic stability" (WHO, 2007, "Overview" section, para. 2). The goals of the IHR are to promote collective defense against the international spread of disease and population health emergencies by addressing diplomatic, political, economic, trade, and business interests. The IHR

EXHIBIT 11.3 • WHO Global Health Collaborations

- Global Outbreak Alert and Response Network (GOARN), which initiates an international disease outbreak alert, technical support, vaccines, drugs, specialists, and equipment, to prevent spread, such as the plague in India, in 1995, which had an economic cost of over $1.7 billion
- Chemical Incident Alert and Response System (ChemiNet): initiates alerts of industrial accidents, chemical, water, sanitation, radionuclear or environmental health emergencies
- Global network of national health systems
- Global Polio Eradication Initiative Network (GPEIN)
- Global Influenza Surveillance Network (GISN)
- FluNet
- H5N1 Avian flu tracking
- XDR-TB drug-resistant tuberculosis tracking
- Containment of 21st-century threats of bioterrorism (anthrax, etc.), SARS, and toxic chemical waste dumping, such as the 2006 illegal dumping of 500 tons of chemical waste in Abidjan, Cote d'Ivoire
- WHO Foreign Policy and Global Health (FPGH) Initiative
- Coordination of responses to natural disasters, with concomitant infectious diseases, malnutrition, mental illness, and displacement of large numbers of people

Source: WHO Health Security (n.d.-a).

lists diseases for mandatory reporting by all countries (polio, smallpox, etc.), specifies responses to radioactive, nuclear, or chemical emergencies, encourages global cooperation in science and technology, and recommends increased workforce and laboratory capacity.

As part of global health security, the WHO established several international collaborations, enumerated in Exhibit 11.3.

The WHO also manages global disease registries, databases, and classification of diseases that are used by members, including the United States, to maintain comparable definitions of health indicators (WHO, 2015). The WHO, with the agreement of member countries, developed Nomenclature Regulations in 1967. The regulations standardize nomenclature (Exhibit 11.4) with respect to morbidity and mortality, and established globally consistent coding, age groupings, territorial regions, and languages for the compilation and publication of health information. All members of the WHO have agreed to use the same nomenclature to collect and publish annual data.

The *International Classification of Diseases (ICD)* is used in the United States to code billing in order to standardize diagnostic categories and thereby to track the incidence and prevalence of disease. The 10th revision of the *ICD* is scheduled to be implemented in 2015. The 11th revision is in progress and due to be released by the WHO in 2017. The *ICD-10* can be downloaded online from the WHO website. A training module is also available (WHO, n.d.-b).

The WHO included the International Classification for Nursing Practice (ICNP) in 1996. It was updated in 2013. The next update is planned for 2015. The ICNP is copyrighted by the International Council of Nurses (ICN),

EXHIBIT 11.4 • WHO Family of International Classification (FIC)

I. WHO Family of International Classification
   • International Classification of Diseases (ICD-10)
   • International Classification of Diseases for Oncology (ICD-O-3)
   • ICD-10 for Mental and Behavioral Disorders: Clinical Descriptions and Diagnostic Guidelines
   • ICD-10 for Mental and Behavioral Disorders Diagnostic Criteria for Research
   • International Classification of Functioning, Disability and Health (ICF)
   • WHODAS 2.0 General Disability Factor
   • International Classification of Health Interventions (ICHI)

II. Family of International Classifications Network

III. Related International Classifications
   • International Classification of Primary Care, second edition (ICPC-2)
   • International Classification of External Causes of Injury (ICECI)
   • Technical aids for persons with disabilities—Classification and terminology (ISO9999)
   • Anatomical Therapeutic Chemical Classification System with Defined Daily Doses (ATC/DDD)
   • International Classification for Nursing Practice (ICNP)

Source: Madden, R., Sykes, C., Ustun, T.B., National Centre for Classification in Health, Australia, Australian Institute of Health and Welfare, & WHO. (n.d.-b)

which ensures the integrity of the classification system. ICNP is translated into several languages and may be downloaded for noncommercial purposes with an authorizing agreement (International Council of Nurses, 2015). The ICNP is designed to enable comparisons of nursing data across countries. It includes nursing diagnoses, nurse-sensitive patient outcomes, and nursing interventions.

The ICNP is a classification system that improves communication between nurses from different countries through standard language. It describes nursing practice in institutional and noninstitutional environments. It also facilitates international nursing research and the promulgation of health policy (ICNP, n.d.). The ICN maintains collaboration with other systems of classification to facilitate cross-mapping of vocabularies and interoperability. The ICN indicates that it has a number of formal agreements to best represent the nursing domain and promote semantic interoperability. ICNP is recognized as a related classification within the WHO Family of International Classifications to promote harmonization with the other WHO classifications.

The International Health Terminology Standards Development Organization (IHTSDO) and the ICN have engaged in a formal Harmonization Agreement to ensure that nursing requirements are adequately captured within the Systematized Nomenclature of Medicine—Clinical Terms (SNOMED CT). In addition to harmonizing ICNP and SNOMED CT, the ICN serves as the international representation for nursing practice to the IHTSDO. The ICN also has Liaison A status with the International Organization for Standardization

(ISO) Technical Committee on Health Informatics (TC215) and is represented at the International Medical Informatics Association through participation in the Nursing Special Interest Group. More recently, the ICN has collaborated with SabaCare to develop linkages between Clinical Care Classification concepts and ICNP concepts (International Council of Nurses, 2015).

As part of the UN, the WHO follows the prescriptions of the UN MDGs, which organize global strategies and priorities in improving health status across countries. UN members committed $2.5 billion in 2013 to accelerate meeting the MDG outcomes by 2015. The MDGs are eight international development goals that were established in 2000 by the UN to reaffirm the commitment of individual nations for a collective responsibility for human dignity, equality, and equity (United Nations General Assembly Declaration, 2000).

UN Millennium Development Goals

The MDGs (Exhibit 11.5) and targets were articulated by the Millennium Declaration of 2000, signed by 189 countries, including 147 heads of states and governments and at least 23 international organizations. The MDGs were further confirmed by the General Assembly of member states at the 2005 World Summit. The goals and targets are interrelated, forming a coherent whole. The MDGs represent an agreement among countries to achieve the MDGs by 2015 and "create an environment—at the national and global levels alike—which is conducive to development and the elimination of poverty" (United Nations General Assembly, 2000, section III, para. 2.).

The eight MDG goals are subdivided into 21 targets, each with measurable health and economic indicators (http://mdgs.un.org/unsd/mdg/Default. aspx). Exhibit 11.6 describes each goal in greater detail with the specific targets for achieving the goals. A conference to review interim progress in meeting the MDG targets was held at the UN in September 2010. A global action plan was adopted to assure progress toward meeting the eight antipoverty goals by 2015, with special emphasis on promoting women's health and children's health, as well as eradicating hunger and disease. *The Millennium Development Goals Report 2014*, approved in New York on 7 July 2014, summarizes the most recent assessment of global and regional progress toward meeting the MDGs.

EXHIBIT 11.5 • Millennium Development Goals

1. Eradicate extreme poverty and hunger.
2. Achieve universal primary education.
3. Promote gender equality and empower women.
4. Reduce child mortality.
5. Improve maternal health.
6. Combat HIV/AIDS, malaria, and other diseases.
7. Ensure environmental sustainability.
8. Develop a global partnership for development.

Source: UNSTATS (n.d.).

EXHIBIT 11.6 • Millennium Development Goals and Targets
Monitoring Progress

MACRO INDICATORS

Goal 1: Eradicate extreme poverty and hunger.

Target 1.A: Halve, between 1990 and 2015, the proportion of people whose income is less than $1 a day.

Target 1.B: Achieve full and productive employment and decent work for all, including women and young people.

Target 1.C: Halve, between 1990 and 2015, the proportion of people who suffer from hunger.

Goal 2: Achieve universal primary education.

Target 2.A: Ensure that, by 2015, children everywhere, boys and girls alike, will be able to complete a full course of primary schooling.

Goal 3: Promote gender equality and empower women.

Target 3.A: Eliminate gender disparity in primary and secondary education, preferably by 2005, and in all levels of education no later than 2015.

Goal 4: Reduce child mortality.

Target 4.A: Reduce by two thirds, between 1990 and 2015, the under-5 mortality rate.

Goal 5: Improve maternal health.

Target 5.A: Reduce by three quarters, between 1990 and 2015, the maternal mortality ratio.

Target 5.B: Achieve, by 2015, universal access to reproductive health.

Goal 6: Combat HIV/AIDS, malaria, and other diseases.

Target 6.A: Have halted by 2015 and begun to reverse the spread of HIV/AIDS.

Target 6.B: Achieve, by 2010, universal access to treatment for HIV/AIDS for all who need it.

Target 6.C: Have halted by 2015 and begun to reverse the incidence of malaria and other major diseases.

Goal 7: Ensure environmental sustainability.

Target 7.A: Integrate the principles of sustainable development into country policies and programmes and reverse the loss of environmental resources.

Target 7.B: Reduce biodiversity loss, achieving, by 2010, a significant reduction in the rate of loss.

Target 7.C: Halve, by 2015, the proportion of people without sustainable access to safe drinking water and basic sanitation.

Goal 8: Develop a global partnership for development.

Target 8.A: Develop further an open, rule-based, predictable, nondiscriminatory trading and financial system, including a commitment to good governance, development, and poverty reduction—both nationally and internationally.

(continued)

EXHIBIT 11.6 • Millennium Development Goals and Targets
Monitoring Progress (*continued*)

Target 8.B: Address the special needs of the least developed countries, including tariff- and quota-free access for the least developed countries' exports; enhanced program of debt relief for heavily indebted poor countries (HIPC) and cancellation of official bilateral debt; and more generous Official Development Assistance (ODA) for countries committed to poverty reduction.

Target 8.C: Address the special needs of landlocked developing countries and small island developing states (through the Programme of Action for the Sustainable Development of Small Island Developing States and the outcome of the 20-second special session of the General Assembly).

Target 8.D: Deal comprehensively with the debt problems of developing countries through national and international measures in order to make debt sustainable in the long term.

Source: United Nations (2015).

In comparison with the initial 2000 assessment, improvement across all goals was achieved by 2014, but continued work is required to meet the 2015 and post-2015 development agenda (United Nations Department of Economic and Social Affairs, n.d.).

Since the MDGs were established, UN member countries have achieved progress on several MDG indicators. China and India have reported the greatest gains in reducing poverty, and Brazil has achieved most of the eight goals. Nepal remains the world's poorest country. However, increased spending in maternal and child health by Nepal resulted in a 50% reduction in maternal mortality between 1998 and 2006. Developing countries still have 21% of their populations living on less than $1.25 a day in 2010 (UN Millennium Development Goals, n.d.). With the USAID investment in global health program collaboration to meet the MDGs, substantial gains have been made in macro population health indicators. Sub-Saharan Africa reports that 43 million more children are in primary education since 1999; child mortality has declined by 35% since 1994, malaria deaths have decreased by 30% since 2004, and 2 billion people have access to clean drinking water (UN Economic and Social Council, n.d.; USAID, n.d.-d). Continued progress in achieving the MDGs requires continued collaboration among nations, global organizations, intergovernmental agencies, local government, and community participation.

Implications for Advanced Practice Nursing

Nursing has become increasingly more active in global health programs by expanding interprofessional and interdependent collaborations. Global health is an essential component in APRN education and practice. Many schools of nursing have formed GHIs to strengthen culturally sensitive nursing education domestically. APRNs work as educators, policy makers, and clinicians in a variety of communities, with different cultural and ethnic groups, as well as with populations that spend extended time in other countries, such as veterans (NLN Global, n.d.). Such programs promote a deeper understanding, in APRN practice, of the complex political, economic, and social factors that affect an individual's health in a community context.

In the future, doctorally prepared nurses will find themselves more and more often in the position of being asked to form strategic partnerships with public and private organizations to strengthen health systems and to deliver culturally competent healthcare. In 2004, the National League for Nursing (NLN) formed the International Nursing Education, Services and Accreditation (INESA) joint taskforce with the National League of Nursing Accreditation Commission (NLNAC). INESA coordinates exchanges between nurse educators from the United States and around the world, and supports the Nursing Education Network of the ICN (National League for Nursing, n.d.). INESA also promotes educating nurses as an ethnic and culturally diverse workforce to meet the challenge of a worldwide nursing shortage and increased migration across nations. The NLNAC serves as a consultant on accreditation issues of nursing education programs in different countries and has developed a free toolkit for nursing faculty traveling abroad (NLNAC, n.d.; NLN, n.d.).

International activities have expanded for nursing faculty to include curriculum development, international collaboration in presentations and publications, consulting in hospital administration, and clinical expertise. Applying U.S. models, concepts, and theories of nursing practice in other nations may not be appropriate or feasible, given varying cultural values and beliefs. Many nursing interventions, practices, licensure requirements, and policies are context-specific and cannot be transferred across cultures. APRNs, as primary care providers, should develop awareness of political and cultural issues that influence individual behaviors, lifestyle, risk factors, and clinical care (Aiken et al., 2008). The multilevel global health model for APRN practice emphasizes cultural sensitivity in engaging in comparative effectiveness programs and interdisciplinary, interprofessional educational interchanges (Kulage, Hickey, & Honig, et al., 2014). APRNs play a leadership role in implementing transcultural changes in healthcare, disseminating science within nursing practice, and collaborating with global partners, such as the WHO.

WHO Collaborating Centers

The WHO has formed collaborating centers with 10 schools of nursing in the United States (WHO Collaborating Centres, n.d.). These collaborating centers bring together experts to solve problems in nursing, to address chronic and communicable diseases, nutrition, mental health, and other areas, and to share data, outcomes, and resolutions with UN member countries. The U.S. schools of nursing have agreed to produce a variety of outputs as part of their collaboration agreement with the WHO (Exhibit 11.7). The U.S. Schools of Nursing WHO Collaborating Centers each focus on such specific themes as clinical training in health promotion, nursing knowledge implementation and dissemination, international nursing development in primary healthcare, and clinical training in home care nursing.

EXHIBIT 11.7 • WHO Evaluation Terms of Reference Outputs between U.S. Schools of Nursing Collaborating Centers and WHO

- Health-workforce information and knowledge base strengthened, and country capacities for policy analysis, planning, implementation, information-sharing, and research built up
- Technical support provided to member states, with a focus on those facing severe health-workforce difficulties in order to improve the production, distribution, skill mix, and retention of the health workforce
- Human resource policies and practices in place to attract and retain top talent, promote learning and professional development, manage performance, and foster ethical behavior
- Management and organization of integrated, population-based health-service delivery through public and nonpublic providers and networks improved; reflecting the primary healthcare strategy; scaling up coverage, equity, quality, and safety of personal and population-based health services; and enhancing health outcomes

Source: WHO. (n.d.-c). WHO Collaborating Centres.

These collaboration initiatives (Exhibit 11.8) promote the work of U.S. nurses in (a) international NGOs of health, (b) best practices in achieving the MDGs, (c) capacity building of nursing human resources, (d) capacity building in nursing education for primary care, (e) training in disease prevention methods, and (f) supporting nurse educational programs in home care and self-management of chronic diseases (World Health Organization Collaborating Centres [WHOCC], n.d.-c). These issues are important for the APRN to consider when planning effective health delivery programs focusing on the individual and community levels, and ensuring that a safety net includes culturally competent health interventions.

The U.S. Surgeon General's Goals of 2000 identified three broad areas that influence population health status and that require public policy and nursing intervention: (a) health practices or health promotion (decreasing risk factors, personal habits such as smoking, lack of physical exercise, poor diet, alcohol abuse), (b) ecological factors or health protection (decreasing occupational and environmental toxic exposures, decreasing accidents), and (c) medical care factors or preventive health services (increasing access to services such as prenatal care, infant programs, family planning, hypertension control) (Campbell, 2004). These goals are reiterated in the macro population health indicators of Healthy USA 2020 and the 2015 UN MDGs, and progress has been made in measuring and addressing these concepts of health inequity and inequality. The APRN can further contribute to the monitoring of inequity in health, as a part of population health practice. With nurse leadership, the lessons learned from the application of effective health strategies in different countries can be shared with an interprofessional team in the United States (McNeal, 2013) and international communities.

EXHIBIT 11.8 • WHO Collaborating Centers With Schools of Nursing, United States (Active Until 2015–2017)

Institution	Title	Terms of Reference
University of Michigan, Ann Arbor, MI	WHO Collaborating Centre for Research and Clinical Training in Health Promotion Nursing	• Collaborate with WHO/PAHO (Pan American Health Organization) to disseminate/share critical information and connect and systematize experiences and good practices of health promotion. • Collaborate with WHO/PAHO to build nursing and local institutional capacity to implement and evaluate individual, family, and community health-promotion interventions. • Collaborate with WHO/PAHO to strengthen nursing/midwifery and local health services education and practice in health promotion. • Collaborate with WHO/PAHO to develop and support nurses' capacity to conduct and implement research on health promotion.
Johns Hopkins School of Nursing, Baltimore, MD	WHO Collaborating Centre for Nursing Information, Knowledge Management and Sharing	• Collaborate with PAHO/WHO to facilitate and promote equitable access to information and scientific knowledge via the Global Alliance for Nursing and Midwifery (GANM) for the promotion and support of global nursing and midwifery communities of practice and other information, communication and technology (ICT)-supported activities. • Collaborate with PAHO/WHO to contribute to the growth, development, and deployment of learning and informed online environments to address the social determinants of health and improve nursing, health, and healthcare globally.
University of Alabama at Birmingham (UAB) Birmingham, AL	WHO Collaborating Centre for International Nursing	• Collaborate with PAHO/WHO to strengthen nursing and midwifery through the development of educational programs and resources to enhance the health of vulnerable families and children. • Collaborate with PAHO and WHO to enhance utilization and dissemination of knowledge resources to strengthen nursing and midwifery capacity, focusing on the health of children and families.

(continued)

EXHIBIT 11.8 • WHO Collaborating Centers With Schools of Nursing, United States (Active Until 2015–2017) (*continued*)

Institution	Title	Terms of Reference
University of Illinois at Chicago, Chicago, IL	WHO Collaborating Centre for International Nursing Development in Primary Healthcare	• To collaborate with WHO/PAHO in the dissemination of WHO/PAHO Primary Healthcare program-based research findings and best practices to address Millennium Development Goals among policy makers, healthcare providers, and consumers. • To collaborate with WHO/PAHO in the facilitation of multidisciplinary research focused on PHC (primary healthcare) education and practice with special emphasis on capacity building of nursing human resources. • To collaborate with WHO/PAHO in developing education mechanisms to develop nursing and other human resources for health for multidisciplinary global PHC practice, education, and research within the PAHO region.
Case Western Reserve University, Cleveland, OH	WHO Collaborating Centre for Research & Clinical Training in Home Care Nursing	• Collaborate with AMRO (Regional Activities in the Americas) to strengthen the development of nursing human resources and other healthcare workers in home care focused on self-management of NCDs (noncommunicable diseases). • Collaborate with AMRO to develop educational programs for nurses and other healthcare workers for the self-management of NCDs in the home and community settings. • Collaborate with AMRO to promote and conduct research to support home care and self-management of NCDs.

Source: WHO (n.d.-c).

SUMMARY

The doctorally prepared advanced practice nurse is well positioned to contribute to the scientific international discourse on subjects related to national (Esperat, Fiandt, McNeal, Heuer, & Denholm, 2011; McNeal, 2012, 2014) and global health initiatives. This chapter has described the seven domains of the global health core competency model developed by the ASPH, and has shown the interrelationship of the ASPH model to the AACN DNP Essentials

V through VII. It is well recognized that the health of a nation is predicated on its ability to have far-reaching influence on the health status of populations around the world. Although U.S. healthcare expenditures are now nearly 20% of the GDP, healthcare outcomes have not improved with rising healthcare costs. Fragmentation of care, lack of access, third-party payer systems, hospital administrative costs, and expense of health-related technologies all have been cited as reasons for the escalating cost of healthcare in this country. Further, with the exponential increase in the immigrant population within the United States and the resultant heightened cross-national border transmission of disease, nursing doctoral programs must address and include global healthcare concepts within the curriculum of study.

Moving beyond the notion that health outcomes are singularly related to the behaviors of the individual, several documents and reports disseminated by the Commission on Social Determinants of Health have changed the focus of the discussion on health outcomes to include those factors associated with the contextual environment in which the individual resides. The WHO construct, which defines the social determinants of health, serves to provide a useful framework on which the APRN can design and implement strategies to address the multifactorial, sociopolitical, economic, ecological, and cultural underpinnings that influence and shape population health. Similarly, the theoretical construct for the Multilevel Model of Global Health supports the approach to analyze and evaluate risk factors and treatment effectiveness at both the individual and community levels. Enhanced knowledge and understanding of the impact of GHIs on health outcomes for communities around the world will provide the APRN with the tools needed to contribute to the national and international dialogues related to population health.

EXERCISES AND DISCUSSION QUESTIONS

Exercise 11.1 You are the executive director for a nurse-managed clinic in an underserved community. A large segment of the community population consists of foreign-born immigrants and refugees from African countries, including Liberia. As the APRN in this leadership role, what resources would you use to develop policies and procedures for the management of an Ebola exposure? Ebola outbreak? What strategies would you implement to develop evidence-based guidelines for practice?

Exercise 11.2 As the program director for an APRN doctoral program of study, you are asked to develop the syllabus for a course on population and global health. Develop the course description, objectives, and weekly topical outline for a course titled "Current and Emerging Trends in Population-Based Global Health."

Exercise 11.3 As an APRN you have been requested to present a paper at a national nursing conference on the design, implementation, and evaluation of a community health clinic. The audience consists of advanced practice clinicians and academicians. List the objectives for the presentation. How would you include the eight recommendations of the IOM Report: "The Future of Nursing" Develop the outline for the presentation to include concepts related to social determinants of health, healthcare access, data collection, and analyses and healthcare outcome evaluation.

Exercise 11.4 One of the important components of the role of the APRN is to influence public policy and to interface with law makers and elected officials in the design and implementation of rules and regulations impacting the health of a nation. Toward that end, how might you develop guidelines for a public policy brief on a current health issue?

REFERENCES

Aiken, L. M., Pelter, M. M., Carlson, V., Marshall, A. P., Cross, R., McKinley, S., & Dracup, K. (2008). Effective strategies for implementing a multicenter international clinical trial. *Journal of Nursing Scholarship, 40*(2), 101–108.

American Association of Colleges of Nursing (AACN). 2014. *Ebola resources for nurse educators.* Retrieved from http://www.aacn.nche.edu/news/articles/2014/ebola-resources

American Immigration Council. (2014). *Refugees: A fact sheet.* Retrieved from http://immigrationpolicy.org/just-facts/refugees-fact-sheet

American Medical Association. (n.d.). *Ebola resource center.* Retrieved from http://www.ama-assn.org/ama/pub/physician-resources/public-health/ebola-resource-center.page

Association of Faculties of Medicine of Canada. (n.d.). *Intervening in individuals or populations?* AFMC Primer on Population Health. Retrieved from http://phprimer.afmc.ca/Part3-PracticeImprovingHealth/Chapter8IllnessPreventionAndHealthPromotion/Interveninginindividualsorinpopulations

Association of Schools of Public Health. (2014). *Global health competency model.* Retrieved from http://www.aspph.org/educate/models/masters-global-health/

Campbell McKeehan, I. (1995). Planning of national primary health care and prevention programs. In E. Gallagher & J. Subedi (Eds.), *Global perspectives on health care* (pp. 174–197). Englewood Cliffs, NJ: Prentice-Hall.

Campbell McKeehan, I. (2000). A multilevel city health profile of Moscow. *Social Science and Medicine, 9*(51), 1295–1312.

Campbell McKeehan, I. (2004). A multilevel evaluation model for health disparity reduction and cultural competency intervention. *Hispanic Health Care International, 1*(3), 1–10.

Campbell McKeehan, I. (2006). An essay on the need to expand and integrate nursing practice educational horizons with information technology and interdisciplinary collaboration [Editorial]. *Journal of Nursing Informatics, 10*(1), Online. Retrieved from http://ojni.org/10%201/irina.htm

Centers for Disease Control and Prevention. (n.d.-b). *Global health—Polio.* Retrieved from http://www.cdc.gov/polio

Centers for Disease Control and Preventions. (2014). *Measles still threatens health security* [Press release]. Retrieved from http://www.cdc.gov/media/releases/2013/p1205-meales-threat.html

Esperat, C., Fiandt, K., McNeal, G., Heuer, L., & Denholm, E. (2011). Nursing innovations: The future of chronic disease management. In *The future of nursing: Leading change, advancing health* (pp. 418–422). Washington, DC: National Academies Press.

Federation for American Immigration Reform (FAIR). (2014). *Estimated cost of K-12 public education for unaccompanied alien children.* Retrieved from http://www.fairus.org/publications/estimated-cost-of-k-12-public-education-for-unaccompanied-alien-children

Frenk, J. (2010). The global health system: Strengthening national health systems as the next step for global progress. *PLoS Med, 7*(1). doi:10.1371/journal.pmed.1000089. Retrieved from http://journals.plos.org/plosmedicine/article?id=10.1371/journal.pmed.1000089

Global Health Observatory, WHO Map Production: Health Statistics and Information Systems, (HIS). WHO (2014). *Total expenditure on health as a percentage of the gross domestic product, 2012*. Retrieved from http://gamapserver.who.int/mapLibrary/Files/Maps/TotPercentGDP_2012.png

Healthy People 2020. (n.d.). *Global health*. Retrieved from http://www.healthypeople.gov/2020/topics-objectives/topic/global-health

Hirsen, J. (2014, June 16). The staging of the illegal immigrant children crisis. NEWSMAX. Retrieved fromhttp://www.newsmax.com/Hirsen/Illegal-Immigrant-Children-border/2014/06/16/id/577295/

Himmelstein, D. U., Jun, M., Busse R. et al., (2014). A comparison of hospital administrative costs in eight nations: U.S. costs exceed all others by far. *Health Affairs, 33*(9):1586–1594.

Immigration in America. (n.d.). *Immigration and Nationality Act of 1965*. Retrieved from http://www.immigrationinamerica.org/594-immigration-and-nationality-act-of-1965.html?newsid=594

International Council of Nurses. (2015). *International classification for nursing practice*. Retrieved from http://www.icn.ch/pillarsprograms/international-classification-for-nursing-practice-icnpr/

Kaiser Health News. (2013, February 13). *Illegal immigrants most helped by Emergency Medicaid Program*. Retrieved from http://www.governing.com/news/state/kh-illegal-immigrants-most-helped-by-emergency-medicaid.html

Kominski, A., Shin, H., & U.S. Census Bureau. (2010, April). *Language acquisition of US children*. Paper presentation at the Annual Meeting of the Population Association of America, Dallas, TX. Retrieved from https://www.census.gov/hhes/socdemo/language/data/acs/Language-Acquisition_presentation.pdf

Kulage, K.M., Hickey, K.T., Honig, J.C., et al. (2014). Establishing a program of global initiatives for nursing education. *J Nurs Educ, 53*(7):371–8.

Lorenzoni, L., Belloni, A., & Sassi, F. (2014). Health-care expenditure and health policy in the USA versus other high-spending OECD countries. *The Lancet, 384*(9937), 83–92.

Madden, R., Sykes, C., Ustun, T.B., National Centre for Classification in Health, Australia, Australian Institute of Health and Welfare, & WHO. (n.d.) *The WHO family of international classifications: Definitions, Scope and purpose*. Retrieved from http://www.who.int/classifications/en

Marmot, M., & Bell, R. (2011). Improving health: Social determinants and personal choice. *American Journal of Preventive Medicine, 40*(1, Suppl. 1), S73–S77.

McKeehan, I. V. (2000). A multilevel city health profile of Moscow. *Social Science and Medicine, 51*(9), 1295–1312.

McNeal, G. J. (2012). The IOM report on the future of nursing: One year later. *ABNF Journal, 23*(1), 3.

McNeal, G. J. (2013). Interprofessional education: An IOM imperative. *ABNF Journal, 24*(3), 69–70.

McNeal, G. J. (2014). Shifting the paradigm: An academic public–private partnership to form a virtual nurse managed clinic. *ABNF Journal, 25*(2), 31–32.

The National Academies. (2013). U.S. health in international perspective: Shorter lives, poorer health. Retrieved from http://sites.nationalacademies.org/cs/groups/dbassesite/documents/webpage/dbasse_080620.pdf

National Association of EMS Physicians. (2014). New travel restrictions (HHS Announcement). Retrieved from http://www.naemsp.org/Pages/Search-Results.aspx?k=travel%20restrictions&cs=This%20Site&u=http%3A%2F%2Fwww.naemsp.org

National Institutes of Health. (n.d.). *NIAID/GSK experimental Ebola vaccine appears safe, prompts immune response*. Retrieved from http://www.niaid.nih.gov/news/newsreleases/2014/Pages/EbolaVaxResults.aspx

National League for Nursing (NLN). (n.d.). *Faculty preparation for global experiences toolkit*. Retrieved from http://www.nln.org/docs/default-source/default-document-library/toolkit_facprepglobexp5a3fb25c78366c709642ff00005f0421.pdf

National League for Nursing Accrediting Commission. (n.d.). Retrieved from http://www.nlnac.org

National Research Council and Institute of Medicine. (2013). General practitioners as a proportion of total doctors in 15 peer countries, 2009. In S.H. Woolf & L. Aron (Eds.), *U.S. health in international perspective: Shorter lives, poorer health* (p. 116). Washington, DC: The National Academies Press. Retrieved from http://www.nap.edu/open book.php?record_id=13497

OECD. (2013). Health at a glance 2013. Retrieved from http://www.oecd.org/els/health-systems/Health-at-a-Glance-2013.pdf

OECD. (2015). OECD work on health. Retrieved from http://www.oecd.org/health/Health-Brochure.pdf

OECD (2013). Health at a glance 2013: OECD indicators. retrieved from http://www.oecd.org/els/health-systems/Health-at-a-Glance-2013.pdf

OECD. (n.d.). *After decline in U.S. health expenditure growth, OECD sees risk of spending uptick in recovery.* Retrieved from http://www.oecd.org/washington/lancet-health-unitedstates.htm

The Organisation for Economic Co-operation and Development. (n.d.-a). *Health policies and data.* Retrieved from http://www.oecd.org/els/health-systems/health-data.htm

The Organisation for Economic Co-operation and Development. (n.d.-b). *History.* Retrieved from http://www.oecd.org/about/history/

Pew Research Center's Hispanic Trends. (n.d.). *Population decline of unauthorized immigrants stalls, may have reversed.* Retrieved from http://www.pewhispanic.org/2013/09/23/population-decline-of-unauthorized-immigrants-stalls-may-have-reversed

Prentice, T., Reinders, L.T., & World Health Report Team. (2007). A safer future: Global health security in the 21st century. (WHO World Health Report). Retrieved from http://www.who.int/whr/2007/whr07_en.pdf

Senate Appropriations Committee. (n.d.). *Chairwoman Mikulski opening statement at full committee hearing on Ebola response.* Retrieved from http://www.appropriations.senate.gov/news/chairwoman-mikulski-opening-statement-full-committee-hearing-ebola-response

Solar, O., & Irwin, A. (2010). *A conceptual framework for action on the social determinants of health* (Discussion Paper 2 for the Commission on Social Determinants of Health). Geneva, Switzerland: World Health Organization.

The United Nations. (n.d.). *The universal declaration of human rights.* Retrieved from http://www.un.org/en/documents/udhr/

United Nations Department of Economic and Social Affairs. (n.d.). *Millennium development goals report 2014.* Retrieved from http://www.un.org/en/development/desa/publications/mdg-report-2014.html

UN Economic and Social Council. (n.d.). Retrieved from http://www.un.org/en/ecosoc/about/mdg.shtml

United Nations General Assembly resolution 555/2, *United Nations millennium declaration,* A/55/L.2 (06 September 2000). Retrieved from http://www.un.org/millennium/declaration/ares552e.htm

United Nations (UN). (2015). Millennium development goals and beyond 2015. Retrieved from http://www.un.org/millenniumgoals/bkgd.shtml

U.S. Agency for International Development. (n.d.-a). USAID Retrieved from http://www.usaid.gov

U.S. Agency for International Development. (n.d.-b). *Afghanistan and Pakistan.* Retrieved from http://www.usaid.gov/where-we-work/afghanistan-and-pakistan

U.S. Agency for International Development. (n.d.-c). *USAID history.* Retrieved from http://www.usaid.gov/who-we-are/usaid-history

U.S. Agency for International Development. (n.d.-d). *Results and data.* Retrieved from http://www.usaid.gov/results-and-data

U.S. Census. (2012). Retrieved from http://www.census.gov/population/foreign/files/cps2012/2012T1.pdf

U.S. Citizenship and Immigration Services. (2015). Refugees. Retrieved from http://www.uscis.gov/humanitarian/refugees-asylum/refugees

U.S. Global Health Programs. (n.d.). *About.* Retrieved from http://www.ghi.gov/about

U.S. Government Interagency Website. (2014). U.S. global health programs. Retrieved from http://www.ghi.gov/index.html

42 U.S.C. (n.d.). *Table of contents.* Retrieved from http://www.gpo.gov/fdsys/search/page-details.action?collectionCode=USCODE&searchPath=Title+42&oldPath=Title+42&isCollapsed=true&selectedYearFrom=2013&ycord=1665&browsePath=Title+42%2F-1&granuleId=USCODE-2013-title42-toc&packageId=USCODE-2013-title42&collapse=true&fromBrowse=true

The White House. (2014). *Fact sheet: U.S. response to the Ebola epidemic in West Africa.* Retrieved from http://www.whitehouse.gov/the-press-office/2014/09/16/fact-sheet-us-response-ebola-epidemic-west-africa

World Health Organization (WHO). (2014). *Global health observatory—Map gallery.* Retrieved from http://gamapserver.who.int/mapLibrary/

World Health Organization (WHO). (n.d.-a). *Health systems financing: The path to universal coverage press kit.* Retrieved from http://www.who.int/whr/2010/media_centre/en/

World Health Organization (WHO). (n.d.-b). The WHO family of international classifications. Retrieved from http://www.who.int/classifications/en/

World Health Organization (WHO). (n.d.-c). World Health Organization Collaborating Centres. Retrieved from http://apps.who.int/whocc/List.aspx?cc_code=USA&

World Health Organization (WHO). (2015). The WHO-FIC Network. Retrieved from http://www.who.int/classifications/network/en/

Index